DENTAL PUBLIC HEALTH

Contemporary Practice for the Dental Hygienist

DENTAL PUBLIC HEALTH

Contemporary Practice for the Dental Hygienist

Second Edition

Christine N. Nathe, RDH, MS
Associate Professor and Graduate Program Director
University of New Mexico
Division of Dental Hygiene

PEARSON
Prentice
Hall

Upper Saddle River, New Jersey 07458

Library of Congress Cataloging-in-Publication Data

Nathe, Christine Nielsen.
  Dental public health : contemporary practice for the
dental hygienist / Christine Nielsen Nathe.—
2nd ed.
      p. ; cm.
  Includes bibliographical references and index.
  ISBN 0-13-113444-2
  1. Dental public health.   2. Dental hygienists.
3. Dental hygiene.
  [DNLM: 1. Dental Care—United States.
2. Dental Hygienists—United States.   3. Delivery of
Health Care—United States.   4. Public Health
Dentistry—United States.   WU 90 N275d 2004]
I. Title.

  RK52.N27 2004
  362.19'76'00973—dc22
                                    2004004785

The procedures described in this textbook are based on consultation with dental authorities. The author and publisher have taken care to make certain that these procedures reflect currently accepted clinical practice; however, they cannot be considered absolute recommendations.

The material in this textbook contains the most current information available at the time of publication. However, federal, state, and local guidelines concerning clinical practices, including, without limitation, those governing infection control and universal precautions, change rapidly. The reader should note, therefore, that new regulations may require changes in some procedures.

It is the responsibility of the reader to familiarize himself or herself with the policies and procedures set by federal, state, and local agencies, as well as the institution or agency where the reader is employed. The authors and the publishers of this textbook disclaim any liability, loss, or risk resulting directly or indirectly from the suggested procedures and theory, from any undetected errors, or from the reader's misunderstanding of the text. It is the reader's responsibility to stay informed of any new changes or recommendations made by any federal, state, and local agency as well as by his or her employing health care institution or agency.

Publisher: Julie Levin Alexander
Publisher's Assistant: Regina Bruno
Senior Acquisitions Editor: Mark Cohen
Associate Editor: Melissa Kerian
Editorial Assistant: Jaquay Felix
Director of Manufacturing and Production:
  Bruce Johnson
Managing Editor for Production: Patrick Walsh
Production Liaison: Cathy O'Connell
Production Editor: Karen Berry/Pine Tree
  Composition, Inc.
Manufacturing Manager: Ilene Sanford
Manufacturing Buyer: Pat Brown

Creative Director: Cheryl Asherman
Senior Design Coordinator: Christopher Weigand
Cover Designer: Kevin Kall
Director of Marketing/Marketing Manager:
  Karen Allman
Channel Marketing Manager: Rachele Strober
Marketing Coordinator: Janet Ryerson
Media Editor: John Jordan
Media Production Manager: Amy Peltier
Media Project Manager: Stephen Hartner
Composition: Pine Tree Composition
Printer/Binder: RR Donnelley & Sons, VA
Cover Printer: Phoenix Color Corp.

Credits and acknowledgments borrowed from other sources and reproduced, with permission, in this textbook appear on appropriate page within text.

Pearson Education LTD.
Pearson Education Singapore, Pte. Ltd
Pearson Education, Canada, Ltd
Pearson Education–Japan
Pearson Education Australia PTY, Limited

Pearson Education North Asia Ltd
Pearson Educaçion de Mexico, S.A. de C.V.
Pearson Education Malaysia, Pte. Ltd
Pearson Education, Upper Saddle River, New Jersey

10 9 8 7 6
ISBN 0-13-113444-2

DEDICATION

This book is dedicated to my husband, Chris Nathe, and our children, Rhen, Marissa, and Chad Nathe, who make every day of my life a joy, and to my parents, John Nielsen and Susan Nielsen, RDH, for their support and example.

In our humanitarian pursuits, we have three encompassing possessions—our time, our talent, and our treasure. Our time, of course, we cannot keep. Only that which we give to others is not lost. We also cannot keep our talent. We must use it or we lose it. Our treasure, at last, is not permanent either. Most of us have lived long enough to know that we really keep only that which we give away.

Author Unknown

CONTENTS

UNIT III: Dental Hygiene Research   193

Chapter II: The Oral Epidemiology of Dental Diseases   195

Chapter 12:   Research in Dental Hygiene   215

Chapter 13:   Biostatistics   233
by Chris French-Beatty, RDH, PhD

Chapter 14:   Evaluation of Scientific Literature and Dental Products   259

UNIT IV: Practical Strategies for Dental Public Health

Chapter 15:   Careers in Dental Public Health

Chapter 16:   Strategies for Creating Dental Hygiene Positions in Dental Public Health Settings

FOREWORD

When Alfred Civilion Fones followed his dream to create within the dental staff a dental therapist whose focus would be the prevention of dental disease, his intention was not merely to have this person perform in dental offices. He recognized from the start that the most effective way to "spread the word" was to direct services, educational and clinical, to groups of people—to the masses. Ideally those groups would be comprised of children who would be taught at an early age the importance of dental health and prevention of dental disease. Where better to interface with children than in grammar schools? And so, in time, what was known as the Bridgeport School Dental Hygiene Corps was established; it was made up of members of Dr. Fones's classes of 1914, 1915, and 1916. Ergo, the first dental hygiene public health program.

I will fast-forward to the early 1950s when I and thirty-three other young women were enrolled at the University of Bridgeport's Fones School of Dental Hygiene in Bridgeport, Connecticut. As part of our field work rotation, we traveled to long established dental clinics throughout the city's schools. I remember being extremely fond of that assignment because I liked interacting with the children. But the real thrill of those trips was coming face-to-face with members of those first classes who were still in charge of the various clinics. These women knew Dr. Fones personally. During lunch hours, they had a captive audience and would relate to us how it all began: the first school in the carriage house adjacent to Dr. Fones's and his father's dental building, and his perseverance and determination in convincing city fathers, the Board of Education, and the Dental Society to allow the early dental hygienists to conduct programs within the schools.

I know how proud and delighted they would be—Dr. Fones and "the pioneers"—to see how dental hygienists have positioned themselves today in various public health settings. And how impressed they would be with Christine Nathe's *Dental Public Health: Contemporary Practice for the Dental Hygienist*. It is a remarkable testimony to the premise that public health dental hygienists have the ability to play a valuable and critical role in the dental health of people everywhere.

Janet Carroll Memoli, RDH, MS
Retired Director, Fones School of Dental Hygiene
Professor Emeritus, University of Bridgeport, Bridgeport, CT

PREFACE

The guiding principles that served as the impetus for the first edition of *Dental Public Health: Contemporary Practice for the Dental Hygienist* remain consistent. The twenty-first century mandates a change in the practice and understanding of dental public health principles. Dental hygienists increasingly are becoming important players in the dental public health arena. In fact, the changes in supervisory status affecting many states will have an unprecedented effect on the practice of dental public health. Moreover, dental hygiene's ability to react proactively to these changes can have a tremendous effect on dental public health within the United States. Additionally, other countries may benefit from dental hygiene's growth within the United States. The dental hygiene practitioners who will be practicing in this new century need information on how to effectively position and practice dental hygiene in the dental public health setting.

Dental Public Health: Contemporary Practice for the Dental Hygienist introduces the student to definitions and discussion on dental public health. Appropriately, the historical development of the profession of dental hygiene, focusing on its inception as a true public health profession, is presented. The prevention modalities encompassing public health dental hygiene are discussed, including fluoridation, dental sealants, fluoride mouthrinse programs, tobacco cessation programs, athletic mouthguards, nutritional counseling, dental screenings, dental health promotion and education activities, and other dental health interventions.

The current status of dental public health delivery in the United States and abroad is discussed, with emphasis on the governmental structures affecting dental hygiene care delivery. Emphasis is placed on the profession's collaboration and partnership with a variety of health care professionals outside of the private dental practice delivery system.

Dental health care personnel issues are discussed, focusing on the shortage and surplus controversies affecting the professions of dental hygiene and dentistry. In addition, factors affecting dental care delivery are presented in detail.

Financing dental care has been added to this edition. Private and governmental programs that fund dental care are discussed in detail. In addition, a detailed overview of the different types of insurance programs in the United States is presented.

Lesson plan development, presentation strategies, and techniques are discussed with guided examples and case studies to aid in student comprehension. Target populations are expanded in this edition, focusing on groups for which dental hygienists frequently provide dental health presentations. Additionally, issues of cultural diversity are reviewed. Program planning and evaluation, utilizing the dental hygiene process of care, are discussed. The topic of program evaluation and the use of dental indices are expanded in this edition.

The oral epidemiology of dental diseases is introduced in this edition. Defined discussions on the current epidemiology of specific dental diseases are presented. Dental hygiene research methodologies are expanded, focusing on the addition of more biostatistical concepts. In addition, easy-to-read tables with explanations on a multitude of research approaches and study designs are included. Case studies of individual research studies and program evaluations aid student understanding. Data analysis makes use of helpful practice problems to increase student understanding. Easy-to-read information on how to effectively evaluate scientific literature and dental products is expanded in this edition.

Strategies on creating dental hygiene positions remain in this edition; moreover, a chapter on existing careers in dental public health is added to enhance the student's understanding of available career opportunities.

Dental hygiene students will be exposed to the "real life" experiences of dental hygienists working in public health settings, including boxed scenarios of the dental hygienist's responsibilities and unique experiences in these settings. A chapter dealing with "how to create" dental hygiene positions in these areas is also presented. This section offers example proposals and helpful strategies to utilize when working to establish a dental hygiene position within a health care organization. A review of dental public health geared toward assisting the student in preparing for the community health section on national boards will remain in the book with the addition of more testlets and a thorough explanation of the correct answers to the questions presented. A glossary of terms is included. An enhanced website is available at www.prenhall.com/nathe.

A website has been designated to accompany this book and can be accessed at www.prenhall.com/nathe. Students can access information on chapter summaries, research slide series manual, test items with answers, and helpful hints for all chapters with concentration on research methods and board review.

Faculty can download a slide series to accompany the textbook and access information on the annual dental public health educator's national workshop and listserve. Faculty can also download the image library that accompanies the text. Moreover, an instructor's manual is available for faculty members teaching dental public health which includes discussion items, simulation activities, and process evaluations for each chapter.

ACKNOWLEDGMENTS

The author wishes to acknowledge the contributions of several individuals, who have greatly influenced the writing of this book. First, the chapter and section contributions from Sue Lloyd, EDH, Administrator, International Federation of Dental Hygienists, London, England, on the international movement of dental hygiene; Chris French-Beatty, RDH, PhD, Professor, Texas Woman's University, Department of Dental Hygiene, Denton, TX on biostatistics; and Meg Zayan, RDH, MPH, Professor and Director, Fones School of Dental Hygiene, University of Bridgeport, Bridgeport, Connecticut on sample test items.

In addition, reviews of the manuscript from dental hygiene students and dental hygiene educators include

Maryellen Beaulieu, RDH, BS, MPH, Ed.D.
Associate Dean/Professor
College of Health Professions
University of New England
Portland, Maine

Lynn Ann Bethel, RDH, BSDH, MPH
Assistant Professor
Mount Ida College
Newton, Massachussetts

Jacqueline N. Brian, L.D.H., M.S.Ed.
Professor
Dental Hygiene
Indiana University–Purdue University
    Fort Wayne
Fort Wayne, Indiana

Janice Brinson, BSDH, MS
Instructor
Department of Dental Hygiene
Tennessee State University
Nashville, Tennessee

Diane L. Bourque, RDH, MS
Chair
Dental Health Programs
Community College of Rhode Island
Lincoln, Rhode Island

Sandra George Burns, RDH, RN, MS
Associate Professor
Dental Hygiene
Ferris State University
Big Rapids, Michigan

Michele M. Edwards, CDA, RDH, MS
Dental Health Programs
Tallahassee Community College
Tallahassee, Florida

Kerry Flynn, RDH, BA
Assistant Professor
Dental Health Services
Palm Beach Community College
Lake Worth, Florida

Theresa M. Grady, RDH, MEd
Program Director
Dental Assisting/Dental Hygiene Program
Community College of Philadelphia
Philadelphia, Pennsylvania

Jamar M. Jackson, RDH, BS, MS
Assistant Professor
Dental Hygiene
Hostos Community College
Bronx, New York

Tara L. Johnson, BSDH, MEd
Assistant Professor
Department of Dental Hygiene
Idaho State University
Pocatello, Idaho

Mary E. Jorstad, RDH, BS, MA
Instructor
Department of Dental Hygiene
Lake Land College
Mattoon, Illinois

Nancy K. Mann, R.D.H., M.S.Ed.
Assistant Professor
Dental Hygiene
Indiana University–Purdue University
    Fort Wayne
Fort Wayne, Indiana

Patricia Mannie, RDH, MS
Instructor
Department of Dental Hygiene
St. Cloud Technical College
St. Cloud, Minnesota

Marian Williams Patton, RDH, EdD
Program Director
Department of Dental Hygiene
Tennessee State University
Nashville, Tennessee

Kari Steinbock, RDH, MS
Instructor
Department of Dental Hygiene
Mt. Hood Community College
Gresham, Oregon

Importantly, support was provided by Demetra Logothetis, Director and Professor, Division of Dental Hygiene, University of New Mexico, and, of course, editorial support and advice from Mark Cohen, senior editor, and Melissa Kerian, associate editor, Prentice Hall. The book would not be possible without support from these individuals.

DENTAL PUBLIC HEALTH

Contemporary Practice for the Dental Hygienist

Unit I

INTRODUCTION TO DENTAL PUBLIC HEALTH

The following excerpt eloquently states the need for the dental public health education of the dental hygienist.

> Although dental problems don't command the instant fears associated with low birth weight, fetal death or cholera, they do have the consequences of wearing down the stamina of children and eating their ambitions. Bleeding gums, impacted teeth and rotting teeth are routine matters for children I have interviewed in the South Bronx. Children get used to feeling constant pain. They go to sleep with it. They go to school with it. Sometimes their teachers are alarmed and try to get them to a clinic. But it's all so slow and heavily encumbered with red tape and waiting lists and missing, lost or canceled welfare cards, that dental care is long delayed. Children live for months with pain that grown-ups would find unendurable. The gradual attrition of accepted pain erodes their energy and aspirations. I have seen children in New York with teeth that look like brownish, broken sticks. I have also seen teenagers who were missing half their teeth. But, to me, most shocking is to see a child with an abscess that has been inflamed for weeks and that he has simply lived with and accepts as part of the routine of life. *

Unfortunately, this statement reflects a problem that exists throughout the world. Dental hygienists do have the skills necessary to help alleviate this problem. Appropriately, this introductory unit focuses on the historical development of dental hygiene as a true public health profession and evidence-based preventive health modalities. The current status of dental care delivery in the United States and abroad is discussed, with emphasis on the government structures and laws affecting dental hygiene delivery.

---

*Kozol, J. *Savage Inequalities: Children in America's Schools.* New York: Crown Publishers, 1991.

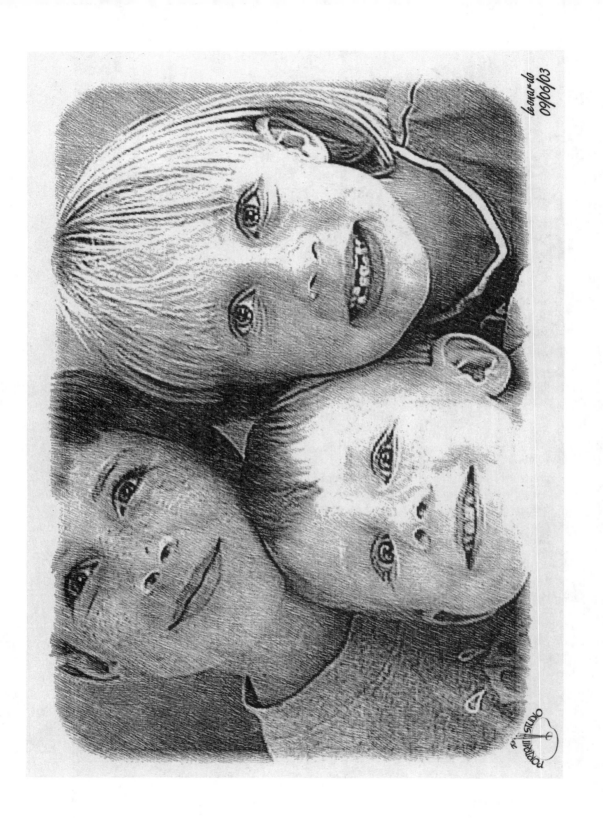

leonardo
09/05/03

PORTRAIT STUDIO

Chapter 1

::

THE PREVENTION MOVEMENT

OBJECTIVES

After studying this chapter the dental hygiene student will be able to:

- describe the history of dental hygiene in relation to dental public health.
- define dental public health.
- list and describe the current public health preventive modalities practiced today.
- defend the need for preventive modalities in dental public health practice.
- define the historical development and mission of the American Dental Hygienists' Association.

COMPETENCIES

After studying this chapter and participating in accompanying course activities and evaluation, the dental hygiene student should be able to:

- promote the values of oral and general health and wellness to the public and organizations within and outside of the profession.
- identify services that promote oral health and prevent oral disease and related conditions.
- be able to influence consumer groups, businesses, and government agencies to support health care issues.

KEY WORDS

Community dental health
Dental hygiene
Dental hygiene treatment
Dental public health
Dental sealants

Fluoridation
Nutritional counseling
Outreach
Tobacco cessation

INTRODUCTION

Dental hygiene as a discipline signals attention to the value placed on the practice of prevention as a health care science. The explosion of dental hygiene in numerous countries is further proof that the practice of prevention is mandatory in health care delivery. Since its inception, dental hygiene as a profession has worked to increase access to dental hygiene care provided by educated dental hygiene professionals throughout the world, decrease barriers to the optimum level of dental hygiene care, and continue to provide care based on the dental hygiene sciences.

As society places an ever-growing demand on self-help, prevention, and wellness, the dental hygiene profession is at the forefront of this prevention movement. In fact, dental hygiene is the only health care profession that is truly focused on preventive health care as its foundation. Further, dental hygiene has historically provided preventive services in a public health forum. Thus, dental hygiene has the scientific and practical background that so adequately complements the dental public health sciences.

HISTORICAL DEVELOPMENT

Although dental hygiene practice dates further back than its cited inception in 1913, the preventive focus of this new profession was emphasized when Dr. Alfred Civilion Fones (Figure 1–1) coined the term dental hygienist.[1] This change in title from dental nurse to dental hygienist placed focus on the necessity of preventive dental hygiene services as a scientifically valid treatment modality. Following research results published on preventive benefits of dental hygiene treatment, dental hygiene was acknowledged as a true college discipline.[2]

Fortunately for the new profession, it was Fones who actually brought the profession into existence, although many individuals saw the need for better oral health. Fones saw dental hygiene as a distinct profession and thought it should be positioned in dental public health, as opposed to working solely in private dental practices. In fact, Fones believed that the dental hygienist could provide education and dental hygiene treatment outside of the dental office, with particular focus on mass pediatric prevention. He emphasized the utilization of dental hygienists as **outreach** workers, to bring patients in need of restorative dental care to private dental practices. See Table 1–1 for more of Fones's thoughts on the dental hygiene profession.

Fones educated the first dental hygienist, Irene Newman (Figure 1–2), for one year before she started treating patients in his practice. Further, he started the Fones School of Dental Hygiene, now within the University of Bridgeport in Bridgeport, Connecticut (Figure 1–3). This school is still educating dental hygienists today (Figure 1–4). Fones initiated the dental hygienist's role in the area of

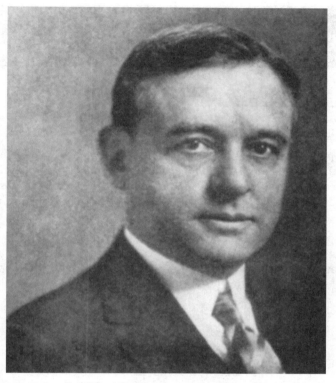

Figure 1–1. Dr. Alfred Civilion Fones, Founder of Dental Hygiene

dental public health by developing curricula for dental hygienists working within the Bridgeport Public School System (Figure 1–5). He actually initiated this program two years before it was adopted. In fact, it was a dentist on the Board of Education that voted against the plan. Deciding that this action was a blessing in disguise, Fones postponed his training course for a year during which he secured instructors and qualified students. Fones was able to secure experienced professors and experts of medicine, basic sciences, public health, and dentistry from Yale University, Harvard University, Columbia University, and the University of Pennsylvania to begin this new college discipline.

Fones stated the following about this avenue for the dental hygienist, "Dental hygiene . . . opens up paths of usefulness, activity and inspiration hitherto undreamed of, allying her with the workers of the world who are helping humanity in masses."[3] Soon, the dental hygienists in Bridgeport were providing care and education to the military after war was declared in 1917 and subsequently emerged in hospitals and numerous factories in Connecticut during the industrial revolution.

Table 1-1. Thoughts from the Writings of Dr. Alfred Fones, Founder of Dental Hygiene, Compared with the U.S. Surgeon General's Report on Oral Health 2000

Recommendations from U.S. Surgeon General's Oral Health in America Report 2000	Excerpts from *Mouth Hygiene* textbook of Dental Hygiene, Editions 1–4, 1916–1934
Change perceptions regarding oral heath and ideas so that oral health becomes an accepted component of general health.	Since the days of Hippocrates, it has been known that infections of dental origin may be accompanied by serious systemic symptoms. The work of the dental hygienist is most important in the prevention of the systemic infection through the avenue of the mouth.
Accelerate the building of the science and evidence base and apply science effectively to improve oral health.	It is no longer a theory that the service of the dental hygienist will better the mouth health and general health of all whom she is permitted to serve.
	The research field in preventive dentistry is gradually widening into a study of constitutional causes that are believed to have an influence on the general health, and consequently on dental health.
Build an effective health infrastructure that meets the oral health needs of all Americans and integrates oral health effectively into general health.	Hundreds of millions of dollars in public and private funds are expended to restore the sick to health, but only a relatively small portion of this amount is spent to maintain the health of well people, even though it is definitely known that the most common physical defects and illnesses are preventable.
	It is not the intention to in any way belittle the efforts being made to aid the sick and needy, nor should such efforts be decreased. The vital point is that we have not commenced to cover the possibilities of true prevention.
Remove known barriers between people and oral health services.	The dental hygienist was created from the realization that mouth hygiene was a necessity and that the average dental practitioner could not give sufficient time to it and that the toothbrush alone would never produce it.

(continued)

Table 1-1. *(continued)*

Recommendations from US Surgeon General's Oral Health in America Report 2000	Excerpts from *Mouth Hygiene* textbook of Dental Hygiene, Editions 1-4. 1916–1934
	The present need of the dental profession in solving the public health problem of mouth hygiene is an immense corps of women workers, educated and trained as dental hygienists, and therefore competent to enter public schools, dental offices, infirmaries, public clinics, sanitariums, factories, and other private corporations, to care for the mouths of the millions who need this educational service.
Use public-private partnerships to improve the oral health of those who still suffer disproportionately from oral disease.	The actual results secured by dental hygienists in private and public services, particularly in public schools, affords incontrovertible proof of the value of the dental hygienists. Those who may still be skeptical are finding it difficult indeed to suggest other means by which similar good results can be accomplished for large groups of people.
	The future of the dental hygienist in public schools work must be determined on a basis of cooperation between the dental profession and the educational authorities.
	The Fones's hygienists who were completing their course in 1917, when war was declared, had the unique experience of completing exams and cleanings and supplying each soldier with a toothbrush and individual instruction in the care of the mouth.

Source: Nathe, C. Dental hygiene's historical roots in modern-day issues. *Contemporary Oral Hygiene* 3 (2003): 24–25.

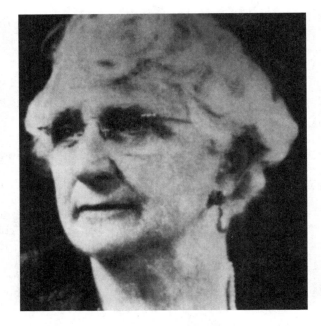

Figure 1–2. Irene Newman, RDH, First Dental Hygienist

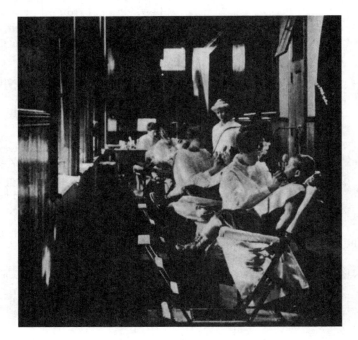

Figure 1–3. Dental Hygiene Supervisors and Clinicians at Work in the Corridors of the Bridgeport Public School System. Source: Fones School of Dental Hygiene, University of Bridgeport.

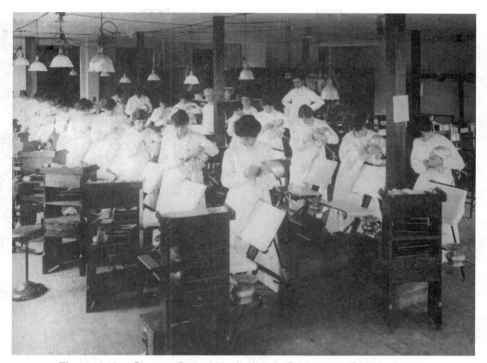

Figure 1–4. Pioneer Dental Hygienists in Bridgeport, Connecticut.
Source: Fones School of Dental Hygiene, University of Bridgeport.

Unfortunately, many state dental organizations were opposed to this new profession. Dr. Fones himself traveled across the country bringing details of the new profession to many other states, which, in the long run, may have actually hurt the profession and the population it serves. Many dental societies thought that dental hygienists might bring an end to the dentistry profession by preventing dental diseases. They were further dismayed about dental hygienists working independently from dentists because they feared it might decrease potential income and shift control from dental practitioners, so they fought to stop its growth. Consequently, many restrictive barriers were signed into law prohibiting the dental hygienist from working in any setting other than a private dental practice with a dentist supervising all treatment. In fact, the American Dental Association and many state dental associations still work diligently at changing state laws and rules and insurance regulations to further restrict access to dental hygiene care and allowing individuals with inadequate educational preparation to provide dental hygiene care.

In hindsight, it may have been more beneficial to society to introduce the new profession to school teachers, school administrators, hospital administrators, and other health care professional organizations. Their support would have increased

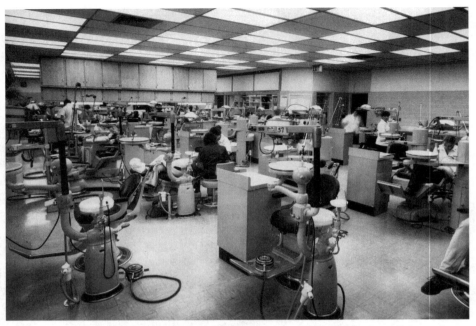

Figure 1–5.   Fones School of Dental Hygiene circa 1970's Bridgeport, Connecticut.
Source: Fones School of Dental Hygiene, University of Bridgeport.

the likelihood of the dental hygienist working as a dental public health practitioner in a variety of settings. Dental hygiene was finally accepted in all states, with a reduced educational standard for dental hygiene practice developed in Alabama.[4]

Chapter 5 discusses the impending access to care issues that resulted from these restrictive practice acts. Fortunately for society, laws are changing, and at least fourteen states now permit the unsupervised practice of dental hygiene in alternative settings, allowing the dental hygienists to work effectively in the public health arena. In fact, in Colorado and New Mexico, dental hygienists are allowed to work independently in all settings.

EVOLUTION OF ORGANIZED DENTAL HYGIENE

The Connecticut Dental Hygienists' Association was formed with nineteen members on graduation day of the first dental hygiene class in Bridgeport, Connecticut, on June 5, 1914. The first president was, fittingly, Irene Newman, the first dental hygienist. The objective of this newly formed association was "to educate the public in, and to advance the cause of Mouth Hygiene for the mutual improvement of its members, and to assist as far as lie within its power in the prevention of disease."[5]

The national association was formed in 1923 in Cleveland, Ohio. Initially, the association was called the American Association of Dental Hygienists, but in 1925 the name officially changed to the American Dental Hygienists' Association (ADHA). Presently, this association is still active, and although the present mission is slightly different, the original objective is forever instilled in its members. The present mission of the ADHA is

to improve the public's total health by working to advance the art and science of dental hygiene by ensuring access to quality oral health care, increasing awareness of the cost-effective benefits of prevention, promoting the highest standards of dental hygiene education, licensure, practice and research and representing and promoting the interests of dental hygienists.[6]

Presently, ADHA represents more than 120,000 registered dental hygienists and works actively in governmental affairs and professional development. Each of the fifty state dental hygiene associations is a constituent member. Constituent organizations serve the components in their jurisdictions by informing them of national policies and programs and actively working on legislative issues.[7] All 375 local dental hygiene associations are known as component organizations. They form the first line of involvement (grass root) for individual members. The components implement community services programs, educational sessions, and offer ideas and information about state and national policies. The board of trustees is comprised of twelve trustees from twelve geographic districts, which represent groups of constituents. The trustees, along with the president, president-elect, vice president, treasurer, and immediate past president, comprise the administrative body of ADHA. The Student American Dental Hygienists' Association (SADHA) is a constituent member of ADHA for student dental hygienists. ADHA publishes the *Journal of Dental Hygiene,* the professional journal; *ACCESS,* the professional magazine; and *Education Update,* the online periodical for dental hygiene educators. Moreover, the ADHA sponsors an annual session in June and national dental health month in October of every year. Last, the ADHA is responsible for development and implementation of the Code of Ethics for Dental Hygienists.

The International Federation of Dental Hygienists is the professional organization that represents dental hygienists from twenty-three countries. It was informally started in 1970, but officially recognized in 1986. The International Federation of Dental Hygienists publishes the *International Journal of Dental Hygiene,* which is the scientific publication of international dental hygiene. Chapter 4 describes this organization in detail. A table that lists the historical development of dental hygiene and its accompanying organizations can be found on the student website.

In addition to the *Journal of Dental Hygiene* and *ACCESS,* the profession has several other publications that deal directly with dental hygienists. Penwell publishes *RDH* magazine monthly. *RDH* is an educational source on professional and clinical issues to all dental hygienists. Montage Media publishes the *Journal of*

Practical Hygiene, which carries articles of clinical interest to the dental hygienists. The *Contemporary Oral Hygiene* periodical is published by Montage Media and emphasizes articles pertaining to the clinical, legal, and public health arena. Belmont Publications publishes the *Dimensions of Dental Hygiene* which focuses on clinical and academic development of the practicing dental hygienist. The *Journal of the Public Health Dentistry,* which is the publication of the American Association of Public Health Dentistry, covers many topics of the dental hygiene sciences. Many other journals, magazines, and Web sites exist that deal with dental hygiene and dental public health, some of which are listed in Appendix A.

DENTAL PUBLIC HEALTH DEFINED

It is important to define the science of dental public health. Although a wide-reaching field of study, dental public health is grounded in distinct concepts. Many times dental public health is termed **community dental health**. Both terms are correct and share similar meanings. Knutson defined public health as:

Public health is people's health. It is concerned with the aggregate health of a group, a community, a state, or a nation. Public health in accordance with this broad definition is not limited to the health of the poor, or to rendering health services or to the nature of the health problems. Nor is it defined by the method of payment for health services or by the type of agency responsible for supplying those services. It is simply a concern for and activity directed toward the improvement and protection of the health of a population group and the aggregate.[8]

Dental public health is defined by the American Board of Dental Public Health and recognized by the American Dental Association as:

the science and art of preventing and controlling dental disease and promoting dental health through organized community efforts. It is the form of dental practice, which serves the community as the patient rather than the individual. It is concerned with the dental health education of the public, with research and the application of the findings of research with the administration of programs of dental care for groups and with the prevention and control of dental disease through a community approach.[9]

Basically, dental public health is the oral health care and education, with an emphasis on the utilization of the dental hygiene sciences, delivered to a population. Many agencies of the federal and state governments fund dental care delivery,

Table 1–2. A Comparison of Aspects of Dental and Dental Public Health Models of Practice

	What the Dental Hygienist Does in Private Practice	**What the Dental Hygienist Does in Public Health**
ASSESSMENT	Conducts initial health assessment by reviewing health and dental history with patient.	Conducts a needs assessment of the target populations.
	Conducts a comprehensive oral examination.	Analyzes needs of the community.
DENTAL HYGIENE DIAGNOSIS	Provides dental hygiene diagnosis of the patients.	Provides dental hygiene diagnosis of the community.
PLANNING	Develops a treatment plan based on the diagnosis, patient interaction, and the priorities and method of payment. Utilizes assessment mechanisms that are measurable.	Develops a program based on the analysis of needs assessment data, priorities and alternatives, community interaction, and the resources available. Utilizes assessment mechanisms that are measurable.
	Selects appropriate health care workers to provide comprehensive care.	Selects appropriate labor to implement program.
IMPLEMENTATION	Implements self-generated treatment plan effectively, changing plan when necessary.	Implements self-generated treatment plan effectively, changing the plan when necessary.
EVALUATION	Evaluation of treatment via dental, gingival, and periodontal evaluations.	Evaluates program via index and community evaluations.

Source: Modified from Young, W., and Striffler, D. *The Dentist, His Practice & the Community.* Philadelphia: W.B. Saunders, 1969.

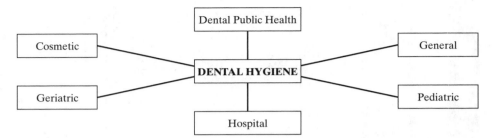

Figure 1–6. Specialties of Dental Hygiene

and Chapter 2 discusses this delivery, as well as the dental labor force needed for this delivery of care.

Because dental practitioners are mostly taught about dental care delivered in the private realm, comparison of dental public health with private dental practice helps to define dental public health. Table 1–2 compares the two types of delivery.

One of the specialties of dental hygiene is dental public health (Figure 1-6). Many dental hygienists choose to work in dental public health settings. Dental public health education is presented to dental hygiene students in all dental hygiene educational programs. The six accepted roles of the dental hygienist as related to dental public health are depicted in Table 1–3.

Table 1–3. Six Roles of the Dental Hygienist as Related to Dental Public Health	
Role of the Dental Hygienist	**Dental Public Health Responsibilities**
Administrator	Develops and coordinates dental public health programs
Change Agent	Lobbies to change laws to increase access to care for the underserved populations
Consumer Advocate	Provides dental health consultation to various target populations
Clinician	Provides clinical care to the population
Educator	Educates and promotes dental health education and issues to various target populations
Researcher	Conducts research germane to the study of health and disease and utilization of the dental hygienist

DENTAL HEALTH PREVENTIVE MODALITIES

Dental hygienists provide diagnostic and therapeutic services aimed at attaining and maintaining oral health. The following modalities have advanced the prevention movement in dental care.

DENTAL HYGIENE TREATMENT

Many postulate that water fluoridation and the recent introduction of dental sealants have had the biggest impact on the dental public health of society. However, little credit has been given to dental hygienists who, since 1913, have undoubtedly made the biggest dent in dental diseases yet witnessed. Interestingly, both *Healthy People 2010, Oral Health in America: A Report of the Surgeon General,* and *A National Call to Action to Promote Oral Health* do not even address the impact dental hygiene has had upon preventive dental care in the United States.[10, 12]

Dental hygienists found more positions around the entire country by the 1970s and have thus had a tremendous impact via the preventive and therapeutic services offered and educational promotion inherent to the practice of dental hygiene. Unfortunately, today in some private dental offices and many dental public health settings, dental hygienists are still not utilized or are underutilized. In a recent survey conducted by the American Dental Association, only 25 percent of responding dentists employ a full-time dental hygienist; furthermore, only 60 percent of dentists employ part-time dental hygienists.[13]

The introduction of **dental hygiene treatment**, which is sometimes referred to as dental cleanings or oral prophylaxes, as well as oral examination and oral hygiene instruction provided by a registered dental hygienist, is likely the reason that Americans experience less oral disease overall. Further, dental hygienists have educated a more oral health-aware consumer. Many postulate that dental hygiene was the forerunner to the prevention movement now seen in the United States.

Dental hygiene as a science has not been documented as a preventive treatment modality, so no research studies have been done to reveal the tremendous benefits to society today. The ADHA is investigating the cost effectiveness and utilization of dental hygienists at the present time, so that in the future, more research can validate the importance of the dental hygienist to societal health.[14]

Fluoridation

Dr. Frederick McKay, a graduate of dental school in Philadelphia who started practicing dentistry in Colorado Springs, Colorado, is partially credited for discovering **fluoridation**. He actually found it accidentally when he was trying to figure out why long-term residents of the area had brown enamel opacities and mottling, commonly referred to as Colorado Brown Stain. In 1908, with funding from the Colorado Springs Dental Society, he began an investigation that ultimately indicated that what he was seeing was dental fluorosis caused by too much naturally occurring fluoride in the water supply.[15] Interestingly, these same patients exhibited far fewer caries than his other patients, thus revealing the preventive benefit of fluoridated water.[16]

By the 1990s, approximately 56 percent of the U.S. population had fluoridated drinking water. In fact, 62 percent of those served by public water systems received fluoridated water.[17] A goal from *Healthy People 2010* targets that 75 percent of the population on piped-water supplies should be serviced with optimally fluoridated water.[10] Figure 1–7 graphically displays the levels of fluoridation by state.

Water fluoridation is the inclusion of fluoride in community water supplies. Although fluoride is present naturally in variable amounts in all soils and existing water supplies, it is also present in animal and plant food consumed by people.[18] Water fluoridation is an excellent method to provide benefits to most people, because everyone drinks and cooks with water. Moreover, fluoridated water is used in the processing and bottling of foods and beverages in many locations. Therefore, it is an effective way to decrease dental caries in a population. It is also cost effective.

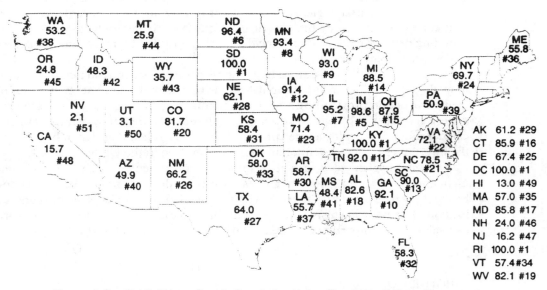

Figure 1–7. Public Water Supply Population Using Fluoridated Water Percentage of Population and State Ranking

Source: B. C. Dyck, Community water fluoridation: From the past toward the year 2000. *Dental Hygienist News* 8 (1995): 3–5.

See the student website for a table depicting direct costs of fluoridation. In addition, the cost per person could be measured against the cost of restoring demineralized tooth structure, which would directly enhance the cost benefit. Further, in areas where it is impossible to fluoridate the water, either because the residents have well water or the opposition to fluoride is overwhelming, schools have the ability to fluoridate the water the school children consume which, of course, benefits the children.

Water fluoridation works both systemically and topically. The systemic effects of water fluoridation occurs as the fluoride is absorbed via the blood plasma and becomes incorporated into the structure of the teeth. On the other hand, fluoridated toothpastes, mouthrinses, professional gels, and water fluoridation work topically, or on the tooth structure. Laboratory and epidemiological research suggests that fluoride prevents dental caries predominately after eruption of the tooth into the mouth, and its actions primarily are topical for both adults and children. These mechanisms include inhibition of demineralization, enhancement of remineralization, and inhibition of bacterial activity in dental plaque.[19]

Fluoridated water has shown to be an effective means of preventing caries in children, from an 8 percent to a 37 percent reduction, and recently studies involving fluoridated water have shown that adults benefit from the topical effect of drinking fluoridated water, reducing caries by about 20 percent to 40 percent.[20] Children benefit from the systemic and topical benefits of fluoride, whereas adults benefit from topical effects.

Water fluoridation is especially beneficial for communities of low socioeconomic status.[21] These communities have a disproportionate burden of dental caries and have less access than higher income communities to dental care services and other sources of fluoride. Therefore, water fluoridation works effectively in these populations.

Table 1–4 provides the recommended levels of fluoride, depending on climate. In a warmer climate less fluoride is needed because people drink more water. Because of the increased use of air conditioning in houses and automobiles, however, this theory may be changing. It is important to note that drinking bottled water is definitely a prevalent practice in the United States, and dental hygienists should be aware that many of these bottles contain no fluoride or have labeling that fails to define the fluoride content. See Table 1–5 for bottled water requirements.

Seldom has there been a measure to protect the public's health which has been so effective, so certain, and so simple. And yet, curiously enough, seldom has a program for safeguarding health evoked an outcry so vehement, so sustained, and so successful in blocking action.[22]

This statement clearly and concisely places into perspective the controversy against fluoridation. Although antifluoridationists have accused water fluoridation of diseases from cancer to AIDS, no credible evidence supports an association between fluoridation and any of these conditions. The U.S. Centers for Disease Control and Prevention has recognized the fluoridation of drinking water as one of ten great public health achievements of the twentieth century. Water fluoridation has

Table 1–4.   Fluoride Levels Recommended by U.S. Public Health Service for Cool and Warm Climates

Annual Average of Maximum Daily Air Temperatures (°F)	Recommended Control Limits of F Concentrations (ppm)		
	Lower	Optimum	Upper
50.0–53.7	1.1	1.2	1.7
53.8–58.3	1.0	1.1	1.6
58.4–63.8	0.9	1.0	1.5
63.9–70.6	0.8	0.9	1.4
70.7–79.2	0.7	0.8	1.3
79.3–90.5	0.6	0.7	1.2

Source: CDC. Engineering and Administrative Recommendations for Water Fluoridation. *Morbidity and Mortality Weekly Review* 44 (RR-13)(2001): 1–40.

helped improve the quality of life in the United States through reduced pain and suffering related to tooth decay, reduced time lost from school and work, and less money spent to restore, remove, or replace decayed teeth. Fluoridation is the single most effective public health measure to prevent tooth decay and improve oral health over a lifetime, for both children and adults. Water fluoridation continues to be a highly cost-effective strategy, even in areas where the overall caries level has declined and the cost of implementing water fluoridation has increased. Compared with the cost of restorative treatment, water fluoridation actually provides cost savings, a rare characteristic for community-based disease prevention strategies.

The only valid opposition ever utilized was that the addition of fluoride to water attacks personal choice. Table 1–6 displays some of the oppositions raised to public water fluoridation.

Defluoridation is the process of removing excess fluoride naturally present in a water supply in order to prevent dental fluorosis. In fact, if the fluoride concentration is high enough, severe skeletal fluorosis can occur, which is seen in some parts of the world. South Carolina, for example, requested the defluoridation of naturally occurring 2.0 ppm fluoride, which would cost an estimated $12 million. The state then found that few of the small communities affected were interested in defluoridating because the degree of fluorosis did not concern them. They did not suffer other ill effects, and they had a lower rate of caries.[23]

Table 1–5.   U.S. Food and Drug Administration (FDA) Fluoride Requirements for Bottled Water Packaged in the United States

Annual Average of Maximum Daily Air Temperature (F) Where the Bottled Water is Sold at Retail	Maximum Fluoride Concentration (mg/L) Allowed in Bottled Water	
	No Fluoride Added to Bottled Water	Fluoride Added to Bottled Water
≤53.7	2.4	1.7
53.8–58.3	2.2	1.5
58.4–63.8	2	1.3
63.9–70.6	1.8	1.2
70.7–79.2	1.6	1
79.3–90.5	1.4	0.8

Note: FDA regulations require that fluoride be listed on the label only if the bottler adds fluoride during processing; the bottler is not required to list the fluoride concentration, which might or might not be optimal. FDA does not allow imported bottled water with no added fluoride to contain >1.4 mg fluoride/L or imported bottled water with added fluoride to contain >0.8 mg fluoride/L.
Source: U.S. Department of Health and Human Services, Food and Drug Administration. 21 CFR Part 165.110. Bottled water. Federal Register 1995;60:57124–30.

Table 1–6.   Some Oppositions to Water Fluoridation

- Violation of personal freedom
- Cause of disease(s) and/or medical conditions: cancer, AIDS, fatigue, etc.
- Forced medication
- Communist plot
- Abuse of police power

In addition to water fluoridation, the effectiveness of other topically applied fluoride is well documented. Fluoridated toothpastes are thought to decrease the prevalence of dental decay by 15 percent to 30 percent.[24] Further, over-the-counter fluoride mouthrinses decrease the prevalence of dental decay by 30 percent to 40 percent.[25] Patients with xerostomia, a high caries rate, orthodontic therapy, or undergoing radiation treatment for cancer can decrease decay by up to 80 percent when utilizing a fluoride gel in a custom-made tray.[26] Fluoride varnishes applied by the dental hygienist increasingly are being used. These measures provide a definite value to the population. Please see Table 1–7 for more information on fluoride modalities.

Dental Sealants

The placement of **dental sealants** is a highly effective means of preventing pit and fissure caries, which are the areas least affected by fluoride. Unfortunately, for a variety of reasons it is currently underutilized in both private and public dental health care delivery systems. Table 1–8 lists various factors that have been reported as contributing to the underutilization of sealants.

Sealants should be placed as soon as possible after the tooth erupts and proper isolation to prevent moisture contamination can be achieved. New diagnostic methods that are specific to site and severity of caries will help make the decision to seal a tooth easier. Some of these new diagnostic modalities include the use of digital imaging systems, fiber-optic transillumination, and light or laser fluorescence.

Indications for dental sealants include newly erupted teeth, deep pits and fissures, history of caries, xerostomia, orthodontics, poor oral hygiene, and incipient caries. Some contraindications for sealants include patient behavior that does not permit a dry field and open occlusal carious lesions.

The average one surface restoration charge is more than double the average sealant charge. In fact, sealants are a cost-effective means to prevent occlusal decay.

Several investigators in several countries have repeatedly demonstrated that caries protection is 100 percent effective in pits and fissures that remain completely sealed. Moreover, studies have confirmed that complete retention rates after one year are 85 percent or better and after five years are at least 50 percent.[27] Sealants are over 65 percent more effective when administered by a dental hygienist utilizing a dental assistant. In fact, some may suggest that sealants should not be placed because of the decrease in effectiveness when one operator is placing without an assistant.

The utilization of dental hygienists with accompanying dental assistants has been shown to be an effective force in public health settings. In fact, many communities have dental hygienists that travel to schools placing dental sealants. In some states dentists are needed to supervise the placement of sealants by dental hygienists, which increases the cost and subsequently decreases cost effectiveness. Moreover, in some states a dentist must approve tooth surfaces before a dental hygienist places a sealant, further increasing the time and decreasing the cost effectiveness of sealant placement.

Table 1–7. Quality of Evidence, Strength of Recommendation, and Target Population of Recommendation for Each Fluoride Modality to Prevent and Control Dental Caries

Modality*	Quality of Evidence (Grade)	Strength of Recommendation (Code)	Target Population[†]
Community water fluoridation	II-1	A	All areas
School water fluoridation	II-3	C	Rural, nonfluoridated areas
Fluoride toothpaste	I	A	All persons
Fluoride mouthrinse	I	A	High risk[§]
Fluoride supplements			
Pregnant women	I	E	None
Children aged <6 years	II-3	C	High risk
Children aged 6–16 years	I	A	High risk
Persons aged >16 years	¶	C	High risk
Fluoride gel	I	A	High risk
Fluoride varnish	I	A	High risk

*Modalities are assumed to be used as directed in terms of dosage and age of user.
[†]Quality of evidence for targeting some modalities to persons at high risk is grade III (i.e., representing the opinion of respected authorities) and is based on considerations of cost-effectiveness that were not included in the studies establishing efficacy or effectiveness.
[§]Populations believed to be at increased risk for dental caries are those with low socioeconomic status or low levels of parental education, those who do not seek regular dental care, and those without dental insurance or access to dental services. Individual factors that possibly increase risk include active dental caries; a history of high caries experience in older siblings or caregivers; root surfaces exposed by gingival recession; high levels of infection with cariogenic bacteria; impaired ability to maintain oral hygiene; malformed enamel or dentin; reduced salivary flow because of medications, radiation treatment, or disease; low salivary buffering capacity (i.e., decreased ability of saliva to neutralize acids); and the wearing of space maintainers, orthodontic appliances, or dental prostheses. Risk can increase if any of these factors are combined with dietary practices conducive to dental caries (i.e., frequent consumption of refined carbohydrates). Risk decreases with adequate exposure to fluoride.
¶No published studies confirm the effectiveness of fluoride supplements in controlling dental caries among persons aged >16 years.
Source: CDC Recommendations for using fluoride to prevent and control dental caries in the United States. *Morbidity and Mortality Weekly Review* 50(RR14)(2001): 1–42.

Table 1–8.   Factors Contributing to the Underutilization of Dental Sealants

1. Perceived lack of data demonstrating efficacy

2. Possibility of sealing decay with subsequent progression of the lesion

3. Lack of retention of sealants

4. Unfamiliarity with technique

5. Difficulty in explaining the rationale and procedure to patients and parents

6. Lack of third-party payment

7. Belief that amalgam restorations are better and more economical

8. Insufficient instruction in curricula for dental personnel

9. Restrictive state practice acts, that is, supervision of dental hygienists

10. Lack of availability of public information about the method and its benefits, and a resulting lack of public awareness

Source: Dental sealants in the prevention of tooth decay. NIH Consensus Statement (December 5–7, 1983): 1–18.

An approach where carious lesions are removed with hand instruments and the resultant cavity and adjoining fissures restored with a dental sealant, usually glass ionomer material, is termed ART (atraumatic restorative treatment). This method of sealing a tooth is used when a provider realizes that there is no restorative option available to the patient. This method is widely used in developing countries and rural areas in developed countries.

Oral Cancer Examinations and Tobacco Cessation

It is well known that tobacco use in any form is dangerous to one's health. The use of tobacco is related to tooth staining, periodontal diseases, and oral and pharyngeal cancer. Oral and pharyngeal cancer is the seventh most common cancer found among white males (fourth most common among black men) and fourteenth most common among women in the United States. The five-year survival rate for oral and pharyngeal cancer is only 52 percent.[28] Only 7 percent of adults in the United States reported having had an oral cancer exam in the past year, which is the recommended interval.[29]

DENTAL HYGIENIST'S SPOTLIGHT
A Day in the Life of Mary Catherine Hollister, RDH, MSPH, Lieutenant Commander, USPHS

After working for eight years in private practice, I moved to an area that had a community health center. My employment there was my introduction to dental public health. I was able to work on some basic programs such as fluoride mouthrinse distribution, classroom education, and Head Start dental office orientation. The concept of treating a group of people all at one time was an exciting one for me. I could impact the dental health of more people in one week through fluoridation or education than I could working chairside in a year. I considered it "treating the nonpatient." By providing fluoride mouthrinse to a whole school, I could reach children who never got a chance to see a dentist. I realized that most public health programs benefited people regardless of their ability to pay for services or their ability to seek dental care. I decided to earn a degree in dental public health.

I was fortunate to be able to attend the University of North Carolina at Chapel Hill. After completing my BS in dental hygiene in their certificate completion program, I was accepted into the School of Public Health in Health Policy and Administration, where I earned my MS in Public Health. Of course, after completing school, one has to find a job. After graduation and considering various employment possibilities, I joined the Public Health Service and became a commissioned officer serving in the Indian Health Service. I am stationed in Gallup, New Mexico, and have the position of Dental Prevention Officer for the Gallup Service Unit.

As prevention officer, I am responsible for the community-based dental prevention programs. These include prenatal education, fluoride varnishes for children age 0 to 5, a school-based sealant program, school fluoride mouthrinse, classroom education, and screening, referral, and education for diabetes patients. Coordinating these programs means establishing baseline information, setting objectives, overseeing the actual programs, and evaluating the progress of each project. Often this work necessitates working with other agencies or nondental health care providers. Our diabetes program, for example, is a multidisciplinary program of many health care providers that give comprehensive care to our patients. Another program that provides fluoride varnish for children age 0 to 5 is a collaborative effort between Women, Infants, and Children (WIC) and the Indian Health Service. Although challenging, these joint projects often achieve far more than one individual or one group could alone.

(continued)

Dental Hygienist's Spotlight   *(continued)*

Public health is a very different type of practice than clinical dental hygiene. A career in dental public health is creative and challenging. It can be discouraging to see little change in disease rates as results are not realized as quickly as in clinical practice. But when community-based prevention works, it really works. Community water fluoridation is being hailed as one of the top ten public health successes. By making fluoride available in the water supply, everyone in the community benefits, and decay rates have been significantly reduced. By following the principles of treating the community as the patient, the public health community can have a positive effect on all citizens.

Dental professionals should conduct oral cancer exams annually and provide educational strategies designed at increasing public awareness of these diseases. Dental hygienists in many states have the opportunity of providing OralCDX, a simple brush biopsy method combined with advanced computer analysis to be used when abnormal tissue presents.[30] This gives the dental hygienist a tool to help increase the referral of oral cancer to oncologists during an early stage, which may improve the prognosis of a disease that has remained unchanged for the last half century.

Moreover, dentists and hygienists can provide counseling to patients to stop tobacco use and limit alcohol use, both of which are associated with oral and pharyngeal cancer. In fact, one study suggested that approximately 90 percent of dentists and dental hygienists ask their patients if they smoke.[31] Unfortunately, many dental professionals stop after they ask the initial question. Programs to help smokers and tobacco chewers quit the habit are plentiful, and many campaigns exist to aid tobacco users. **Tobacco cessation** programs are implemented in many dental public health and private dental settings. Tobacco cessation programs encourage patients to quit tobacco utilization by emphasizing four steps of intervention: asking patients about their tobacco use, advising patients to stop using tobacco products, assisting patients in taking steps to stop, and arranging patient follow-up services.[32] Dental hygienists are in a unique position to influence the population on this addictive drug.

Nutritional Counseling

In *Mouth Hygiene,* the first textbook for dental hygienists, the author states that the two great factors for the prevention of dental pathology are normal nutrition and mouth cleanliness.[33] With this in mind, it is necessary for the dental hygienist to incorporate **nutritional counseling** into all regimens related to oral health care. In fact, oral health is a major contributor to good nutrition. The oral cavity is the pathway to the body, and disturbances in the mouth can profoundly affect diet and ultimately nutritional status. Conversely, good nutrition provides the foundation for good oral health. Diet plays a major role in the etiology or prevention of dental caries, and is an important supporting factor in other oral infections.

The American Dental Hygienists' Association recommends that dental hygienists maintain a current knowledge of nutrition recommendations and that they relate to general and oral health and disease and effectively educate and counsel their patients about proper nutrition and oral health.[7] Further, the American Dietetic Association states that collaboration is necessary between dietetics and dental professionals for oral health promotion and diseases prevention and intervention.[34]

The dental hygienist should continue to manage nutritional issues by presenting nutritional and dental health topics to populations and referrals to appropriate health care workers. In addition, it is important that dental hygienists work with dietitians in community endeavors aimed at educating and promoting the importance of a healthy diet in oral health and, consequently, total health.

Xylitol

Xylitol is a sugar substitute that has shown promising results in reducing tooth decay and ear infections. Xylitol is found in berries, fruit, vegetables, mushrooms, and birch wood. Xylitol can be delivered in teeth via mints, gums and lozenges to help reduce dental decay. After taking xylitol, bacteria do not adsorb well on the surface of the teeth and the amount of plaque decreases. Dental public health programs aimed at decreasing dental decay in children have started utilizing xylitol lozenges.

Mass Education and Promotion

Chapter 6 includes an in-depth look into dental health education and promotion, which is an important topic because of the primary goal of the dental hygienist to improve oral health. One of the most important functions of the dental hygienist is to provide dental health education and promotion of dental health to the public. For these reasons it is important for the dental hygienist to be well versed as an educator and public speaker.

Many dental supply companies have developed mass educational materials for specific target populations. These materials are helpful to the dental hygienist and can be utilized by teachers and health care workers. Moreover, many popular children's books and videos about dental health issues are available, which of course, increase public awareness.

The other areas in which consumers are provided dental education and promotion is by advertising in written form and through television. Many times television sitcoms discuss dental issues and even the role of dental hygienists. Sometime this information is correct; however, oftentimes the population will be given inaccurate information by these mass messages, and therefore it is important for the dental hygienist to help provide correct information to the population.

SUMMARY

Dental hygiene historically was initiated as a public health profession. In fact, dental hygiene was the forerunner of the prevention movement now prevalent in public health care. It is vitally important to the public that dental hygienists be educated in the dental public health sciences. Furthermore, refined skills in program planning, dental health education and promotion, and oral epidimiology are necessary for dental hygienists in all aspects of the dental hygiene sciences. Dental hygienists must work as advocates for various dental public measures and further expand the practice to the entire public. Dental hygiene will continue to strive to meet the needs of the public by educating dental hygienists to provide effective dental public health care.

REFERENCES

[1]Fones, A. C. Origin and history. *Journal of the American Dental Hygienists' Association* 3 (1929): 9–10.

[2]Motley, W. E. *History of the American Dental Hygienists' Association 1923–1982.* Chicago: American Dental Hygienists' Association, 1983.

[3]Fones, A. C. *Mouth Hygiene,* 2d ed. Philadelphia: Lea and Febriger, 1916.

[4]Goldenberg, S. Alabama dental hygiene program, what it is, what it does. Bensden, PA, 1987.

[5]History of the Connecticut Dental Hygienists' Association. *Journal of the American Dental Hygienists' Association* 5 (1931): 26.

[6]American Dental Hygienists' Association Membercard, ADHA. Chicago, 2000.

[7]http://www.adha.org.

[8]Knutson, J. W. What is public health? In W. J. Pelton, J. M. Wison, eds. *Dentistry in Public Health,* 2d ed. Philadelphia: W. B. Saunders, 1955.

[9]American Board of Dental Public Health. *Guidelines for Graduate Education in Dental Public Health.* Ann Arbor, MI: American Board of Dental Public Health, 1970.

[10]U.S. Public Health Service. *Healthy People 2010.* National health promotion and disease prevention objectives. Conference edition. Washington, DC: U.S. Dept. of Health and Human Services, 2000.

[11]U.S. Department of Health and Human Services. *Oral Health in America: A Report of the Surgeon General.* Rockville, MD: U.S. Department of Health and

Human Services, National Institute of Dental and Craniofacial Research, National Institutes of Health, 2000.

[12]U.S. Department of Health and Human Services. *A National Call to Action to Promote Oral Health.* Rockville, MD: U.S. Department of Health and Human Services, Public Health Service, Centers for Disease Control and Prevention, National Institutes of Health, National Institute of Dental and Craniofacial Research. NIH Publication No. 03-5303 May 2003.

[13]Nathe, C., M. Darby, D. Bauman, and D. Shuman. Too few resumes. *RDH* 17 (1997): 18–29.

[14]American Dental Hygienists' Association Council on Research Meeting Minutes. Chicago: American Dental Hygienists' Association, 1999.

[15]The relation of mottled enamel to caries. *American Dental Association Journal* 15 (1928): 1429–37.

[16]Striffler, D. F. et al. *Dentistry, Dental Practice, and the Community,* 2d ed. Philadelphia: W. B. Saunders, 1983.

[17]Centers for Disease Control and Prevention. Achievements in Public Health, 1990–1999: Fluoridation of Drinking Water to Prevent Dental Caries. *Morbidity and Mortality Weekly Report* 48 (1999): 933–40.

[18]Dyck, B. C. Community water fluoridation: From the past toward the year 2000. *Dental Hygienist News* 8 (1995): 3–5.

[19]Centers for Disease Control and Prevention. *Fluoridation census 1992.* Atlanta, GA: U.S. Department of Health and Human Services, National Center for Prevention Services, Division of Oral Health, 1993.

[20]Newbrun, E. Effectiveness of water fluoridation. *Journal of Public Health Dentistry* 49 (1989): 279–89.

[21]Riley, J. C., M. A. Lennon, and R. P. Ellwood. The effect of water fluoridation and social inequalities on dental caries in 5-year-old children. *International Journal of Epidemiology* 28 (1999): 300–305.

[22]Paul, B. D. et al. Trigger for community conflict: The case of fluoridation. *Journal of Sociology Issues* 17 (1961): 1–84.

[23]Newburn, E. *Fluoride and Dental Caries.* Springfield, IL: Charles C. Thomas, 1986; National Research Council. *Health Effects of Ingested Fluoride.* Washington, DC: National Academy Press, 1993.

[24]Richards, A., and D. W. Banting. Fluoride toothpastes in Fejerskov, O., Ekstrand, J., Burt, B. A, eds. *Fluoride in Dentistry,* 2d ed. Copenhagen: Munksgaard, 1996, pp. 328–46.

[25]National Fluoride Task Force of NFDH. A guide to the use of fluorides for the prevention of dental caries. *Journal of the American Dental Association* 113 (1986): 503.

[26]Englander, H. R., P. H. Keyes, and M. Gestwicki. Clinical anticaries effect of repeated topical sodium fluoride applications by mouthpieces. *Journal of the American Dental Association* 75 (1967): 638.

[27]Dental sealants in the prevention of tooth decay. NIH Consensus Statement (December 5–7, 1983): 1–18.

[28]American Cancer Society. *Cancer Facts and Figures 1998*. Atlanta, GA: American Cancer Society, 1998.

[29]Horowitz, A. M., and P. A. Nourjah. Patterns of screening for oral cancer among U.S. adults. *Journal of Public Health Dentistry* 56 (1996): 331–35.

[30]http://www.oralcdx.com.

[31]Tobacco control activities in U.S. dental practices. *Journal of the American Dental Association* 18 (1997): 172.

[32]Wood, G. Office-based training in tobacco cessation for dental professionals. *Journal of the American Dental Association* 128 (1997): 216.

[33]Fones, A. C. *Mouth Hygiene*. Philadelphia: Lea and Febiger, 1916.

[34]http://www.eatright.org.

Get Connected

Multimedia Extension Activities

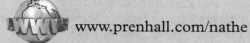 www.prenhall.com/nathe

Use the above address to access the free, interactive companion web site created specifically to accompany this textbook. Here you will find an array of self study material to help you gain a richer understanding of the concepts presented in this chapter.

Chapter 2

DENTAL CARE DELIVERY IN THE UNITED STATES

OBJECTIVES

After studying this chapter, the dental hygiene student will be able to:

- describe the state of dental health in the United States.
- list the government agencies related to dental hygiene.
- compare the federal, state, and local presence of government in dental care delivery.
- define the dental hygienist employment opportunity ratio.
- describe dental hygiene labor force issues.
- define need, supply, demand, and utilization.

COMPETENCIES

After studying this chapter and participating in the accompanying course activities, the dental hygienist student should be competent in the following:

- promote the values of oral and general health and wellness to the public and organizations within and outside the profession.
- be able to influence consumer groups, business, and government agencies to support health care issues.
- provide dental hygiene services in a variety of settings including offices, hospitals, clinics, extended care facilities, community programs and schools.

KEY TERMS

Dental care delivery	Medicaid
Demand	Need
Department of Health and Human Services	SCHIP
Head Start	Supply
Malpractice	Workforce
	Utilization

www.prenhall.com/nathe

INTRODUCTION

Dental care delivery in the United States involves many different private and government entities. Although most dental hygienists are employed through private-practice dentists, many dental hygiene positions are available in government organizations. When discussing dental public health care, it is necessary to define dental public health and to present the dental care delivery system currently existing in the United States. Chapter 4 discusses dental care delivery systems in other countries.

Although dental diseases are preventable, dental health in the United States remains an issue. In fact, it has been postulated that oral health is a major unmet need in this country.[1] And although more than 80 percent of seventeen-year-old children experience dental decay, the burden of this disease is not evenly distributed.[2] A startling statistic revealed that more than 80 percent of dental decay was found in 25 percent of the population.[3] Moreover, these children are from lower-income households, ethnic minorities, and many times have special needs.

The consequences of this widespread problem are alarming. More than half (57 percent) of parents report unmet dental needs of their children, which is nearly five times the number reporting the need for eyelgasses.[4] Untreated dental diseases result in children who have constant pain, difficulty eating, difficulty speaking, chronic infections, increased use of pain medicine, and embarrassment over the esthetic condition of their teeth. Moreover, emergency room and operating room staffs regularly see large numbers of children presenting with unrelenting toothaches and caries beyond dental office management.[5] Emergency visits usually consist of antibiotic therapies and can require hospitalization if not treated in an effective manner.[6] Research has linked periodontal diseases to heart and lung disease; diabetes; premature, low-birthweight babies; and a number of other systemic diseases.

Unfortunately, the individuals who most need dental care are not receiving it. Dental hygiene treatment can help alleviate this problem, specifically in states where dental hygienists can provide care as outreach workers.

FACTORS AFFECTING DENTAL PUBLIC HEALTH

Many different issues face dental public health and impact the care that dental hygienists deliver. Probably the number one issue facing dental care delivery in the United States today is access to dental care. This issue is widespread; many individuals do not have adequate access to care. The reasons vary, but in many states dental hygienists are restricted to providing care with the supervision of dentists. Moreover, many individuals lack the financial resources or transportation needed for dental care services. In fact, numerous barriers to care exist in the United States and are discussed in detail in chapter 8.

The introduction of professional dental hygiene care, fluoride, and dental sealants, more than any other factors, have influenced the reduction in dental caries rates. The related demographic information depicts an interesting correlation. The socioeconomic status of an individual affects the access and provision of dental care. Socioeconomic status can be defined as an individual's comparative status in social and economic standing within a community. Specifically, the lower the socioeconomic status of the individual, the increased frequency of untreated dental caries. Children from lower-income and ethnic minority households and children with special health care needs are more likely to experience tooth decay and have higher levels of untreated tooth decay compared with children from more economically advantaged households. This correlation again points to the inadequate accessibility of dental hygiene and dental care.

The increased number of dental hygienists has certainly been a benefit to dental disease prevention. One sure sign is seen in the growing aging population, where the advent of dental hygiene and fluoride has subsequently increased the number of teeth lasting a lifetime. Further, medical science has increased life expectancies for the elderly and otherwise medically compromised individuals. Accordingly, dental hygiene science has evolved in treating these patients with often debilitating diseases.

Malpractice has also had a direct impact on dental care delivery and quality. The first medical malpractice suit was won in 1976, thus the advent of patient's rights and medical and dental malpractice.[7] Patients are able to sue if the provider does not adequately diagnose and treat periodontal diseases. Moreover, dental hygienists should carry malpractice insurance due to the increase in malpractice suits filed. Although supervised and employed by a dentist in most states, dental hygienists are liable for all treatment they render or fail to render.

The introduction of dental insurance has increased the number of paying patients seeking preventive care in private dental offices. The impact of managed dental care insurance programs is being watched carefully by all dental providers and dental professional organizations. Although insurance may have increased the number of patients seeking dental treatment, it also has influenced the quality and quantity of services provided in many situations.

DELIVERY OF DENTAL CARE IN THE UNITED STATES

Dental care delivery in the United States is provided for the most part in private dental practices. Figure 2–1 depicts the vehicles involved in the delivery of dental care. Providers of dental care include dental hygienists, dentists, dental assistants, and dental technicians. Even though the government plays a small role in funding and regulating dental care delivery, most patients receive treatment from private dental practitioners utilizing employer-paid dental insurance.

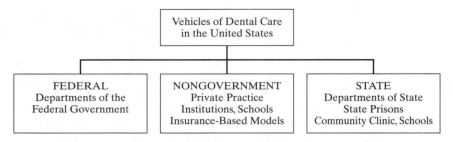

Figure 2–1. Dental Care Delivery in the United States

Dental care delivery is impacted by many federal and state governmental entities. State practice acts and rules and regulations are responsible for governing the practice of dental hygiene in specific states, which is discussed further in chapter 5.

FEDERAL AND STATE STRUCTURE OF DENTAL PUBLIC HEALTH

Federal Influence

The executive branch of the federal government has direct impact on dental care delivery. The department obviously responsible for many entities of dental care is the **Department of Health and Human Ser-vices** (HHS).

Department of Health and Human Services

The HHS is the government's principal agency for protecting the health of all Americans and providing essential human services, especially for those who are least able to help themselves. The HHS includes more than 300 programs, covering a wide spectrum of activities. Some highlights can be seen in Table 2–1. HHS is the largest grant-making agency in the federal government, providing approximately 60,000 grants per year. These grants provide funding for specific health or human service programs. HHS works closely with state and local governments, and many HHS-funded services are provided at the local level by state or county agencies, or through private sector grantees. The eleven HHS operating divisions depicted in Figure 2–2 administer the department's programs. In addition to the services they deliver, the HHS programs provide for equitable treatment of beneficiaries nationwide, and they enable the collection of national health and other data. The secretary of the department, who is appointed by the president of the United States, directs the HHS. HHS has two operating divisions, the Public Health Service Operating Division and the Human Services Operating Divisions.

Table 2–1.   Activities of the Department of Health and Human Services

- Medical and social science research
- Preventing outbreak of infectious diseases, including immunization services
- Assuring food and drug safety
- Medicare (health insurance for elderly and disabled)
- Medicaid (health, including dental, insurance for low-income people)
- Financial assistance for low-income families
- Child support enforcement
- Improving maternal and infant health
- Early Head Start and Head Start (prenatal, infant, and preschool education and services)
- Preventing child and domestic violence
- Substance abuse treatment and prevention
- Services for older Americans, including home-delivered meals
- Comprehensive health services delivery for Native Americans and Alaska Natives

Public Health Service Divisions

The National Institutes of Health (NIH) is the government's medical research organization, supporting some 35,000 research projects nationwide in diseases such as cancer, Alzheimer's, diabetes, arthritis, cardiovascular diseases, and AIDS. NIH has seventeen separate health institutes, including the National Institute of Dental and Craniofacial Research, which focuses on research in the oral health sciences. The NIH is headquartered in Bethesda, Maryland.

The Food and Drug Administration (FDA) assures the safety of foods and cosmetics and the safety and efficacy of pharmaceuticals, biological products, and medical devices. FDA was established in 1906 and is headquartered in Rockville, Maryland. Specifically, this division is responsible for the regulation of dental materials, dental equipment, and over-the-counter dental care products.

The Centers for Disease Control and Prevention (CDC) provides a system of health surveillance to monitor and prevent outbreak of diseases and maintains national health statistics. In addition, the CDC provides for immunization services and guards against international disease transmission. It was established in 1946

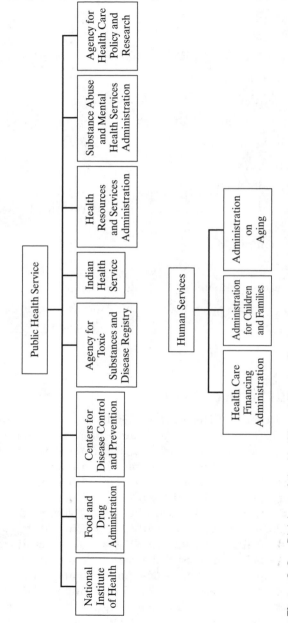

Figure 2-2. Divisions of the Health and Human Services

and is located in Atlanta, Georgia. The CDC plays a major role in preparing guidelines for the prevention of oral diseases.

Federal Health Services for Indians began in the early nineteenth century when U.S. Army physicians took steps to curb small pox and contagious disease among tribes living in the vicinity of military posts. By 1880, the first federal hospital was built in Oklahoma. By 1913, the first dental services were provided with dentists visiting reservations and schools.[8]

The Indian Health Service (IHS) provides 1.5 million Native Americans, including Alaskan Natives, with medical and dental care. In addition, it assists thirty-four urban Native American health centers. IHS was established in 1955. Dental hygienists and dentists can work for the IHS as Public Health Service Commissioned Officers, civil servants, or independent contractors. In many IHS settings dental assistants provide some dental hygiene services, including the provision of dental scalings and polishing to the Native American population. This is legally accepted because state laws do not have to be practiced in all clinics.

In addition to the IHS dental services, many individual tribes offer dental services. In fact, tribal dental clinics are common in many locations, and tribes hire dental hygienists, dentists, and dental assistants to work within the tribal clinics. Tribal clinics are governed by each of the more than 547 federally recognized tribes.

The Health Resources and Services Administration (HRSA) helps provide health resources for medically underserved populations. It entails a nationwide network of community health centers, migrant health centers, and primary care programs. HRSA works to build the health care workforce and maintains the National Health Service Corps. This agency provides services to people with AIDS through the Ryan White CARE Act, oversees the organ transplantation system, works to decrease infant mortality, and improve children's health. Dental hygienists may serve with the National Health Service Corps.

The Substance Abuse and Mental Health Services Administration (SAMHSA), Agency for Health Care Policy and Research (AHCPR), and Agency for Toxic Substances and Disease Registry (ATSDR) are also housed organizationally with the Public Health Service Operating Division.

Human Services Divisions

The Administration on Aging (AOA) is the principal agency designated to carry out the provisions of the Older Americans Act of 1965 and is responsible for enhancing and supporting the older population's independence. Additionally, the AOA is involved in dental education in geriatric dental care.

The Administration for Children and Families (ACF) is responsible for federal programs that promote the economic and social well-being of families, children, individuals, and communities and is responsible for the Early Head Start and Head Start programs, which provide educational social, medical, dental, nutrition, and mental health services to pregnant mothers and children up to five years old from low-income families.

The Centers for Medicare & Medicaid Services (CMS), which was formerly known as the Health Care Financing Administration (HCFA), is the federal agency responsible for administering the Medicare, **Medicaid, SCHIP** (State Children's Health Insurance), HIPAA (Health Insurance Portability and Accountability Act), CLIA (Clinical Laboratory Improvement Amendments), and several other health-related programs. CMS is responsible for overseeing the federal portion of the Medicaid program and has full responsibility to the Medicare program. Medicare funds cover medical care for the elderly and disabled. In specific cases, Medicare may provide reimbursement for dental procedures carried out in the hospital on elderly or disabled individuals, but generally Medicare does not fund dental care. Medicaid is the program that traditionally funds dental care in the indigent population and is administered by states. Medicaid insurance can be paid to dentists and, in some states, dental hygienists in private practice or community clinical settings. These two federal health care programs are the largest and account for about 80 percent of annual federal health care expenditures. Additionally, CMS runs the State Children's Health Insurance Program (SCHIP). SCHIP is the largest effort by Congress since Medicaid was enacted thirty-two years ago to provide health insurance to vulnerable children throughout the United States. Enacted as part of the Balanced Budget Act of 1997, it addresses the program of 10 million medically uninsured children. SCHIP is distinct from Medicaid in that it entitles states, but not individual children, to federal allotments to purchase child health assistance; it pays a 30 percent larger share of program costs than Medicaid, and it gives states a great deal more latitude in program design, including eligibility, benefits, cost sharing, and administration.

The Public Health Services (PHS) Commissioned Corps is directed by the U.S. Surgeon General. The Public Health Service works toward improving and advancing the health of our nation's people. The PHS Commissioned Corps was established in 1889 when Congress officially organized the commissioned corps along military lines with titles and pay corresponding to the Army and Navy grades. Officers are currently commissioned in eleven professional categories representing the breadth of health care professionals.

Many other departments additionally have impact on dental health, including the Departments of Agriculture, Defense, Education, Justice, Labor, State, Treasury, and Veteran's Affairs. Food, nutrition counseling, and access to health and dental services are provided to low-income women, infants, and children under the Special Supplemental Nutrition Program for Women, Infants, and Children, known as WIC. The Food and Nutrition Services of the Department of Agriculture administer WIC at the federal level. WIC actually provides federal grants to states for state WIC programs. Most state WIC programs provide vouchers that participants use at authorized food stores. Specifically, WIC programs collaborate with dental hygiene programs and community dental clinics to offer dental screenings and dental health education.

The Department of Defense oversees the dental care of military dental personnel and their dependents. Dentists in the military and enlisted dental technicians often deliver this care. One interesting facet of dental care delivery in the military is that in some military branch dental settings, enlisted dental technicians provide supragingival scalings and coronal polishing, which are termed prophylaxis, without graduating from an accredited dental hygiene program and taking the national and regional dental hygiene board examinations. Dental hygienists may work as a civil servant or independent contractor for the Department of Defense, and dental hygienists with bachelor of science degrees may work as military officers (see Table 2–2). Dependents, including spouses and children, generally receive care through the dental providers participating in the dental insurance program provided to them through military benefits.

The Department of Justice is responsible for the Federal Bureau of Prisons and the dental care provided to inmates incarcerated in this system. Dentists and dental hygienists may work as U.S. Public Health Service officers in federal prisons, civil servants, or under independent contracts. Settings can vary from prison camps (minor offenders) to maximum-security prisons. In the United States, inmates have a constitutional right to health care, thus, the need for dental hygiene services. Providing dental hygiene to this population decreases cost through a decrease in restorative services needed.

Table 2–2. Federal Dental Hygiene Positions

Department	Position
Agriculture	Women, Infant, Children (WIC) Program Dental Hygiene Educator
Defense	Dental Hygienist at a Military Base
Justice	Dental Hygienist at a Federal Prison
Health and Human Service	PHS Commissioned Officer
	Early Head Start and Head Start
	Centers for Disease Control and Prevention
	Research/Administrative Position
	National Institute of Dental and Craniofacial Research
Peace Corps	Dental Hygienist in a developing country.
State	Civil Servant Position with Military, VA Hospital, or other governmental agency
Veteran's Affairs	Dental Hygienist at a Veteran's Affairs (VA) Hospital

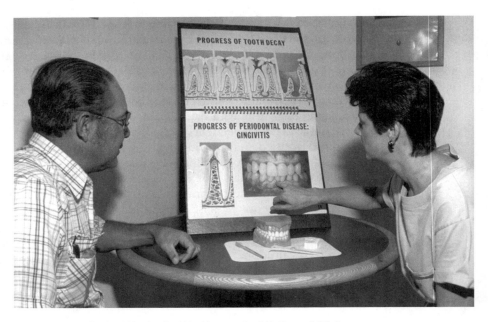

Figure 2–3. Dental Hygienist Working at the VA Dental Clinic

Many dental hygienists practice in settings of the Department of Veteran's Affairs (VA). Dentists, dental hygienists, assistants, and technicians are usually employed in civil servant positions (Figure 2–3). Veterans with service-connected dental disabilities are treated in these facilities. Occasionally, military members who have left military service but did not complete dental care are served through the VA dental services. In addition, veterans who live within the long-term care facilities at the individual VA Medical Centers are offered dental services. Dental hygienists in this setting have a variety of responsibilities, including education of patients and nurses and clinical treatment within the dental clinic and bedside.

The Bureau of Labor Statistics (BLS), which is organizationally housed within the Department of Labor, is the principal fact-finding agency for the federal government in the broad field of labor, economics, and statistics, which impacts dental care delivery. The BLS is an independent national statistical agency that collects, processes, analyzes, and disseminates essential statistical data to the American public, the U.S. Congress and other federal agencies, state and local governments, business, and labor. Specifically, the BLS forecasts dental and dental hygiene labor force for future years.

As previously discussed, the State Department employs persons in Civil Services positions. Many dental hygienists work as civil servants in federal prisons, military settings, and VA hospitals. Civil service positions for dental hygienists pay quite low and, many times these settings will contract with dental hygienists unable to work for the civil service pay. To qualify for a civil service position, a candidate must be a U.S. citizen and undergo a thorough background investigation to receive a security clearance.

The Department of Treasury is responsible for the manufacturing and labeling of alcohol and tobacco products and the health of the members of the Coast Guard.

The Department of Education's mission is to ensure equal access to education and to promote educational excellence for all Americans.

The Peace Corps was formally initiated in 1961 and is an independent agency within the executive branch of the U.S. government. The president of the United States appoints the Peace Corps director and deputy director, and the appointments must be confirmed by the U.S. Senate. The Senate Foreign Relations Committee is charged with general oversight of the activities and programs of the Peace Corps, and the House Committee on International Relations serves a similar function. Dental hygienists can provide dental hygiene treatment and education as a peace corps worker.

State Influence

All states, including Washington, D.C., and U.S. territories, utilize departments that are focused on providing health and human services to those in need. Many departments have different names but all state departments of health services share a similar mission. Appendix D lists these state departments.

Specifically, these departments include dental divisions. Dental divisions are directed by dental hygienists and dentists in many states. State dental departments work as dental consultants within the state environment and strive to promote dental health. Many state departments work to implement water fluoridation within communities, school-based prevention programs, school sealant programs, and fluoride mouthrinse programs.

Medicaid programs are usually operated through the human services division of the state health department. Often Medicaid programs are operated by a third party, generally an insurance company. Many state health departments are in charge of the SCHIPS program as well.

Many states provide dental care within community clinics (Figure 2–4). Some of these clinics are private, and many are nonprofit but utilize state and sometimes federal funds in addition to sliding scale reimbursements and Medicaid reimbursements to operate. In some states community clinics are owned and operated through the state. Many states dental clinics can be federally qualified heath centers (FQHCs), which means that they would qualify for enhanced reimbursement from Medicaid and other benefits. FQHCs must serve an underserved area or population, offer a sliding fee scale, provide comprehensive services, have an ongoing quality assurance program, and have a governing board of directors. Although some of these clinics are in an urban (metropolitan) setting, many of these clinics serve in rural or frontier settings where the population is underserved.

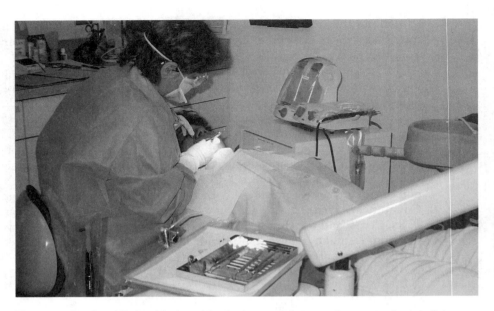

Figure 2–4.   A public health dental hygienist providing care in a state dental clinic.

State prison systems are separate from the Federal Bureau of Prisons, but also provide dental care to inmates. State prisons can be operated by the state or private organizations. Dental hygienists often work in these settings.

States may also have tribal dental clinics. These clinics are operated within the state but usually follow guidelines established within the tribe. In some instances, the IHS will provide assistance. Dental hygienists are often employed in these settings and may provide care in migrant clinics as well.

Many states provide dental care to the elderly and developmentally disabled in institutionalized dental clinic settings. Care to these groups is difficult to obtain in private dental practices due to the difficulty in transportation, low reimbursement rates, specialization needed to treat these populations, and refusal by providers to accept Medicaid insurance.

DENTAL HEALTH CARE PERSONNEL

In the United States pluralism is the way of organizing and providing health care services.[9] In fact the dental care delivery system is a mixture of organizations, practitioners, financing mechanisms, and innovative approaches to health services

DENTAL HYGIENIST'S SPOTLIGHT
Kathleen Mangskau, RDH, MPA

Kathleen Mangskau, RDH, MPA, is the administrator of the Tobacco Prevention and Control Program, North Dakota Department of Health. Kathleen administers the statewide tobacco prevention and control program designed to reduce the health and economic consequences of tobacco use in the state. She supervises the tobacco control team at the state level that includes four additional staff. Kathleen oversees grants and contracts to over fifty agencies and individuals to carry out the goals and objectives of the cooperative agreement with the Centers for Disease Control and Prevention, Office of Smoking and Health, and administers the funds from the Tobacco Master Settlement Agreement that are appropriated to tobacco control.

Kathleen's responsibilities as the tobacco program administrator include overseeing assessment of the tobacco control problem in the state, promoting policy and environmental change and assurance of services. Assessment data are used for program planning, surveillance, and evaluation of programs. Policy efforts include recommending and reviewing legislation and related rules and providing testimony before the State Legislature and interim committees on tobacco-related issues. Assurance activities include health promotion efforts, such as community interventions and media advocacy efforts, to denormalize tobacco use. Kathleen also serves as a liaison to other agencies and organizations on tobacco control issues. She has the fiscal responsibility for seeking out grants and preparing and monitoring program budgets and contracts.

Kathleen served as the director of the Oral Health Program, North Dakota Department of Health, for sixteen years prior to her role in tobacco control. She

(continued)

Dental Hygienist's Spotlight *(continued)*

administered the statewide oral health program designed to improve the oral health of the residents of the state. She oversaw a network of eight regional oral health consultants providing services at the local level.

Kathleen served as the president of the Association of State and Territorial Dental Directors from 1998–2000. She was the first dental hygienist and the first female to serve as president of the organization. Kathleen is a strong advocate for oral health at the state and national level. She was instrumental in getting oral health questions on a number of national surveys, including the Behavioral Risk Factor Surveillance System and the Youth Risk Behavior Survey. She has been involved in the development and review of the oral health objectives for the Healthy People 2010 Health Objectives for the Nation and has served as a reviewer for the Surgeon General's Report on Oral Health.

Kathleen spent fourteen years as a clinical dental hygienist prior to joining public health in 1985. She believes her clinical experience and background as a state dental director provided a framework for her new role in tobacco control. "I have always liked challenge and change and that is what attracted me to public health. In my role as a tobacco program administrator, I have new opportunities and challenges each day. I

like to try new approaches and be able to impact population based health services. Public health provides tremendous opportunities for dental hygienists to initiate innovative approaches to health promotion and disease prevention efforts and expand dental hygiene practice." Tobacco use has a significant impact on oral health. She says, "Oral health professionals should be involved in preventing and reducing tobacco use. Each dental visit provides an opportunity to talk to patients about tobacco use and prevent initiation and promote quitting." Kathleen has also served as a consultant and reviewer for Head Start programs and state oral health programs, as adjunct faculty for the North Dakota AIDS Education and Training Center, and has published a number of articles on oral health in North Dakota.

Kathleen earned an Associate of Science Degree in Dental Hygiene in 1971 from the North Dakota State College of Science, Wahpeton, ND; a Bachelor of Science Degree in Business Administration in 1991 from the University of Mary, Bismarck, ND; and a Master of Public Administration Degree in 1996 from the University of North Dakota, Grand Forks, ND. Kathleen is a 2002 graduate of the National Public Health Leadership Institute, University of North Carolina at Chapel Hill.

planning. Those concerned with planning for health labor force requirements attach a specific meaning to the concepts of **need, demand, utilization,** and **supply.** Need can be defined as a normative, professional judgment as to the amount and kind of health care services required to attain or maintain health. The particular frequency or desired frequency of dental care from a population is demand, and the quantity of dental care services available can be termed supply. Utilization is the number of dental care services actually consumed, not just desired, which can be of importance when speculating on the available supply of personnel to meet the demand and/or need. One example of the difference between need and demand is demonstrated with children's hockey teams. Players on these teams have high rates of oral-facial injuries and concussions, and professional recommendations mandate custom-made mouthguards; however, many young hockey players across the country do not wear mouthguards. Obviously the need (mouthguards) is present, but the demand by the consumer is not. Now, assume that the demand by the consumers is great, but not enough available dental providers (supply) in these communities are available to fabricate these mouthguards. This scenario would change the equation by not having the supply to meet the demand and the need.

The federal guidelines forecast the number of dentists needed for a population, without mention of the necessary dental hygienist labor force. Adequate dental capacity as suggested by the National Health Manpower Shortage Area is designated as 1 dentist per 2,000 population.[10] Further, the appropriate dentist to population ratio for the special consideration population such as a state facility or reservation has been estimated at 1 dentist per 4,000 population, and the HHS states that the appropriate dentist to population ratio is 1 dentist per 5,000.

Dental Hygiene Workforce Issues

Dentists in many states report local shortages in dental hygiene labor force, although no published data can be found confirming such a shortage.[11] Even though the ADHA has issued a report suggesting an adequate supply of dental hygienists, the ADA continues to support these anecdotal claims.[12] The reason may be that the proposed solutions to remedy this anecdotal dental hygiene labor shortage include preceptorship training for dental hygienists and the generation of additional dental hygiene programs. History reveals that these solutions are ineffective at increasing the supply of dental hygienists.[13] In fact, these solutions may have hidden motives, including increasing the labor supply, which subsequently decreases the workers' salaries.

Many state dental associations propose the initiation of preceptorship training or alternative training for dental hygienists as a way of easing a reported shortage. Presently, Alabama is the only state that utilizes the preceptorship training method to prepare dental hygienists. Moreover, a 1990 study revealed that Alabama exhibits a dental hygiene shortage, which indicates that preceptorship training has done little to maintain an adequate labor force in dental hygiene in Alabama.[14]

Many state dental associations propose the development of additional dental hygiene programs as another strategy for solving the perceived dental hygiene shortages. However, data suggest that more dental hygiene programs do not translate into an increase in enrollment and graduates. Interestingly, the data suggest that the increase of dental hygiene programs leads to a decrease in dental hygienists' salaries.[15]

Few would argue that before a problem can be solved it must be identified and defined. Considering the logic of that statement, the first step in dealing with a labor force issue is to assess the labor distribution.

The term **workforce** shortage often is used loosely to describe a variety of situations, some of which generally are not considered actual shortages. Various labor force situations may involve the supply and geographic location of workers, the going wage rate, employer demand for workers, and consumer utilization of the product or service.[16] In fact the Institute of Medicine stated:

Reported vacancies should be viewed with caution because they do not always represent a shortage. If, through one mechanism or another, wages are kept below the level that would bring demand and supply into equilibrium, employer demand will always exceed the number of allied health personnel who want to work at the going wage. Such excess demand cannot really be characterized as a shortage but rather as an imperfection in the operation of the market.[17]

The dental hygiene labor paradigm describes the steps necessary in studying the dental hygiene labor force (Figure 2–5). Interestingly, most occupations can study labor supply using a worker-to-population ratio. Dental hygienists though are unable to provide care to the population in many states without the supervision of a dentist. So the supply of dental hygienists is directly linked to the number of dentists available to employ them. In fact, even when dental hygienists may practice independently, a dentist is needed for referrals. Numerous studies have suggested that the most common dental hygienist-to-dentist employment ratio is 1:2.[18] In fact, in a recent survey conducted by the American Dental Association, only 25 percent of responding dentists reported employing a dental hygienist full time, while approximately 60 percent reported employing a part-time dental hygienist.[19] In other words, for every two dentists, one dentist employs or would like to employ one full-time dental hygienist. The significance of this ratio to dental hygiene labor force is that for every dental hygienist in the workforce, there should be two dentists. States facing labor issue threats may utilize this ratio when studying dental hygiene labor force. Unfortunately, dental hygiene labor force became an issue before it could be documented as a problem.

Figure 2–5.   Paradigm for Studying Dental Hygiene Labor Force Issues

Step One: Demand

→ Identify the dental hygiene employment opportunities in your jurisdiction, by

→ Identifying the hygienist to dentist employment ratio if restrictive legislative barriers exist to prevent access to care (the national ratio of 1:2 can be used), or

→ Identify the dental hygienist to population employment ratio if your jurisdiction enables dental hygienists to practice without restrictive barriers.

Step Two: Supply

→ Obtain a list of licensed dental hygienists and dentists residing in your jurisdiction.

→ Utilize counties within the state to determine locality distributions.

→ Segregate the supply of dental hygienists and dentists by zip codes and place into the respective counties.

→ An optional step which may be useful would be to utilize the past data or conduct a survey to identify the practicing status of dental hygienists and dentists.

Step Three: Labor Force

→ Calculate the frequency distribution of dental hygienists and dentists in the jurisdiction.

→ Calculate the ratio of dental hygienists to dentists in the locality.

→ Compare these ratios to dental hygiene and dental employment ratio.

→ Depict the surplus and deficit status of dental hygienists in the counties.

→ If you have the practicing status of dental hygienists and dentists, you may utilize the practicing status of dental professionals in these aforementioned frequency distributions and ratios.

Source: Nathe, C., M. Darby, D. Bauman, and D. Shuman. Too few resumes. *RDH* 17 (1997): 18–29.

SUMMARY

Many issues face dental care delivery; in fact, the delivery of dental care in the United States has proven ineffective in providing care to all segments of the population. Dental hygiene positions in public health settings that exist in many interdisciplinary settings can help alleviate the unbalanced delivery of dental care. The intricacies of the governmental structure in relation to dental hygiene care is fascinating, and many opportunities exist for dental hygiene employment. Dental hygienists should be cautious about dental hygiene labor shortage claims and be able to effectively discuss labor force issues.

Note

Much of the information on the federal government was taken directly from the Web sites http://www.hhs.gov, http://www.ed.gov, http://www.va.gov, http://fns1 .usda.gov, and http://www.dol.gov.

REFERENCES

[1]Mangskau, K. The roles of state policymakers in promoting healthy families. Minneapolis: Looking Forward Conference, June 25–27, 1999.

[2]Collins, R. J. Celebrating the year of oral health: Changing public expectation and challenges for the profession. *Journal of American College of Dentistry* 61 (1994): 6–12.

[3]Kaste, L. M., R. H. Selwitz, R. J. Oldakowski et al. Coronal caries in the primary and permanent dentition of children and adolescents 1–17 years of age. *Journal of Dental Research* 75 (1996): 631–41.

[4]*Healthy People 2000 Review 1997.* Hyattsville, MD: U.S. Department of Health and Human Services, National Center for Health Statistics, 1997.

[5]Wilson, S., G. A. Smith, J. Preish, and P. S. Casamassimo. Nontraumatic dental emergencies in a pediatric emergency department. *Clinical Pediatrics* 36 (1997): 333–37; Sheller, B., B. J. Williams, and S. M. Lombardi. Diagnosis and treatment of dental caries-related emergencies in children's hospital. *Pediatric Dentistry* 19 (1997): 470–75.

[6]Mangskau, K. The roles of state policymakers in promoting healthy families. Minneapolis, MN: Looking Forward Conference, June 25–27, 1999.

[7]Boyce, J. S. Risk management: An introduction for the dental practice. *Dental Hygiene* 181 (1987): 504–507.

[8]Gundrum, C. Dental hygiene in the Indian Health Service with information from Ann Witherspoon. Albuquerque: Presentation at University of New Mexico, November 3, 1999.

[9]DeFriese, G., and B. Barker. *Assessing Dental Manpower Requirements.* Cambridge, MA: Ballinger Publishing, 1982.

[10]Health Resources and Service Administration guidelines on designation of population groups with health manpower shortages. Bethesda, MD: U.S. Department of Health and Human Services, 1995.

[11]Nathe, C., M. Darby, D. Bauman, and D. Shuman. Too few resumes. *RDH* 17 (1997): 18–29.

[12]Manpower Needs Assessment Status Report. Chicago: American Dental Hygienists' Association, 1999.

[13]Goral, V. Trends in dental hygiene education. *Advisor* 8 (1988): 19–21.

[14]Academy of General Dentistry membership survey: Confirms shortage of dental staff. AGD Impact, 1990.

[15]Lazar, V. Dental hygienists in the United States: Results of an ADA survey. *Journal of the American Dental Association* 128 (1997): 651–53.

[16]Sargent, J. Labor shortages: Menace or mirage? *Occupation Outlook Quarterly* 4 (1988): 27–33.

[17]Institute of Medicine, National Academy of Sciences. *Allied Health Services: Avoiding Crisis.* Washington, DC, 1989.

[18]Nathe, C., M. Darby, D. Bauman, and D. Shuman. Too few resumes. *RDH* 17 (1997): 18–29.

[19]American Dental Association. *Dental Health Policy Analysis Series: 1999 Workforce Needs Assessment Survey.* Chicago: American Dental Association, 2000.

Get Connected

Multimedia Extension Activities

 www.prenhall.com/nathe

Use the above address to access the free, interactive companion web site created specifically to accompany this textbook. Here you will find an array of self study material to help you gain a richer understanding of the concepts presented in this chapter.

Chapter 3

∙∙∙

FINANCING OF DENTAL CARE

OBJECTIVES

After studying this chapter, the dental hygiene student will be able to:

- describe current methods of payment for dental care.
- define and apply terminology associated with financing dental care.
- list the different insurance plans available for dental care.
- describe the role of the government in financing dental care.

COMPETENCIES

After studying this chapter and participating in accompanying course activities, the dental hygiene student should be competent in the following:

- evaluate reimbursement mechanisms and their impact on the patient's access to oral health care.

KEY WORDS

Barter	Health maintenance organization
Capitation	Preferred provider
Encounter	Usual, customary, reasonable (UCR) fee
Fee for service	

www.prenhall.com/nathe

INTRODUCTION

Historically, the financing of dental care was the responsibility of the patient in need of treatment and the dental practitioner involved in managing his/her dental practice. However, in today's economy, the financing of dental care in the United States involves both the private and public sectors. In fact, numerous entities are involved in the financing of dental care. In this chapter, the private and public relationships in financing dental care are discussed.

Of the total health care expenditures in the United States in 1996, only 4.6 percent were spent on dental services. Moreover, of the total expenditures for dental care, nearly 96 percent were paid for by private funds, whether by the patient (93 percent) or by the health insurance (51 percent). Interestingly, only 4 percent of all dental expenditures were paid by federal, state, or local governments.[1] Figures 3–1 to 3–3 depict health and dental expenditures in the United States.[2,3]

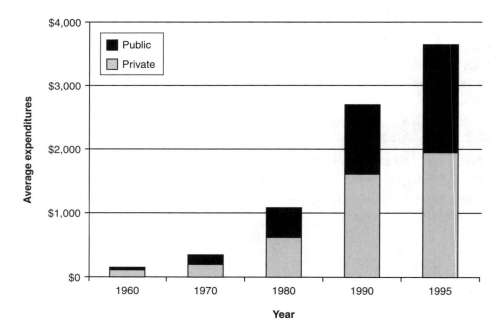

Figure 3–1. Per capita national health expenditures, showing the proportionate expenditure of private and public funds, United States, selected years 1960–1995.

Source: Levit, K. R., H. C. Lazenby, and B. R. Braden. National health expenditures. *Health Care Financing Rev* 18(1996): 175–82.

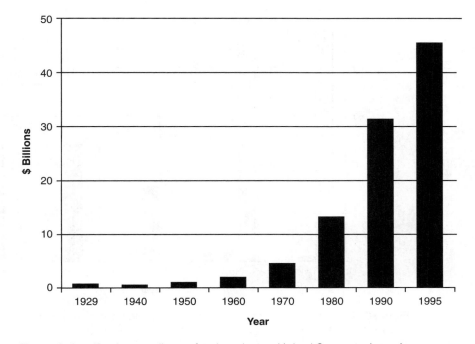

Figure 3–2. Total expenditures for dental care, United States, selected years 1929–1995.

Source: Cooper, B. S., and N. L. Worthington. National health expenditures, 1929–72. *Soc Security Bull* 36 no. 3(1973): 19, 40; Levit, K. R., H. C. Lazenby, and B. R. Braden. National health expenditures. *Health Care Financing Rev* 18(1996):175–82.

PAYMENT METHODS

Generally, there are four types of payment methods used in dental care delivery. These include the **fee-for-service** arrangements, **capitation** plans, **encounter** fee plans and the **barter** system (Table 3–1). Although these reimbursement mechanisms are all unique in different parts of the country, the similarities are discussed.

The *fee-for-service* arrangement is the most commonly used method in the United States at the present time. A fee-for-service arrangement in which the fee scale is developed for a service is the traditional method of billing. Patients are charged for services performed by a dental hygienist, dentist, or denturist.

Basically, a dental practice sets a fee, and the patient and/or third party (insurance company) pays the fee. The fees that are set are referred to as a **usual, customary, and reasonable (UCR) fee.** Usual implies that the fee is what is

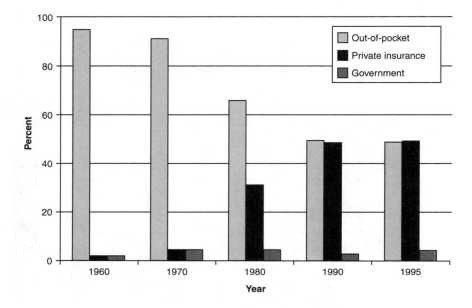

Figure 3–3. Proportions of total dental care expenditures paid by consumers out-of-pocket, by private insurance, and by government funds, United States, selected years 1960–1995.

Source: Levit, K. R., H. C. Lazenby, and B. R. Braden. National health expenditures. *Health Care Financing Rev* 18(1996): 175–82.

Table 3–1.	Types of Payment Methods

Payment Method	Definition
Fee-for-service	Fee scale is developed for all services provided by the dental provider and a payment is then developed for the service(s) rendered. This is the most common payment method used in the United States.
Capitation	The dental provider contracts with a program to provide all or most dental services to the program's subscribers in return for payment on a per capita basis.
Barter System	Dental provider and patient negotiate payment by exchanging goods or services without utilizing money.
Encounter	Payment is based on the office visit and is always the same regardless of the service(s) rendered.

most often charged by the dental provider for a given dental or dental hygiene service. Customary means a range of fees charged by dental providers with similar training and service within a specific and limited geographic area as determined by the administrator of a dental plan, based on submitted fees. Customary is an established maximum benefit payable. Reasonable meets the usual and customary and is justifiable.

Some clinics that try to make services more affordable for patients with a low income will institute a sliding fee scale. This implies that the fees for services may be decreased depending on the patient's income and family's size. This type of reduced fee program is available through federal grants.

Indemnity plans are fee-for-service traditional insurance plans that operate by means of a submittal and reimbursement method. Basically, the dental practitioner provides a service, and then either the bill is given to the patient to submit to an insurance company for reimbursement after the patient has paid the dental practice or the bill is submitted to the insurance company for direct reimbursement to the dental practice.

Many times in a fee-for-service payment method a discounted fee may be identified for a target population. An example may be a dental office has a 10 percent lower fee for senior citizens or a lowered fee scale for participants in a prepaid group.

A copayment is a portion of the cost of each service that is paid by the patient, in other words, the part of the payment not covered by the third party. It is used to discourage overuse of services.

A fee-for-service plan would tend to provide an incentive for the dental provider to provide all necessary treatment. Generally, fee-for-service plans increase production in an office because providers are paid on the amount of services that are produced. Most dental practices accept fee-for-service plans.

A *capitation* method of payment is a plan in which a dental provider contracts with a third party to provide all or most of the dental services to subscribers in return for payment on a per capita basis. The fee is a fixed monthly payment paid to a dental provider by a third party based upon the number of patients assigned for treatment. Moreover, the dental provider receives the fees whether or not the patients use the care.

Capitation plans are typically provided by dental managed care organizations. Managed care organizations were developed in medical care in 1973 by the HMO Act. There are claims that **Health Maintenance Organizations** (HMOs) actually reduce health care costs for participants by reducing hospitalization and the use of costly services. Many dental organizations are not supportive of dental managed care plans because of the reduction in reimbursement and the decrease in control of providers' recommended treatment. Organized dental hygiene has maintained a positive relationship with dental managed care.

In many instances, capitation plans actually decrease the productiveness of a dental practice. For example, if a dental practice receives a set amount of money each month, which is dependent on the number of patients signed up with that dental practice, there is little incentive to provide preventive treatment to these patients. In other words, if a practice gets paid whether providing treatment or not, the practice may choose not to provide treatment to capitation plan members, but instead to schedule as many fee-for-service plan members. This way the office could collect the monthly stipend from the capitation plan, while still collecting fees for services provided to fee-for-service plans.

The *encounter* arrangement basically is payment for each encounter. If a patient came in on one day for an exam and prophylaxis and the next day for two amalgam restorations and the next day for a class V glass ionomer restoration, each encounter would generate the same reimbursement fee. The encounter arrangment may tend to decrease productivity.

The *barter system* may be used in the private sector. Typically the dental provider and the patient negotiate payment by exchanging goods and services without using money. This is still in place in many United States private dental offices, particularly in rural areas. An example would be that the dental provider may provide dental care and the patient may in return provide carpentry service.

INSURANCE PLANS

Dental service corporations are legally constituted nonprofit organizations incorporated on a state by state basis often sponsored by the state dental societies. They negotiate and administer programs for employer groups and have a contractual relationship with dentists to provide care to eligible beneficiaries using agreed upon fees. Generally, dental providers accept a discounted payment as payment in full, in recognition that many people seek care because of the dental coverage arrangement. Regular audits and inspections of patient charts occur. An example of a dental service corporation would be Delta Dental Plan. Delta Dental currently is the largest dental benefits carrier in the United States. Delta Dental is operated on an individual state basis, but care is provided nationally as plans are united through the Delta Dental Plans Association. Figure 3–4 depicts a typical example of explanation of a dental service corporation's "Summary of Covered Dental Services."

Health service corporations offer limited dental coverage as part of their hospital-surgical-medical policies. A common example of a health service corporation is Blue Cross/Blue Shield.

Moreover, many dental practices in the United States are involved in **preferred provider** organizations (PPOs). PPOs are defined as contractual agreements between practitioners and their insurers to provide dental care services for lower than average fees. Providers participate in these contracts because it allows competition for patients.

Individual practice associations (IPA) are legal entities organized for individual participating dental providers to enter into contracts collectively to provide prepaid dental services to enroll. They may contract directly with a group purchase or

I. SUMMARY OF COVERED DENTAL SERVICES

DIAGNOSTIC & PREVENTIVE SERVICES	Delta Dental Pays: 100%* no deductible	You Pay: 0%*

- Oral Examinations - twice in a calendar year
- Cleanings - twice in a calendar year
- X-rays: Full mouth - once every 3 years / Bitewing - twice in a calendar year
- Topical Fluoride - through age 18, twice in a calendar year
- Emergency Treatment - for relief of pain
- Space Maintainers - through age 15, 5 year limitation
- Sealants - through age 15, permanent molars only, 3 year limitation

RESTORATIVE SERVICES (Fillings)	Delta Dental Pays: 85%* after deductible	You Pay: 15%*

- Amalgam fillings on posterior teeth
- Composite resin fillings for anterior teeth only
- Stainless steel crowns

BASIC SERVICES	Delta Dental Pays: 85%* after deductible	You Pay: 15%*

- Extractions - surgical and non-surgical extractions
- Oral Surgery - maxillofacial surgical procedures of the oral cavity
- Periodontics - nonsurgical and surgical
- Endodontics - pulp therapy and root canal filling
- General Anesthesia - intravenous sedation and general anesthesia, when dentally necessary and administered by a licensed provider for a covered oral surgery procedure

MAJOR SERVICES	Delta Dental Pays: 50%* after deductible	You Pay: 50%*

- Crowns and Cast Restorations - when teeth cannot be restored with amalgam or composite resin restorations
- Prosthodontics - procedures for construction or repair of fixed bridges, partials or complete dentures

ORTHODONTIC SERVICES	Delta Dental Pays: 50%* after deductible	You Pay: 50%*

- Procedures using appliances to treat poor alignment of teeth and/or jaws which significantly interferes with their function
- Coverage is for enrolled adults and dependent children

DEDUCTIBLE	You Pay: $25 per enrolled person $50 aggregate per family

- You pay a deductible for each enrolled person each benefit period up to a maximum aggregate deductible per family.
- The benefit period for your group is July 1 to June 30.
- You do not have to pay a deductible for DIAGNOSTIC AND PREVENTIVE SERVICES or ORTHODONTIC SERVICES. Payments for services described under DIAGNOSTIC AND PREVENTIVE SERVICES or ORTHODONTIC SERVICES will not be credited toward the deductible.

MAXIMUM	Delta Dental Pays: $1500 per enrolled person

- Delta will pay up to a maximum amount for covered services each benefit period per enrolled person.
- The benefit period for your group is July 1 to June 30.
- Any amount for covered dental services that exceed the maximum benefit amount during the benefit period is the responsibility of the enrolled person.

ORTHODONTIC MAXIMUM	Delta Dental Pays: $1000 per enrolled person

- Delta will pay up to a separate maximum per lifetime per enrolled dependent for covered Orthodontic Services.
- Coverage is for enrolled adults and dependent children.

* Applied to the lesser of the Delta Maximum Approved Amount or the Delta Premier dentist's billed amount.

Obtaining services from a nonparticipating dentist may result in higher out-of-pocket expenses.

Please note: You are not eligible for benefits prior to your individual effective date or following your termination date.

This is a summary of benefits. To fully understand the coverage provided, please read the sections of this handbook that describe: How the Plan Works; Eligibility and Enrollment; Benefits, Limitations and Exclusions; Definitions.

Figure 3–4. Summary of Covered Dental Services

Table 3–2. Types of Insurance Plans

Insurance Plans	Definition	Examples
Dental Service Corporations	A not-for-profit organization that negotiates and provides dental care contracts. Corporated on a state-by-state basis and sponsored by a constituent dental society to negotiate and administer programs.	Delta Dental Plans
Health Service Corporations	Offer limited dental coverage as part of their hospital-surgical-medical policies.	Blue Cross/Blue Shield
Preferred Providers Organization (PPO)	Dental providers and third-party contract with employer of dental benefits to offer services at reduced prices.	Aetna U.S. Healthcare Dental PPO
Individual Practice Association (IPA)	Legal entities organized for dental providers to enter into contracts collectively to provide prepaid dental services to enrolled groups.	MD Individual Practice Associates, Inc.
Commercial Insurance Plan	Operate for-profit and designed as an indemnity plan.	Unicare 200
Prepaid Group Practice	Large group practices that contract to groups of subscribers.	Golden West Dental and Vision
Health Maintenance Organization (HMO)	Developed in 1973 by the HMO Act. Allowed federal funds to provide an alternative to customary fee-for-service payment. Initially designed to decrease health care costs. Comprehensive prepaid health plan.	Presbyterian Health Plan
Capitatation Plan	Per capita payment from a defined population and specific dental providers selected. Payment made to provider regardless of use.	Concordia Plus

with an insurance carrier. This is usually referred to as managed care and is a capitation type method of reimbursement.

Capitation programs, sometimes referred to as Dental HMO plans, are a type of managed care plan. In these types of plans, the dentist is paid a fixed amount (usually monthly) per capita (per patient) or family rather than for actual treatment provided. In return, the dentist agrees to provide specific types of treatment to patients at no charge (for some treatments there may be a patient copayment).

Concordia Plus is an example of a prepaid dental plan that focuses on preventive care and the early diagnosis of dental problems. Under Concordia Plus, members select a primary dental office (PDO) from a contracted and credentialed network of providers. The PDO handles the member's dental care needs, including referrals to specialists whenever necessary. Each member can select his or her own PDO from the Concordia Plus network of participating dentists.

HMOs do not typically provide coverage for routine dental care. They are primarily concerned with providing coverage for medical care. (Please see Table 3–2 for types of insurance plans.)

DENTAL BILLING

Dental providers bill for dental procedures utilizing a dental claim form. See Figure 3–5 for an example fee slip and Figure 3–6 for an example claim form. Dental procedures generally are billed utilizing certain procedures definitions. The American Dental Association's (ADA) Code on Dental Procedures and Nomenclature is contained in the CDT-4 user guide. The maintenance of these codes is the responsibility of the Council on Dental Benefit Programs with consultation from Blue Cross and Blue Shield Association, the Health Insurance Association of America, the Health Care Financing Association, National Electronic Information Corporation, and the American Dental Association recognized dental specialty organizations. The ADA updates the user guide approximately every five years. CDT codes are five-character, alpha-numeric configurations (e.g., D2110). Figure 3–7 is a page with definitions of billable oral exams.

If a patient is self-pay, the procedures are generally paid for immediately after the dental appointment. However, many dental offices have payment plans for patients, and some use specific dental credit cards as a financial plan for patients. When a patient is covered by insurance, the claim form is mailed to the insurance company either electronically or by hard copy. The insurance company then makes the decision on payment. The insurance company will then create an explanation of benefits (see Figure 3–8) to the patient and the provider with accompanying payment or denial of payment with explanation.

UNIVERSITY OF NEW MEXICO
DIVISION OF DENTAL HYGIENE

I. DIAGNOSTIC SERVICES			
00120	Periodic Oral Evaluation		
00140	Limited Oral Evaluation (Emergency)		
00150	Initial Comprehensive Oral Evaluation		
RADIOGRAPHS		TOOTH	ARCH
00210	Intraoral Comp Series-Inc. BW		
00220	Intraoral Periapical-1st Film		
00230	Intraoral P.A.-Ea. Addl. Film		
00240	Intraoral Occlusal Film		
00270	Bitewing-Single Film		
00272	Bitewing-Two Films		
00274	Bitewings-Four Films		
00330	Panoramic Film		
II. PREVENTATIVE SERVICES		TOOTH	
01110	Prophylaxis - Adult		
01120	Prophylaxis - Child		
01203	Topical Floride - Child (without Prophy)		
* 01204	Topical Floride - Adult (without Prophy)		
01351	Sealant - Per Tooth (multiple teeth)		
01510	Space Maint-Fixed-Unilateral		
01515	Space Maint-Fixed-Bilateral		
01550	Re-cement Space Maintainer		
III. RESTORATIVE SERVICES		TOOTH	SURFACE
02140	Amalgam-1 Surface, Prim. or Perm.		
02150	Amalgam-2 Surfaces, Prim. or Perm.		
02160	Amalgam-3 Surfaces, Prim. or Perm.		
02161	Amalgam-4+ Surfaces, Prim. or Perm.		
02330	Resin-based comp.-1 Surface, Anterior		
02331	Resin-based comp.-2 Surfaces, Anterior		
02332	Resin-based comp.-3 Surfaces, Anterior		
02335	Resin-based comp-4+ Surfaces or Incisal, Ant.		
02390	Resin-based composite crown, Anterior		
02391	Resin-based composite-1 Surface, Posterior		
02392	Resin-based composite-2 Surfaces, Posterior		
02393	Resin-based composite-3 Surfaces, Posterior		
02394	Resin-based composite-4+ Surfaces, Posterior		
CROWNS		TOOTH	SURFACE
* 02710	Crown Resin (Indirect/Laboratory)		
02740	Crown-Porc/Ceramic Substrate		
02750	Crown-Porc. High Noble Metal		
* 02751	Crown-Porcelain to Base Metal		
* 02752	Crown-Porcelain to Nobel Metal		
02790	Crown-Full Cast. High Noble Metal		
* 02791	Crown-Full Cast. Base Metal		
* 02792	Crown-Full Cast. Nobel Metal		
02910	Recement Inlay		
02920	Re-cement Crown		
02930	Stainless Steel Crown-Primary		
02931	Stainless Steel Crown-Permanent		
02932	Prefabricated Resin Crown		
02940	Sedative Filling		
02950	Crown Buildup, including any pins		
02951	Pin Retention, per tooth, in addt'n to restoration		
02952	Cast Post & Core, in addt'n to crown		
02954	Prefab Post & Core, in addt'n to crown		
* 02960	Crown Repair by report		
06930	Recement Fixed Partial Denture (Bridge)		
IV. ENDODONTIC SERVICES		TOOTH	
03220	Therapeutic Pulpotomy		
* 03310	Anterior RCT (Exel. Rest.)		
* 03320	Biscuspid RCT (Excl. Rest.)		
* 03330	Molar RCT (Excl. Rest.)		
03410	Apicoectomy-Anterior		
03421	Apicoectomy/Periadicular Bicuspid		
03425	Apicoectomy/Periadicular Molar		

Con't. ENDODONTIC SERVICES		TOOTH	
03426	Apicoectomy/Periadicular ea. Addt'l root		
03430	Retrograde Filling, Per Root		
03450	Root Amputation, Per Root		
V. PERIDONTAL SERVICES		TOOTH	QUAD
* 04210	Gingivectomy Or Gingivoplasty (Per Quad)		
04320	Provisional Splinting, Intracoronal		
04321	Provisional Splinting, Extracoronal		
* 04341	Scaling & Root Planing, 4+ teeth, Per Quad		
* 04342	Scaling & Root Planing, 1-3 teeth, Per Quad		
* 04910	Periodontal Maintenance		
VI. REMOVABLE PROSTHODONTIC SERVICES			
* 05110	Complete Denture-Maxillary		
* 05120	Complete Denture-Mandibular		
* 05130	Immediate Denture-Maxillary		
* 05140	Immediate Denture-mandibular		
* 05211	Maxillary Partial-Resin Base		
* 05212	Mandibular Partial-Resin Base		
* 05213	Maxillary Partial-Cast Metal Framework		
* 05214	Mandibular Partial-Cast Metal Framework		
05410	Adjust Complete Denture-Maxillary		
05411	Adjust Complete Denture-Mandibular		
05421	Adjust Partial-Maxillary		
05422	Adjust Partial-Mandibular		
X. ORAL SURGERY SERVICES		TOOTH	QUAD
07111	Coronal Remnants-Deciduous Tooth		
07140	Extraction, Erupted Tooth or Exposed Root		
07210	Extraction, Surgical Removal-Erupted Tooth		
07220	Extraction-Impacted Tooth-Soft Tissue		
07230	Extraction-Impacted Tooth-Partial Bony		
07240	Extraction-Impacted Tooth-Full Bony		
07241	Extraction-Unusual Tooth-Full Bony w/ compl.		
07250	Extraction-Residual Root-Surgical		
07270	Tooth Reimplantation-Accident (Avulsed)		
07281	Surgical Exposure to Aid Eruption		
07285	Biopsy of Oral Tissue-Hard		
07286	Biopsy of Oral Tissue-Soft		
07320	Alveoloplasty-No Extractions-Per Quad		
07510	I & D Intraoral Abscess		
07520	I & D Extraoral Abscess		
07960	Frenulectomy		
XII. ADJUNCTIVE GENERAL SERVICES		TOOTH	
09110	Palliative (Emerg) Treatment-Minor Procedure		
09410	House Call (nursing home visits)		
09420	Hospital Call		
09630	Other Drugs and Medicaments, by report		
0359Y	DD Dental Special Needs		
OTHER SERVICES RENDERED (NOT LISTED ABOVE)			

Location: _____ Tax ID#: 00-0000001

Provider: _____

Date of Service: _____ / _____ / _____

PATIENT IDENTIFICATION

Last	First	I.

* Services allowed by Medicaid, but must be pre-authorized

Figure 3–5. University of New Mexico Division of Dental Hygiene Fee Slip

DENTAL CLAIM FORM

1.	2.	3. Carrier Name and Address
☐ Dentist's pre-treatment estimate ☒ Dentist's statement of actual services Provider ID #	☐ Medicaid Claim ☐ EPSDT Prior Authorization # Patient ID #	**Fones Dental of New Mexico** **2500 Newman Blvd.** **Bridgeport, CT 06601**

PATIENT COVERAGE INFORMATION

4. Patient Name **Marissa A. Nathe**	5. Relationship to employee ☐ Self ☐ Child **Child** ☐ Spouse ☐ Other	6. Sex M F F	7. Patient birthdate MM DD YY **07/02/1995**	8. If full time student school city

9. Employee/subscriber name and address **Christine N. Nathe** **1234 Main St.** **Albuquerque NM 87120**	10. Employee/subscriber dental plan I.D. number **123-45-6789**	11. Employee/subscriber birthdate MM DD YY **02/05/1966**	12. Employer (company)	13. Group number

14. Is patient covered by another dental plan? **No** Is patient covered by a medical plan? yes no	15-a. Name and address of carrier(s)	15-b. Group no.(s)	16. Name and address of other employer

17-a. Employee/subscriber name (if different than patient's)	17-b. Employee/subscriber dental plan I.D. number	17-c. Employee subscriber birthdate MM DD YY	18. Relationship to patient ☐ Self ☐ Parent ☐ Spouse ☐ Other

19. I have reviewed the following treatment plan and fees. I agree to be responsible for all charges for dental services and materials not paid by my dental benefit plan, unless the treating dentist or dental practice has a contractual agreement with my plan prohibiting all or a portion of such charges. To the extent permitted under applicable law, I authorize release of any information relating to this claim. > **SIGNATURE ON FILE** **09/04/2003** Signed (Patient or parent if minor) Date	20. I hereby authorize payment of the dental benefits otherwise payable to me directly to the below named dental entity. > **SIGNATURE ON FILE** **09/04/2003** Signed (Employee/subscriber) Date

BILLING DENTIST

21. Name of Billing Dentist or Dental Entity **Dental Hygiene DH0000** **University of New Mexico Dental Hygiene**	30. Is treatment result of occupational illness or injury?	No	Yes	If yes, enter brief description and dates.
	N			

22. Address where payment should be remitted **2320 Tucker NE, Novitski Hall**	31. Is treatment result of auto accident? **N**

23. City, State, Zip **Albuquerque, NM 87131-1391**	32. Other accident? **N**

24. Dentist SSN or T.I.N. **00-0000000**	25. Dentist License no. **DH-1230**	26. Dentist phone no. **(505)555-4106**	33. If prosthesis, is this initial placement? **N**	(if no, reason for replacement)	34. Date prior placement

27. First visit date current series	28. Place of treatment Office Hosp. ECF Other **X**	29. Radiographs or models enclosed?	No **N**	Yes	How many? **0**	35. Is treatment for orthodontics? **N**	If services already commenced enter:	Date appliances placed	Mos. treat. remaining **0**

36. Identify missing teeth with 'X'	37. Examination and treatment plan - List in order from tooth no. 1 through tooth no. 32 - Using charting system shown.						For administrative use only
	Tooth # or letter	Surface	Description of service (including x-rays, prophylaxis, materials used, etc.)		Date of service performed Mo. Day Year	Procedure number	Fee	

(Tooth chart diagram: Facial / Right / Left / Lingual / Facial)

			Description of service	Date of service	Procedure number	Fee	
			Periodic Oral Evaluation	10/26/2001	00120	30.00	
			Prophylaxis, Child	10/26/2001	01120	50.00	
			Topical Fluor.(not proph)Child	10/26/2001	01203	20.00	

38. Remarks for unusual services

39. I hereby certify that the procedures as indicated by date have been completed and that the fees submitted are the actual fees I have charged and intend to collect for those procedures. > **Christine Nathe, R.D.H** **DH-1230** **09/04/2003** Signed (Treating Dentist) License no. Date	41. Total Fee Charged **100.00**
	42. Payment by other plan

40. Address where treatment was performed **2320 Tucker NE, Novitski Hall** **Albuquerque, NM 87131-1391** City, State, Zip	Max Allowable	
	Deductible	
	Carrier %	

Carrier Pays	
Patient Pays	

Figure 3–6. Dental Claim Form

● new procedure code   ▲ revised code   ✖ revised descriptor

D0120 periodic oral evaluation
✖   An evaluation performed on a patient of record to determine any changes in the patient's dental and medical health status since a previous comprehensive or periodic evaluation. This includes periodontal screening and may require interpretation of information acquired through additional diagnostic procedures. Report additional diagnostic procedures separately.

D0140 limited oral evaluation — problem focused
✖   An evaluation limited to a specific oral health problem or complaint. This may require interpretation of information acquired through additional diagnostic procedures. Report additional diagnostic procedures separately. Definitive procedures may be required on the same date as the evaluation.

Typically, patients receiving this type of evaluation present with a specific problem and/or dental emergencies, trauma, acute infections, etc.

▲ D0150 comprehensive oral evaluation — new or established patient
      Typically used by a general dentist and/or a specialist when evaluating a patient comprehensively. It is a thorough evaluation and recording of the extraoral and intraoral hard and soft tissues. It may require interpretation of information acquired through additional diagnostic procedures. Additional diagnostic procedures should be reported separately.

This would include the evaluation and recording of the patient's dental and medical history and a general health assessment. It may typically include the evaluation and recording of dental caries, missing or unerupted teeth, restorations, occlusal relationships, periodontal conditions (including periodontal charting), hard and soft tissue anomalies, oral cancer screening, etc.

D0160 detailed and extensive oral evaluation — problem focused, by report
      A detailed and extensive problem focused evaluation entails extensive diagnostic and cognitive modalities based on the findings of a comprehensive oral evaluation. Integration of more extensive diagnostic modalities to develop a treatment plan for a specific problem is required. The condition requiring this type of evaluation should be described and documented.

Examples of conditions requiring this type of evaluation may include dentofacial anomalies, complicated perio-prosthetic conditions, complex temporomandibular dysfunction, facial pain of unknown origin, severe systemic diseases requiring multidisciplinary consultation, etc.

Figure 3–7. Source: American Dental Assoc., CDT-4. 2002. Chicago: American Dental Association. CDT-4 Definitions of Billable Oral Exams.

FONES DENTAL

Fones Dental

2500 Newman Blvd.
Bridgeport, CT 06601
555-3161 or 1-555-375-3320

Explanation of Benefits
(THIS IS NOT A BILL)

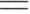

Check No.:	NO CHECK
Issue Date:	08-25-2003

Patient Name: CHAD NATHE

Receipt Date: 08-20-2003

Relationship Code: 03
Subscriber Name: CHRISTIN NATHE
Dentist: Alfred Fones, DDS

Document No.: 0123
Document Type: 1

Pay To: S=Subscriber
P=Provider

IMPORTANT NOTICE: Payment for these services is determined in accordance with the specific terms of your dental plan and/or Fones Dental's agreements with its participating dentists.

Tooth Code	Date of Service	Procedure Code	Procedure Description	Submitted Amount	Approved Amount	Allowed Amount	Deductible	% Co-Pay	Patient Payment	Plan Payment	Pay To
GROUP NO:	000123		NAME: Dental Hygiene Corp.								
SUBGROUP NO:	0001		NAME: Dental Hygiene Corp.								
	08/05/03	D1120	CLEANING	60.00	60.00	.00	.00		.00	60.00	P
POLICY CODE:		966									
	08/05/03	D1203	FLUORIDE	24.00	24.00	.00	.00		.00	24.00	P
POLICY CODE:		966									
			TOTAL	84.00	84.00	.00	.00		.00	84.00	

THE FOLLOWING POLICIES ARE APPLIED TO EXPLAIN BENEFITS PAYABLE AND ARE NOT INTENDED TO
ALTER THE TREATMENT PLAN DETERMINED BY THE DENTIST AND PATIENT:
966. THE PATIENT'S DENTAL COVERAGE WAS NOT IN EFFECT WHEN THIS SERVICE WAS
PERFORMED OR SUBMITTED FOR PREDETERMINATION. PLEASE VERIFY THE CLAIM
WAS SUBMITTED TO THE PROPER CARRIER BASED ON THE DATE OF SERVICE AND
THE CORRECT SOCIAL SECURITY NUMBER WAS PROVIDED.

Payment for these services is determined in accordance with the specific terms of your dental plan and/or Fones Dental's agreements with its participating dentists. For inquiries regarding participating dentists, please call the number above. Fones Dental's payment decisions do not qualify as dental or medical advice. You must make all decisions about the desirability or necessity of dental procedures and services with your dentist.
If your claim was denied in whole or in part so that you must pay some amount of the claim, upon a written request and free of charge, we will provide you with a copy of any internal rule, guideline or protocol or, if applicable, an explanation of the scientific or clinical judgment relied upon in deciding your claim. If you think Fones Dental incorrectly denied all or part of your claim, you may ask to have the claim reviewed. Your written request for a formal review must be sent within 180 days of your receipt of this EOB to the address on the upper-left hand corner. You may submit any additional materials you believe support your claim. A decision will be made no later than 30 days from the date we receive your request. Refer to your Dental Benefit Handbook for a complete description of Fones Dental's Claims Appeal process. You are not required to file a formal appeal to Fones Dental prior to arbitration or taking civil action.

Insurance fraud significantly increases the cost of
health care. If you are aware of any false information
submitted to Fones Dental, you can help us lower
these costs by calling our toll-free hotline. You do not
need to identify yourself Only ANTI-FRAUD calls
can be accepted on this line.

ANTI-FRAUD TOLL-FREE HOTLINE
1-800-000-0000

I|ılılıılıılllılılIlıılıllılıılIIllIlIlıılılılıl
#BWNCYPW
#S0041334569NM6#
CHRISTIN NATHE
1234 MAIN ST
ALBUQUERQUE NM 87120-6066

PAGE   1 OF 1

Figure 3–8.   Explanation of Benefits Form

GOVERNMENT ROLE IN FUNDING DENTAL CARE

The federal, state, and local government's share of expenses for dental care has continued to be approximately 4 percent. Basically, the federal government provides funding for dental care delivery in two programs for the express purpose of improving the nation's capacity to provide improved oral health care. The government funds programs that provide research, disease prevention, and control (i.e., water fluoridation, fluoride mouthrinse programs—swish and spit, dental sealants in schools, etc.); the planning and development of dental programs; education of dental professionals (via scholarship, loan forgiveness programs, and financial aid—see Chapter 15 for more information on current government incentives for dental hygiene students); and regulation by means of quality assurance programs and assessment.

The federal government provides funding to programs concerned with the provision of dental care services such as the United States Public Health Service and the National Health Service Corps. Additionally, the federal government funds dental services for federal prisoners, military personnel, Veterans with dental service-connected disabilities, the Indian Health Service, and Head Start and Early Head Start children. Dental hygienists may be eligible for loan repayment programs when practicing in these settings.

Federal block grants, primarily the Maternal and Children's Health Services (MCHS) Block Grant Title V and Preventive Health and Human Services, usually are utilized as Preventive Block Grants and may cover dental services for children. Many dental clinics utilize federal and state grants to help cover the operational costs for the clinic.

State governments generally fund dental services for inmates of state prisons and state dental departments. Many times the state may contract with a private agency to deliver dental services. The state dental departments may be utilized as a consultative agency providing state and private programs consulting skills in developing and managing dental health programs. State dental clinics are established in some states and offer dental services to a select target population, which usually includes, children, patients with special needs, older adults, and indigent patients. Dental treatment for children with craniofacial deformities, cleft lip and palate, and certain other conditions is funded by state and federal money.

Local governments may provide dental care via school and/or community clinics. In many instances the funding for these clinics are derived from federal, state, private, and local government entities. Funding for water fluoridation usually falls under the auspices of local government.

Medicaid Dental Coverage

Moreover, the federal government funds dental services under the auspices of Medicaid and a limited amount of funding for dental services limited to those that are medically necessary, such as oral/maxillofacial needs related to a medical condition

DENTAL HYGIENIST'S SPOTLIGHT
Ginny Berger, RDH

ACC Consultants Inc. was founded by Ginny Berger, RDH, in 1993 as a temporary staffing company for the dental practices throughout New Mexico. Ginny graduated in 1976 from the University of New Mexico. After applying to provide temporary dental hygiene services with an existing temporary employment service, she realized the current service was not owned by anyone with any experience in the dental profession and the level of professionalism was not what she had hoped, so instead of taking a position with the company she formed her own.

Dental hygiene had provided a great opportunity in the health care field and was professionally satisfying. However, after graduation the "glass ceiling" is inevitable as the money is good but advancement nearly impossible. Lack of benefits and infrequent pay raises for the profession pushed her to develop a company to provide an environment with health insurance benefits, 401K, dental insurance, and so on to colleagues by eliminating the office politics and offering some flexibility in hours and opportunities in a variety of workplaces.

Through the staffing business, the Public Health Dept of New Mexico contracted with her company to supply staff to the state dental sealant program. Developing relationships with Dr. Calderone, the dental director of New Mexico at the time, and discussing the needs of underserved children, a plan was developed to partly privatize the state sealant program.

At the same time, the needs of the other neglected population—geriatrics—became a concern. There were no oral health care services being provided to this population. Ginny contacted the state Medicaid office and Ken Padilla, DDS, dental director of Medicaid at the time, was instrumental in helping develop a program to address the needs of the long-term care population. He was able to ascertain a provider number for ACC Consultants Inc., and the company was on its way to meeting its mission of "enhancing the quality of life in our communities by promoting and providing access to oral health care and education."

ACC Consultants Inc. now provides school-based programs to over seventy-five schools and eighty long-term care facilities and has expanded services to include prison systems. ACC Consultants Inc. employs over seventy-five professionals committed to providing quality oral health care and education.

Table 3–3.　Financing Dental Care Terminology

Benefits: the amount that the insurance entity will pay for covered dental services described in their policy.

Capitation: a dental provider gets paid a specified dollar amount, for a given time period, to take care of the dental needs of a specified group of people.

Civilian Health and Medical Program of the Uniformed Services (CHAMPUS): medical benefits for military personnel, dependents, and retired military.

Claims Processing: The entire process of entering the procedures rendered until payment is collected or denial is determined.

Commercial Insurance Plans: An insurance plan that operates for a profit.

Contract: The insurance contract between the insurance entity and the group.

Copayment: A portion of the costs of each service which is paid by the patient.

Deductible: The amount an individual enrolled in the insurance plan must pay toward covered services before the insurance entity begins paying.

Dental Claim: A claim for payment made by the patient for a dental procedure that was rendered.

Dental Claim Form: The standard dental form utilized to file a claim or request authorization for a procedure.

Dental Necessity: A service provided by a dental provider that has been determined as a generally acceptable dental practice for the diagnosis and treatment of an individual.

Early and Periodic Screening, Diagnosis and Treatment (EPSDT): Persons under twenty-one years of age must be covered by Medicaid for medical, dental, and vision care.

Exclusive Provider Arrangement (EPA): Dental care providers contracts with an employer (which eliminates the third party) and negotiates the fees for services offered to the employer's employees.

Explanation of Benefits: A form sent to the patient and provider explaining the payment for procedures or denial of payment for procedures rendered.

Fee Slip: Form utilized by the dental provider that details the services rendered.

Managed Care: Refers to the integration of health care delivery and financing.

Medicaid (Title XIX): Money from federal, state, and local taxes pays bills for certain groups of people, including low-income, aged, blind, disabled, and member of families with dependent children.

(continued)

Table 3–3. *(continued)*

Medicare (Title XVIII): A federal insurance program from trust fund to pay medical bills of all people over sixty-five.

Preexisting Condition: The condition of the mouth that exists prior to the patient being covered by an insurance entity.

Premium: The monthly amount due to the insurance entity by the group or the individual.

Procedure Number: The number given to a specific procedure as designated in the *Codes on Dental Procedures and Nomenclature* published by the ADA.

Provider: A legally licensed dental hygienist or dentist who is operating within his/her scope of practice.

Prepaid Group Practice: A large group of dental providers contract to groups of patients.

Single Procedure: A specific procedure designated by a specific code.

Sound Natural Teeth: Teeth that are either primary or permanent that have adequate hard and soft tissue support.

State Children Health Insurance Program (SCHIP): A federal program that was created by the federal government to cover individuals that have incomes too high to qualify for state medical assistance but cannot obtain private insurance. All states participate, but some do not cover dental.

Three-Party System: The dental provider renders the service and a sponsor of the patient pays for the service. Insurance company or employer pays the dental provider for the service.

Two-Party System: The dental providers render the service, and the patient pays the dental provider for the service.

UCR (usual, customary, and reasonable fee): The fee that reflects the average dental provider fee per service in the immediate local.

under the auspices of Medicare. As discussed in Chapter 2, Medicaid, which is Title 19 of the Social Security Act, is a federal program, enacted in 1965, that distributes funds to states for the provision of health care services to the indigent. Dental care is an option, depending on the state, and requires additional funding from the state.

Each individual state decides whether to offer Medicaid dental insurance as a traditional fee-for-service plan or a capitation agreement. In many states, Medicaid insurance is actually operated by private insurance agencies.

Medicaid dental benefits are different in all states. This is due to the fact states have the freedom to apply the federal money in a variety of ways. Some states actually only provide coverage to children under the age of twenty-one, while other states choose to insure all low-income individuals regardless of age. If states offer coverage only to children, they have more money to spend on these individuals and are able to pay providers UCR rates. However, many individuals are left with no dental coverage. States may choose this option because, theoretically, more providers would be motivated to see children covered by Medicaid insurance because the rates were comparable to most dental insurances.

Although many states may fund dental care to the indigent population via Medicaid, the population covered by Medicaid may have difficulty accessing dental care. Many dental providers choose not to enroll as Medicaid providers so that they do not have to accept patients with Medicaid insurance. Many cite factors such as frequently missed appointments, difficult treatment issues, low reimbursement rates, too much bureaucratic paperwork, and not wanting Medicaid patients in the waiting room with other patients. This tremendously effects access to care for these patients. (Please see Table 3–3 for a list of financing dental care terms.)

SUMMARY

Dental care in the United States is still mostly a private sector endeavor. However, the federal, state, and local governments are involved in funding dental care to certain populations. The government also funds dental research and education of dental providers. Dental insurance plans have made routine dental care affordable to most individuals. In order to become a consumer advocate, dental hygienists must understand dental funding in both private and public organizations.

REFERENCES

[1]1988–1991: First three years of the third national health and nutrition examination survey. *Journal of Dental Research* (special research) 75 (February 1996).

[2]Levit, K. R., H. C. Lazenby, and B. R. Branden. National health expenditures. *Health Care Financing Review* 18(1996): 175–82.

[3]Cooper, B. S., and N. L. Worthington. National health expenditures, 1929–1972. *Social Security Bulletin* 36 no. 3 (1973): 19–40.

Get Connected

Multimedia Extension Activities

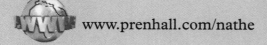 www.prenhall.com/nathe

Use the above address to access the free, interactive companion web site created specifically to accompany this textbook. Here you will find an array of self study material to help you gain a richer understanding of the concepts presented in this chapter.

Chapter 4

∙∙

DENTAL CARE DELIVERY AROUND THE WORLD

by Sue Lloyd, EDH, EDT

OBJECTIVES

After studying this chapter, the dental hygiene student will be able to:

- describe the evolution of dental hygiene in other countries.
- define the roles of dental hygienists in other countries.
- describe the demographics and educational preparation of dental hygienists in other countries.
- compare dental public health programs in other countries.
- list and define the international professional organizations involving dental hygiene.
- discuss the regulation of dental hygienists in other countries.

COMPETENCIES

After studying this chapter and participating in the accompanying class activities, the dental hygiene student should be competent in the following:

- promote the values of oral and general health and wellness to the public and organizations within and outside of the profession.
- be able to influence consumer groups, businesses, and government agencies to support health care issues.

KEY WORDS

Dental hygiene movement   Dental therapists
Dental nurses   World Health Organization (WHO)

INTRODUCTION

The methods in which dental care is provided on a global basis differ widely. Variations between industrialized nations and developing nations are obvious. Specifically, delivery systems are affected by political, cultural, and socioeconomic factors and can change frequently. Some countries have no set oral health policy, and in others highly structured policies are practiced. Dental hygienists place oral health as a priority issue, but for many countries oral health is low on the list. Government health policies too often exclude oral health, or it is hidden in the text among nutrition or general health policies. Even in these enlightened times, oral health promotion is often the "Cinderella" of dentistry. Gathering data around the world shows a lack in national dental health promotion programs and a growing belief that oral health promotion campaigns do not achieve the desired effect. In the United Kingdom, active research is underway to develop systems of measuring the effectiveness of oral health promotion.[1]

The World Health Organization (WHO) Oral Health Unit in conjunction with the Fédération Dentaire Internationale (FDI) recommended the establishment of specific oral health goals in 1979 at the WHO Assembly. The Assembly adopted a resolution calling for the attainment of Health for All by the Year 2000 (see Table 4–1).

It is important to gather global data in order to forecast disease trends. The WHO maintains such information in the Global Oral Data Bank. These data are further combined with information from the WHO Country Profiles Project and are available to administrators for planning and evaluation of oral care services.[2]

Table 4–1. WHO Goals for "Health for All" by the Year 2000

By the age of 5–6 years	50% should be caries free
By the age of 12 years	DMFT should be less than 3
By the age of 18 years	85% should have retained all their teeth
By the age of 34–44 years	A 50% reduction in the number of persons with no teeth
By the age of 65 + years	25% reduction in the number of persons with fewer than 20 teeth

PERIODONTAL DISEASES

Collection of periodontal disease data was extremely difficult until the development of the Community Periodontal Index of Treatment Needs (CPITN). This periodontal index has quickly achieved worldwide acceptance. With the CPITN tool, the epidemiology of periodontal diseases has now moved on to a new level. The CPITN records periodontal diseases in terms of four clinical signs:

1. Bleeding from the gums
2. Presence of calculus
3. Presence of shallow periodontal pockets
4. Presence of deep periodontal pockets

Interestingly, the compiled data show frequency patterns and severity of disease that has surprised epidemiologists. Far from proving that periodontal diseases are rampant in developing countries, the surveys show that the percentage of people who have deep pockets is quite low. The good news is that far fewer of the population suffer from severe forms of periodontal diseases than was previously thought. Those requiring complex surgery and treatment are far from common.

No apparent difference was observed in frequency between developing and industrialized countries for the severe forms of the disease. What has been found, however, is that the early, less severe forms of periodontitis are much more prevalent in developing countries. The data have also shown what was once theorized: that early untreated periodontitis does not always progress into more severe forms of the disease.

What is required to control the incidence of periodontal diseases is a simple program of oral hygiene and regular, professional prophylaxis provided by a dental hygienist or dental therapist. It is also interesting to note that those populations showing high scores for bleeding on probing and calculus are in countries where dental hygienists are either few or nonexistent.

DENTAL CARIES

Data collection for measuring the extent of caries in a population is carried out by means of an index called the Decayed, Missing, and Filled Teeth (DMFT for permanent teeth, deft for deciduous teeth). This simple, rapid, and universally applied measurement has been widely used for several decades. The key ages for data collection are 12 years, 35–44 years, and 651 years. A DMFT between 0.0 and 1.1 is considered low, and a figure of 6.6 or more is high. A moderate DMFT is between 2.78 and 4.4.

The dental hygienist's role is primarily to promote oral health and prevent dental disease. As evident by the global incidence of both dental caries and periodontal diseases, much remains to be accomplished. The methods in which dental hygiene services are delivered also differ from country to country and what is a problem in one country is not always a problem in another. For example, the conditions and priorities for oral health in Latvia are not the same as those in the United Kingdom. These issues should be taken into consideration when planning and implementing dental public health programs.

In order to reduce the incidence of caries, some countries have introduced mass population fluoridation programs. This approach has resulted in a drop in the DMFT, but even so, mass fluoridation is regarded as a controversial issue in many countries. Interestingly, Denmark did have a program, but the cost per person was considered too high for the perceived benefits and has been discontinued.

This chapter focuses on the many ways the dental hygienist influences dental delivery systems within the global dental public health arena.

HISTORICAL PERSPECTIVE OF THE GLOBAL DENTAL HYGIENE MOVEMENT

Dental hygiene is a comparatively young profession. Dental hygiene started in the United States as discussed in chapter 1. Although records going back to 1819 show oral hygiene being recommended to patients on a daily basis, it was not until 1843 that the **dental hygiene movement** began emerging. In 1913 the term dental hygienist was first used, and Dr. Alfred C. Fones started the first courses for dental hygienists in Bridgeport, Connecticut. The profession has steadily progressed, and many schools of dental hygiene around the world have based their curriculum on the American style of training. Certainly, it can be said that training programs in other countries have aspired to achieve the same quality as the American style and career structure. In 1923 the first meeting of the American Dental Hygienists' Association (ADHA) was held. In 1925 its constitution and bylaws were adopted, followed by a code of ethics in 1926. The establishment of the ADHA encouraged most countries involved in training and employing hygienists to set up national associations of dental hygienists, many of whom have joined the International Federation of Dental Hygienists (IFDH), which is discussed later in this chapter.

A survey of fourteen countries, excluding the United States, was conducted recently to look at aspects of the work of the dental hygienist with particular reference to dental public health.[3] The countries included were Australia, Canada, Denmark, Germany, Italy, Israel, Japan, the Netherlands, New Zealand, Norway, Portugal, South Korea, Switzerland, and the United Kingdom. Other than the

United States, England recorded one of the earliest histories of establishing the profession of dental hygiene. Its beginnings came in the form of training of dental hygienists in 1942 to ensure that pilots in the Royal Air Force (RAF), flying fighter planes during World War II, had good dental health and were not troubled by dental pain, which can occur when flying at high altitudes, particularly in unpressurized aircraft.

At that time the RAF had dentists who had an interest in oral hygiene and had trained further in periodontics in the United States after having heard about the training programs involving dental hygienists. These pioneering, enthusiastic dentists were instrumental in urging the British government's Department of Health to start training "civilian" hygienists at the Eastman Dental Institute, London, in 1949, after the war had ended. A number of schools around the world were influenced by the British example, such as those in Australia, New Zealand, and Nigeria (once, all members of the British Commonwealth). The School in Nigeria, in fact, was set up by one of the first civilian hygienists, Vera Creaton, who originally trained in the RAF and then taught at the Eastman Dental Institute. For many years the school, which was a school for training dental therapists, ran parallel with the British courses and was regulated by the General Dental Council (GDC) of the United Kingdom. However, since then the Nigerian course has devised its own method of training dental hygienists and is run independent of the GDC.

As with many other allied health professions, dental hygienists are as much influenced by dentists as nursing professionals are by the doctors who work with them. However, in most countries, dental hygienists are not allowed to practice without a dentist either being present or giving the dental hygienist a treatment plan to follow when treating a patient. In many countries dentists have exerted a great deal of pressure on the dental hygienist movement to comply with their own ideals and goals. They have been most reluctant to relinquish their considerable influence over the practice of the dental hygienist in spite of advances in the implementation of oral health promotion and the teaching programs that are now in place. The dental hygienist is educated as a health care professional and an expert in promoting oral hygiene and preventing dental diseases.

DEMOGRAPHICS AND THE DENTAL HYGIENIST

In a perfect world the ratio of dental hygienists to dentists and the general population would be even and adequate. Unfortunately, it is not always so. Some countries have too many dental professionals and others too few. Large countries such as Australia and Canada have populations that are mainly gathered in cities with small numbers scattered in rural areas, which reduces some of the population segment's accessibility to dental services. Other countries have large populations in relation to land mass with perhaps more dental personnel than needed. Labor surveys are always open to different interpretation and are not regularly conducted. The last global survey seems to have been conducted by the FDI and published in 1990.[4] A new survey is needed now in the twenty-first century to enable the dental profession to get a clear view of its situation.

One study revealed that Germany came out lowest of the league with fewer than 90 hygienists to serve a population of 81 million. The number of dentists is 55,000, which provides a ratio of one hygienist to 647 dentists or one hygienist to 952,941 potential patients. The highest number of hygienists was in Japan with 157,941 to 85,518 dentists, or a ratio of almost two hygienists for every dentist. The population stands at 126 million and provides one hygienist for 1,242 people. The least populated country was New Zealand with only 4 million people, 120 hygienists, and 1,200 dentists, which provides a ratio of 1 hygienist to every 10 dentists. The ratio of hygienists to the general population is 1 to 33,333. Even in the most heavily populated countries with a good supply of dental hygienists, it still may be difficult to reach patients on a one-to-one basis, and other means of promotion must also be considered. (See Table 4–2.)

Countries such as India, Pakistan, and Thailand train students in basic oral health education and oral hygiene instruction. They are trained to demonstrate toothbrushing and encourage individuals to adopt a preventive attitude toward dental diseases. Once trained, the students tend to be employed by the government to work in public dental health clinics and to go out to villages and either train the health staff (nurses/doctors) to supervise oral hygiene or to teach the village population in groups themselves.

In other countries, such as Belize, Chile, and Mexico, which have few or no hygienists or other dental professionals working on dental public health, the caries incidence is climbing. This trend can be theorized to be due to the access to more sugar and processed foods, carbonated drinks, and little education about the dental problems such products can cause.

In countries where populations have been influenced by oral health promotion, programs are now showing a decline in the incidence of caries but often demonstrate a high incidence of periodontal disease. In the United Kingdom, in 1996–97, the average DMFT was recorded as 1.1, but still, in 1991 the percentage of people (15–19 years) showing bleeding on probing was 36 percent, and 49 percent demonstrated the presence of calculus (using the CPITN index of probing).

In Tajikistan (formally part of the Soviet Union) in 1990 the average DMFT was 1.2, but the periodontal condition in 1987 was showing pocket depths of 4–5 mm. To those with an interest in oral health promotion, these statistics clearly show a great need to educate populations in the benefits of effective oral hygiene practices to maintain healthy oral tissues, as well as to prevent dental decay.

Even industrialized countries where the caries incidence is low are now beginning to show trends of increasing caries in inner cities and among ethnic minorities. This worrisome trend has no explanations other than theories attributing the cause to changing diets and lifestyles for these groups.

Table 4–2. Number of Qualified Dental Hygienists and Dentists and Country Population			
Country	**Population (estimate)**	**Number of Qualified Dental Hygienists**	**Number of Dentists**
Australia	18,750,982	330	7,700
Canada	27,000,000	13,500	25,000–30,000
Denmark	5,000,000	1,150	6,000
Germany	81,000,000	85	55,000
Italy	58,000,000	1,050	6,000
Israel	5,500,000	620	7,000
Japan	126,000,000	157,861	85,518
The Netherlands	15,000,000	1,900	7,500
New Zealand	4,000,000	120	1,200
Norway	4,350,000	1,200	3,800
Portugal	10,000,000	129	2,000+
South Korea	46,858,000	15,567	15,950
Switzerland	7,000,000	1,600	4,000
United Kingdom	58,000,000	3,800	29,000
United States	281,400,000	150,000	140,000

Source: Lloyd, Sue. Survey into training, international oral health promotion and dental delivery systems by the dental hygienist (1999).

DENTAL HYGIENE EDUCATION

Not surprisingly the number of training schools reflects the number of hygienists in the country as depicted in Table 4–3. Basic entry qualifications are similar around the world. Each dental hygiene program requires a high standard of high school matriculation. Candidates must be over eighteen years of age. In addition, some schools have adopted a two-tier entry level. It requires the candidate either to

Table 4–3. Training Schools by Country	
Country	**Number of Training Schools**
Australia	5
Canada	25
Denmark	2
Germany	0
Italy	16
Israel	2
Japan	135
Latvia	1
The Netherlands	4
New Zealand	1
Norway	3
Portugal	1
South Korea	23
Sweden	11
Switzerland	4
United Kingdom	17
United States	273

Source: Lloyd, Sue. Survey into training, international oral health promotion, and dental delivery systems by the dental hygienist (1999).

demonstrate a high standard of matriculation or have studied and qualified as a dental assistant and have a good standard of matriculation.

The length and types of training vary. In most countries the length of study is 2 years. Denmark has a 2.5-year course of study. Italy, the Netherlands, Portugal, and Switzerland offer 3-year courses. The 3-year courses may provide degree status rather than diploma status, which all the 2-year courses offer. The few exceptions include Lithuania, which now offers a 4-year baccalaureate degree in public health and a certificate in dental hygiene.[5] However qualified, dental hygienists have no further opportunities for career development in dental hygiene. Australia offers courses ranging from 5 months plus 1-year preceptorship in the Armed Forces to a 3-year baccalaureate degree that include a module in oral health promotion.

All students complete examinations at the end of their courses to obtain a national qualification. In the larger countries, such as Australia and Canada, state/province examinations (sometimes called "Boards") are also required.

THE ROLE OF THE DENTAL HYGIENIST

As previously stated, the role of the dental hygienist is to promote oral health and prevent dental diseases. This task can be done in a variety of ways. All hygienists are involved in dental health education that emphasizes motivational education. Approaches to dental health education have changed considerably since Fones first established his school. In recent years education has made use of behavioral sciences, including sociology, psychology, and communication. Motivation and planning achievable oral health programs for patients have become the main goal in dental public health program development.

Without motivation and compliance the patient cannot achieve the goals set for improving oral hygiene. In past years emphasis was placed on clinical skills and scaling techniques with the result that the patient left the treatment room with very clean teeth and healthy gums only to return some months later in a similar state to that when they first presented to the hygienist.

All dental hygienists carry out basic scaling and root planing tasks, followed by prophylaxis. In addition, most also apply concentrated fluoride products to the teeth and provide dental sealants as needed.

It is interesting to note that some countries allow hygienists to train in specific techniques or tasks, which allow them greater flexibility when working. Among these extra tasks are impression taking, taking radiographs, giving local anesthesia, and planning their own treatments for patients.

Other roles for hygienists may be overlooked in favor of the more traditional clinician's role. Darby and Walsh list these roles as administrator/manager; change agent (facilitating changes in legislation and promoting oral health care for communities); client advocate (protecting and supporting client's rights and well-being); educator/oral health promoter; and researcher. These roles may be expanded and followed more closely by individuals with a particular interest in their chosen field.[6]

The United States and Canada seem to offer the best routes for career development, but other countries are developing their own approaches. The future for dental hygienists certainly holds great potential in their exciting and worthwhile profession.

ACCESS TO DENTAL HYGIENE CARE

For most people in industrialized countries, going to the dentist and seeing a dental hygienist is relatively easy, although costly. Surveys reveal that cost is a major factor in preventing people from accessing dental care. Generally, free dental treatment is provided only for children and the ages of the child varies. The best options are in Australia, New Zealand, Denmark, and the United Kingdom. All covered children are zero to eighteen years of age and students in full-time education (United Kingdom). In Norway, children are treated free in clinics funded by the government. Often conditions dictate who qualifies for such treatment, which also reduces accessibility. Free treatment is available in both private and public health settings, and the hygienist may work in both environments. Medical insurance covering dental treatment is available in some countries, for example, Australia, Canada, and Denmark. In Japan it is compulsory. Others, such as Norway, Portugal, and South Korea, offer no insurance option; all treatment has to be paid by the patient.

Many countries, as indicated in Table 4–4, have community and school dental services within the public health program, and hygienists play a significant part in providing these services. Some hygienists are actively involved in clinical work, and others work solely in oral health promotion. In Norway, the majority of hygienists work in the community dental services.

It is difficult to find out how much money governments allocate to their public dental health services, because the amount is often included within the total health budgets. Generally, though, it seems that public dental health is not perceived as a priority service in many countries. Dental hygienists can play a major role in influencing health services to attach more importance to their dental public health programs. Preventing dental diseases translates into cost savings in the long term to any government or individual. In addition the quality of life is improved for the individual.

Some hygienists are able to undertake voluntary work in the dental public health sector. Many are involved with oral health promotion with children and oral hygiene instruction to disadvantaged groups in the community.

DENTAL PUBLIC HEALTH PROGRAMS AND CAMPAIGNS

Most countries have some public dental health services that are administered by states or provinces within the country. Dental hygienists are part of the group of dental professionals responsible for oral health promotion. In some countries, such as Germany and the United Kingdom, specifically trained oral health promoters run programs. In the United Kingdom, this person is often a dental professional (dental hygienist, dental therapist, or dental assistant). In the United Kingdom, a

Table 4–4. Location of Dental Hygienists Working in Dental Public Health

Country	Community Dental Services	Hospital	School Dental Services	Industry	Armed Forces	Education
Australia	✓	✓	*	*	*	*
Canada	*	*	*	*	*	✓
Denmark	✓	✓	✓		✓	✓
Germany	x	x	x	✓	x	✓
Italy	*	*	*	*	*	✓
Israel	*	✓	*	x	✓	✓
Japan	✓	*	*	*	*	*
The Netherlands	✓	✓	x	✓	x	✓
New Zealand	*	*	*	*	*	✓
Norway	✓	✓	✓	✓	x	✓
Portugal	✓	✓	✓	✓	x	✓
South Korea	✓	✓	*	*	*	✓
Switzerland	✓	✓	✓	✓	x	✓
United Kingdom	✓	✓	✓	✓	✓	✓
United States	✓	✓	✓	✓	✓	✓

✓ Working in this sector
* Not stated
x Not working in this sector
Source: Lloyd, Sue. Survey into training, international oral health promotion, and dental delivery systems by the dental hygienist (1999).

DENTAL HYGIENIST'S SPOTLIGHT
A Day in the Life of Til Van Der Sanden-Stoelinga,
IFDH President

In 1970 I graduated from the School of Dental Hygiene of the University of Utecht (first class), after a two-year course.

I immediately started work in the field of oral health promotion, at that time still called dental health education.

In the Netherlands we were confronted with a terrible increase of caries from the beginning of the twentieth century until the late 1960s: from 37 percent caries-free twelve-year-old children in 1913, to 1.4 percent in 1967. At the age of eighteen, the situation was even worse. Out of 1,000 eighteen-year-old boys serving in the Dutch army, only four boys had a caries-free set of teeth.

This situation led to two important initiatives. The Department of Preventive Dentistry, which already existed, and the Dutch Ivory Cross (Het Ivoren Kruis), the institute for dental health education, started the promotion of fluoridation of the drinking water and initiating local dental health education programs. Being an employee of the Ivory Cross, I was involved with this from the beginning.

Unfortunately, in 1973 the fluoridation of drinking water was no longer a priority, although it proved to be the best way of getting healthy teeth. For reasons of principle, cultural, and religious nature, fluoridation of the drinking water was forbidden by law. So, dental health education became more important. One of my roles in this was, together with people of municipalities, school dental health services, commu-

nity health services, and so on, to develop strategies to reach children aged zero to twelve years old and their parents. Another aspect of my task was to facilitate the work of dental hygienists and educators working in school dental health services by means of special courses (teaching the teachers). The third part of my job was to design educational materials. All kinds of educational materials were distributed in schools and dental practices.

Plaque control was recognized as one of the most important factors to decrease dental caries, together with the change of food habits (sugar intake). Dental awareness of the people increased over the years, and they began to brush their teeth on a regular basis. Between 1980 and 1994, the use of toothpaste increased from 0.2 to 0.4 liter per capita per year. Moreover, the fact that fluoride could decrease dental caries became common knowledge. Manufacturers of toothpaste started to make toothpaste with fluoride on a wide scale. In the meantime, the Ivory Cross developed standards for those toothpastes, the size of toothbrushes, and the use of fluoride tablets. Today 98 percent of all toothpastes contains fluoride.

In the 1980s and 1990s, other influences were recognized as being important for the reduction of caries, such as biological factors, cultural factors, income, level of education, and the social setting. We also changed the channels

(continued)

Dental Hygienist's Spotlight *(continued)*

of education: more and more other professionals, such as teachers, nurses, and other health professionals (now called primary intermediaries), became partners in our work. Moreover, health education changed in health promotion. Last but not least, changes in society and health structure induced changes in the relationship between health promoters and the public. For example, school health dental services are gone. Dental hygienists got a role as municipal public health service workers, and they are seen as important "vehicles" in supporting the primary intermediaries.

In the 1990s, the average number of decayed, missing, and filled teeth of six-year-old Dutch children is four. This number is stabilizing. At the age of twelve, 74 percent of the children are caries free, but still another 26 percent of these children are developing caries.

Although the use of fluoridated toothpaste is probably the main cause of the lower caries prevalence, if we had not changed people's attitudes toward dental health in the first place, toothpaste manufacturers would not have thought to produce these fluoridated toothpaste so early and on such a wide scale.

The situation is far better than in 1967, but we cannot lean back and relax; we still have work to do. In the first place, it is evident that for those people who do not have caries at the moment, a constant and structural stream of oral health promotion is still of great importance to stimulate and motivate this group. In the second place, we have to face the fact that, as in most industrialized countries, there are still people who develop caries or other oral diseases,

most of them belonging to the so-called risk groups. In our country, these groups consist of the elderly, those who consume many soft drinks, people with a low social economic status (including migrant groups), and toddlers constantly sucking on their baby bottles.

About ten years ago, the Ivory Cross (and later on the Netherlands Institute of Health Promotion and Disease Prevention, in which the Ivory Cross has been incorporated since 1996) started several nationwide projects for special groups concentrating on a specific subject. We know, among others:

- Project Collective Information on oral hygiene for Turkish and Moroccan immigrants
- Campaign against baby caries
- Project Collective Implementation of a new fluoride advice

The most important differences with the initiatives in the 1970s are both the intermediaries (as we call the health providers, carers, and counselors now) and the public as the ultimate target group are involved in the development of the projects. For both target groups, we develop materials at the same time, but with a different nature, for example, fact files for the intermediaries and attention-getting posters and brochures for the public. Mass media is used when new ideas have to be implemented.

I am still involved in this kind of work, and although the nature of the work is the same, I have changed with the changing society. The emancipation of the public and one's own responsibility for his life and health are especially important to me.

Certificate in Oral Health Promotion is open to all qualified dental personnel who wish to work in the field of oral health promotion. A part-time course leads to a formal qualification. In addition to government agencies running oral health promotion programs, nongovernmental agencies such as national dental health foundations, dental organizations, and professional associations are often involved.

Many governments are, however, reducing their financial support for national oral health promotion programs, in part because market research shows that such campaigns have little long-term effect on the public's oral health behavior. In the United Kingdom, emphasis is on evaluation of all major oral health promotion programs. This type of evaluation is quite difficult to devise, and new models are being researched to provide objectivity and quantitative analysis rather than the qualitative analysis such promotions have been subjected to in the past. It has led to more sophisticated planning before a dental public health program is launched. The goals and objectives are formally worked out along with final evaluation processes prior to submitting a bid to the public health provider of funding. It will be interesting to follow results in the coming years.

Encouragingly, many countries have had significant dental public health campaigns in the last five years. Some of the major campaigns are Japan's "8020" campaign, which focuses on retaining twenty teeth by eighty years of age; South Korea's "10 Principles of Dental Health" poster campaign; the Netherlands' extensively documented "Bottle It Up, Take a Cup" campaign to reduce the incidence of nursing caries; and the United Kingdom's "Early Years" campaign that reflects similar principles as those of the Netherlands. These campaigns are presented in Table 4–5.

ORAL HEALTH POLICIES

Few countries have formal, national published oral health policies or strategies that are provided by the government. Examples from Japan, South Korea, and the United Kingdom are provided in Table 4–6. Denmark, Germany, Norway, and Portugal also have policies in place. They range from statements about entitlement to dental treatment to strategies explaining in detail about what the government is striving to achieve. An Oral Health Strategy for Europe is under consideration and has been put forward by the Council of European Dental Officers. This ambitious project will need excellent collaboration to be implemented.

Mass fluoridation programs were popular at one time; however, research has shown that they have reduced in number, due in part to the success that fluoride toothpaste has had on reducing caries. Still many developing countries need help to control dental disease.[7] Populations in developing countries may not be able to afford expensive fluoride dentifrices. With changing living conditions and lifestyles, an increase in dental caries has been reported in several developing countries. Seven countries reported that mass fluoridation is still available either nationally or on a local basis. The majority supply either water or salt fluoridation.

Table 4–5.	Significant Dental Health Campaigns Introduced in the Past 5 Years
Country	**Dental Health Campaign**
Australia	Commonwealth dental health program to provide dental treatment at an agreed set fee (now discontinued)
	Pensioner denture service, similar to commonwealth program (now discontinued)
Japan	"8020" campaign
	National campaign administered by the Ministry of Health and Welfare
The Netherlands	"Bottle It Up, Take a Cup" campaign to prevent nursing caries
South Korea	"10 Principles for Dental Health"
United Kingdom	"Early Years" campaign, to prevent nursing caries and encourage better nutrition and oral health
United States	"Smiles within Reach" campaign of ADHA and Oral-B for children "Access to Care" campaign by ADHA

Source: Lloyd, Sue. Survey into training, international oral health promotion, and dental delivery systems by the dental hygienist (1999) and www.adha.org.

LOBBYING GROUPS

A minority of so-called "lobbying" groups promote oral hygiene in a few countries. From the survey it appears that the United Kingdom is the most active country with several groups focusing on sugars: Action and Information on Sugars (AIS); Chuck Sweets off the Checkout campaign; Toothfriendly UK. The Food Commission and the Food Labeling Group embrace all food issues, including sugars and oral hygiene. Such groups campaign to have clearer, less misleading labels on foods and drinks containing sugars and less misleading advertisements, especially those targeted at children, including the way the food and drink industry infiltrate the education system.

Toothfriendly Sweets International (TSI) provides the confectionery industry with the means of informing the public that their candies are safe for teeth.[8] It

Country	National Oral Health Policy
	Table 4–6. National Oral Health Policies
Japan	Policy for the mentally and physically disadvantaged Prevention of dental disease campaigns for adults over 40 years of age
South Korea	Provide education on oral health to everyone
United Kingdom	1. Scientific Basis of Dental Health Education, a policy document 2. Oral Health Strategy: By the year 2003 • 70% of 5-year-olds will have no caries experience • on average, 5-year-olds should have no more than 1 DEFT • on average, 12-year-olds should have no more than 1 DMFT • The percentage of dentate adults over 45 with at least one 6 mm + periodontal pocket should be reduced to 10% (currently approx. 17%)

Source: Lloyd, Sue. Survey into training, international oral health promotion, and dental delivery systems by the dental hygienist (1999).

licenses products that can prove, through means of an independent scientific test, that their product does not harm teeth. The logo is a happy, smiling tooth covered by a protective umbrella as seen in Figure 4–1. A number of Toothfriendly organizations round the world are affiliated with TSI and not only license products but also actively campaign to publicize the role sugar plays in the caries process. A selection of lobbying groups is listed in Table 4–7.

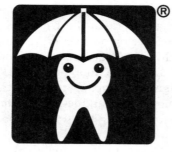

Figure 4–1.   Toothfriendly Logo

Table 4–7 Known Lobbying Groups by Country	
Country	**Lobby Groups**
Germany	Toothfriendly Germany (Aktion Zahnfreundlich e.v.) for sugarfree confectionery and drinks
New Zealand	New Zealand Dental Health Foundation
Switzerland	Toothfriendly Switzerland (Aktion Zahnfreundlich Sussugkeiten) for sugarfree confectionery and drinks
United Kingdom	Action and Information on Sugars (watchdog on misinformation on sugars through poor labeling and advertising) The Food Commission (watchdog on food industry includes sugar issues) Chuck Sweets off the Checkout Toothfriendly UK for sugarfree confectionery and drinks

Many countries offer oral health promotion annual events. Only Japan is run by the government's Ministry of Health and Welfare; other countries are organized by National Dental and Dental Hygiene Associations and National Dental Health Foundations. Table 4–8 presents the oral health promotional activities in different countries.

INTERNATIONAL DENTAL PROFESSIONAL ORGANIZATIONS

The International Federation of Dental Hygienists (IFDH), developed from the International Liaison Committee (ILC), was established in 1970 and included representatives from Canada, Japan, the Netherlands, Norway, Sweden, the United Kingdom, and the United States. In 1986 the IFDH replaced the ILC during the 10th International Symposium in Dental Hygiene in Oslo, Norway. Such an organization had been promoted by a number of people, including the late Dr. G. H. Leatherman, executive director of the FDI. The American Dental Hygienists' Association was also instrumental in establishing the federation. Both Leatherman and the ADHA infused the organization with enthusiasm and dedication for the dental hygiene profession. The objectives for the federation are listed in Table 4–9.

Members are national dental hygiene associations that can meet the criteria for membership. Members can appoint two delegates as their representatives on the Board. An executive committee runs the federation on a daily basis. Policies are

Table 4–8.   Oral Health Promotion Action Days/Weeks/Month by Country

Country	OHP Day/Week/Month	Title
Australia	Week	National Dental Health Week
Canada	Month of April	Dental Health Month
	Month of October	National Dental Health Campaign
Germany	Day (September 25)	National Dental Health Day
Italy	Month of October	Dental Health Month
Japan	Week June 4–8	Dental Hygiene Week
	Day (November 8)	Good Teeth Day
New Zealand	Week	Dental Health Week
South Korea	Day (June 9)	Dental Health Day
United Kingdom	Week in May	Smile Week
United States	Month of October	National Dental Hygiene Month

**Table 4–9.   Objectives of the International Federation
of Dental Hygienists**

- To promote access to quality preventive oral health services to all peoples.
- To represent and advance the profession of dental hygiene on a nongovernmental, worldwide basis.
- To promote and coordinate the exchange of knowledge and information about the profession, and its education and practice.
- To raise the level of awareness of the public that oral disease can be prevented through proven regimens.

Source: International Federation of Dental Hygienists, *Contact International* 14 (2000): 6.

based on those agreed by the house of delegates and implemented by the executive committee. A regular publication, the *International Journal of Dental Hygiene,* is published quarterly and contains peer-reviewed scientific articles and international issues involving dental hygiene.

IFDH is a strong and growing organization with twenty-three countries currently members: Australia, Austria, Canada, Colombia, Denmark, Finland, Germany, Israel, Italy, Japan, Latvia, the Netherlands, New Zealand, Nigeria, Norway, Portugal, South Africa, South Korea, Spain, Sweden, Switzerland, the United Kingdom, and the United States. In addition a European group, affiliated to IFDH, meets from time-to-time to discuss European matters. This organization is useful in the light of directives from Brussels and the free movement of workers across the European Union.

With the emergence of developing countries training dental hygienists comes the hope that more associations will join the federation to form a truly worldwide network. IFDH promotes access to quality preventive oral services and strives to raise public awareness about the prevention of dental disease. IFDH also has forged strong links with international organizations who have similar outlooks on oral health promotion such as FDI and WHO (Oral Health Unit).[9]

The Fédération Dentaire International (FDI), the World Dental Federation, was founded in 1900, in Paris, France. It is one of the oldest international health organizations. Its objectives are provided in Table 4–10. It has member associations in eighty-two countries and has established Standing Commissions and Programs on a number of dental-related issues including oral health. FDI was admitted into official relations with WHO in 1948 and collaborates with WHO on planning and development of global goals for oral health.

Table 4–10.   Fédération Dentaire Internationale (FDI) Objectives

- To be the authoritative, professional, independent, worldwide voice of dentistry.
- To support the principle that all people should have access to the best possible care to achieve optimal oral health.
- To support and promote the interests of the member associations and their members.
- To contribute internationally to the development and dissemination of policies, standards, and information related to all aspects of oral health care.

Source: www.fdi.org.uk; 2000.

FDI has also had a long-standing official relationship with the International Organization for Standardization (ISO). One aspect of this relationship is the development of international standards of dental materials and equipment.[10]

The **World Health Organization (WHO)** was established on April 7, 1948 (now called World Health Day) and is headquartered in Geneva, Switzerland. WHO is a self-governing, specialized, multilateral agency within the United Nations headed by a director general and governed by an Executive Board representing more than thirty countries. It is responsible for public health and international health issues. Because of information gathered from the community health programs of almost 200 countries, it has the ability to make many projects logistically possible. WHO's objective was the attainment of health for all by the year 2000.

The Oral Health Unit within WHO maintains the Global Oral Data Bank. It is a means of accumulating initial and future standard statistics on the oral health status of the world's populations' statistics from more than 170 countries which is available through the data bank. The Oral Health Unit has established the Oral Health Program to encourage oral health care and the prevention of dental disease on a global basis.[11] Its goals are presented in Table 4–11. In spite of success in helping to improve oral health in most of the industrialized countries, unsolved and ongoing problems still exist in many communities all over the world.

The International Association of Dental Research (IADR) is an organization with the mission to advance research and increase knowledge for the improvement of oral health worldwide. It consists of divisions and sections that establish and support programs to promote oral health research and IADR activities. IADR collaborates with other international dental associations, industry, health agencies, and scientific and educational professional organizations. IADR holds conferences all over the world. It has no permanent headquarters for the association but rests with the incumbent president.[12]

INTERNATIONAL OVERVIEW OF LAW

The International Federation of Dental Hygienists (IFDH) uses the following definition of a dental hygienist: a health professional who graduated from an accredited school of dental hygiene, and who, through clinical services, education, consultative planning, and evaluation endeavors, seeks to prevent oral disease, provides treatment for existing disease, and assists people in maintaining an optimum level of oral health. Dental hygienists are health professionals whose primary concern is the promotion of total health through the prevention of disease.

On an international basis, it is clear that dental hygienists are educated in accredited establishments to the same high standards. Prior to dental hygiene education admission, all prospective students must have received the equivalent of a high school education. Standards achieved are expected to be above average before admitting the student to a dental hygiene program. Equal opportunities exist for both

Table 4–11.   WHO Oral Health Program Activities

- Information collection and methods development

- Monitoring changes in oral diseases and outcomes of oral care

- Maintenance of the Global Oral Data Bank

- Situation analyses for country oral care services development

- Development and testing epidemiological methods

- Country Profile development: providing detailed up-to-date information about oral disease and oral care systems and services, oral care personnel, legislation, and information related to oral diseases and provision of services (sugar consumption, fluoride exposure, use of oral hygiene products, tobacco use, and HIV and Hepatitis B infections)

- Implementation and evaluation of Community Preventive Programs Affordable Oral Care demonstrating and assessing community preventive programs using fluoride in water, salt and milk, in toothpastes and other vehicles. Development, testing, and dissemination of minimal oral care approaches including altraumatic restorative treatment (ART)

- Public education, promotion of appropriate oral health messages in schools, work places, practices in the community

- Advocacy and legislation promotion and dissemination of information about appropriate legislation favoring oral health promotion and community disease preventive activities (e.g., tax exemption for fluoridated toothpastes)

These activities are being implemented in close collaboration with the WHO Regional Advisers for Oral Health and with more than 41 WHO collaborating centers around the world.

men and women, but traditionally dental hygienists have been women. Their larger numbers are partially due to the methods in which hygienists have been selected for admission and partially due to poor salary scales in the past. Fortunately, this situation is changing.

RELATED DENTAL PROFESSIONALS

Other classes of dental health care practitioners provide care in addition to the dental hygienist, dentist, and dental assistant. **Dental therapists,** referred to as school dental nurses in New Zealand, are allowed to undertake all the tasks that a dental hygienist can do and may also restore both the permanent and primary dentition and extract primary teeth.

Dental therapists work mostly in the United Kingdom, New Zealand, and Nigeria. In the United Kingdom, many programs are now training students who will graduate as a dually qualified professional: a dental hygienist and a dental therapist. Courses are being combined to facilitate training a more flexible dental provider. The trend in the United Kingdom is toward an expansion of duties and is based on the recommendations of the Nuffield Report published in 1993. The report put forward the view that the United Kingdom needed an oral health therapist who would be multiskilled and could work in a flexible way. Until recently, the dental therapist was only allowed to practice within the community dental services. The General Dental Council, the regulatory body in the United Kingdom, recently approved dental therapists working in all environments. This move will provide greater accessibility to dental care for many more people in the United Kingdom.

Other professionals working closely with dental hygienists are dental assistants, referred to as **dental nurses** in the United Kingdom. In Japan, for example, dental hygienists provide dental assistant duties. Dental assistants have to train to high standards, qualify, and be registered before being considered a professional member of the dental team. In some countries, however, their skills may not be rated so highly and are not recognized by regulatory authorities. Many receive only on-the-job (preceptorship) training with no formal education to reinforce the practical aspect. Consequently, the standard of training is inconsistent.

A formally trained and registered professional is more likely to receive public confidence. Nonregulation and deregulation allow greater opportunity for negligent care by nonprofessionals with no recourse to an authority should the need arise. Fortunately, this risk is being recognized slowly by countries endeavoring to standardize training. Society has the right to expect their dental health needs be provided by educated and qualified personnel.

Developing countries have training programs that provide oral health care workers who are suited to the needs of the indigenous population. Little can be gained by training a highly skilled professional to undertake complex clinical tasks when the population requires simple oral hygiene techniques and oral health promotion programs.

In this context IFDH, representing the views of its members, considers it unprofessional to call such oral health care workers dental hygienists. The title is protected in a number of countries and has an international definition. Prophylaxis assistants, prophylaxis nurses, and oral health care workers are often termed dental hygienists, but such labeling is to be discouraged because they do not fulfill the criteria that define a dental hygienist.

Orthodontic auxiliaries are trained in Canada, Australia, and soon in the United Kingdom. Such workers are already qualified as a dental assistant and take a postgraduate course in orthodontics. They assist orthodontists in technical tasks by making and fitting bands, taking impressions, and fitting arch wires. They also ensure that the patient undergoing treatment maintains a high standard of oral hygiene.

REGULATION

Countries have different means of regulating dental hygienists. Some, including some provinces of Canada, Sweden, and Portugal, allow self-regulation as provided by the national association of dental hygienists. Other countries have dental boards, the government (Ministry of Health), dental councils, and dental or dental hygiene associations. In Switzerland, the training is the responsibility of the Swiss Red Cross, and regulation is the responsibility of the dental association.

New Zealand has no regulatory body at all. Section 11 of the Dental Health Act states that any person under the direction of a dentist who is present on the premises at which the work is carried out may

- Remove deposits from the teeth
- Apply materials to the teeth for the purpose of preventing disease
- Give advice on dental health

Australia may also be thinking of deregulating but no further information is available at this time. Table 4–12 presents the regulation of dental hygienists in various countries.

INDEPENDENT PRACTICE

The definition of independent practice in one country is not necessarily the same in another. Countries allowing full independent practice are greater than those permitting hygienists to run a referral practice. Canada (British Columbia), Denmark, the Netherlands, Norway, Sweden, and some parts (cantons) of Switzerland allow hygienists to run their own practices. In the United Kingdom, dental hygienists may own and run their own practices but may only work to the treatment plan of a referring dentist and must not directly accept payment for services from the patient. The dental hygienist has to invoice the referring dentist who invoices the patient. The General Dental Council of the United Kingdom believes this system still maintains the links with the dentist that a team member requires. It also means that the dentist maintains full control over the treatment provided. Dental hygienists in Italy may not run their own practices but are allowed to recruit their own patients to the dentist's practice where they work.

Table 4–12. Regulation of Dental Hygienists	
Country	**Regulating Authority**
Australia	Dental Board
Canada	5 provinces are self-regulating (representing 90% of dental hygienists) 5 provinces by Dental Board
Denmark	Board of Health
Germany	No formal regulating body
Italy	Ministry of Health
Israel	Dental Board
Japan	No information available
The Netherlands	Dental Association/Dental Hygienists' Association/Dental Assistants Association
New Zealand	Not regulated
Norway	Dental Health Act
Portugal	Dental Hygienists' Association
South Korea	Medical Technician Law of the Korean government
Switzerland	Dental Association
United Kingdom	Dentists' Act administered by the General Dental Council of the United Kingdom
United States	Individual State Boards

Source: Lloyd, Sue. Survey into training, international oral health promotion, and dental delivery systems by the dental hygienist (1999).

Surprisingly, relatively few numbers of hygienists work in this manner. Financial considerations have to been given to buying expensive equipment, and leasing/buying premises mean large financial commitments that possibly appeal to few. Practitioners must also take on the responsibility of office maintenance and administration. But independent practice has its benefits too: flexible working times, flexible vacation time, and being the "boss," as well as additional options and the choice of how and where to practice. Table 4–13 displays the option of independent practice per country.

Table 4–13. Incidence of Independent Practice by Country	
Country	**Independent Practice Allowed?**
Australia	No
Canada	British Columbia only
Denmark	Yes
Germany	No information available
Italy	Partial independence in that direct recruitment of clients is allowed
Israel	No
Japan	No
The Netherlands	Yes
New Zealand	No
Norway	Yes
Portugal	No
South Korea	No
Sweden	Yes
Switzerland	4 cantons
United Kingdom	Yes, but "referral practice only"
United States	Yes, in selected states

Source: Lloyd, Sue. Survey into training, international oral health promotion, and dental delivery systems by the dental hygienist (1999).

PORTABILITY OF LICENSURE

Many hygienists would like to be able to travel and work in countries other than their own. Unfortunately this option is difficult. In large countries such as Australia, Canada, and the United States not only are national qualifications required, but also state or province qualifications. Although a certain amount of freedom is granted by allowing resident hygienists to work in a number of states/provinces with one type of qualification when wishing to move on, another state examination will be required.

Within the European Union (EU) countries, an equivalency ruling exists; it permits the regulatory body to assess whether training in one EU country is equivalent to another. If agreed, then the dental hygienist is permitted to work. One drawback is often not the training but the inability to speak the language of the country in which they wish to work. Of course, hygienists are only permitted to work in those European countries that recognize them. For example, France, Belgium, Greece, and Cyprus do not recognize dental hygienists.

The Fédération Dentaire Internationale has devised general principles for the equivalency of dental degrees and is developing general guidelines and model protocols for the evaluation of dental education programs that meet acceptable standards of outcome assessment. Also the FDI is developing the professional dental experience and professional conduct required of candidates seeking the right to practice in another state, country, or region. The IFDH has set up an advisory service with information sheets for hygienists interested in working in other countries.

A general rule of thumb, apart from EU countries, is that any dental hygienists wishing to work in countries other than their own have to retrain for a prerequisite time and complete the national or state examination. These requirements are not merely to provide barriers to portability of licensure but to ensure that the relevant tasks are familiar to the hygienist and that cultural difficulties and working practices are well understood.

FUTURE OF DENTAL HYGIENE

Dental hygiene has come a long way in a relatively short time. The progress from the inception by Dr. Fones to the professorships and eminent scholars in dental hygiene represents a great advance.

In conjunction, legislation has also advanced. The responsibilities that dental hygienists are required to fulfill change from time to time as dental research discovers new treatments and preventive techniques and what the public requires. A forward-thinking legislative body will take these advances into account when drawing up or revising regulations.

A real step forward, recently, from the General Dental Council of the United Kingdom (May 1999) was the move to the concept of the dental team by endorsing the statutory regulations of all members of the team. In addition the council agreed that the term dental auxiliary would be replaced by professional complementary to dentistry (PCD). The GDC believes that this term more accurately reflects the professional nature of the health care worker. The modifications also mean a big change in the representational structure within the regulatory body. Until now, one person has represented dental auxiliaries on the council for many years. The new changes will mean that following registration of dental assistants (nurses) and dental technicians, the system will need to be adjusted so that all

PCDs are represented. These and similar changes are in direct contrast to countries such as New Zealand that advocate no regulation.

It is certainly an area to observe. It makes sense for hygienists to be involved in regulations covering their work because they are the professionals involved and are perhaps more likely to press for implementation of more science-based responsibilities to improve oral health than dentists and government officials alone.

SUMMARY

This chapter has attempted to give an overview of dental delivery systems and the ways in which dental hygienists are involved in dental public health on a global basis. It is by no means extensive and has covered a sample of countries only. Its intention is to help the reader gain insight into how dental public health activities are run in countries other than his or her own.

Dental hygienists should be flexible in their approach to delivering oral hygiene. Many countries lack basic facilities for sophisticated oral health promotion programs and are not able to utilize a dental hygienist in the traditional role.

Oral health issues are not recognized as health problems in many countries, and as such periodontal diseases and oral hygiene are neglected and programs are nonexistent or underfunded. Oral health should embrace other health issues in order to make a case for priority funding in national health programs. The use of tobacco and its often-devastating effects on the oral tissues as well as general health should be emphasized and tackled. Nutrition and diet are prominent issues that dental hygienists can address in their efforts to prevent dental disease.

It is an exciting time for dental hygienists, and the profession will continue to grow in importance and status within the dental team. Today's technology will greatly assist oral health care teams to identify population groups needing the expert input of the dental hygienist. It is possible to greatly reduce oral disease on a global basis if dental public health systems make maximum use of their dental hygienists.

REFERENCES

[1]Watts, Elizabeth, and David Locker. Effectiveness of oral health promotion: A review. *Health Effectiveness Reviews* no. 7. London: Health Education Authority, 1997.

[2]http://www.who.int.

[3]Lloyd, Sue. A survey on training, international health promotion and dental delivery systems. Unpublished paper. London, 1999.

[4]FDI Basic Facts 1990. Dentistry round the world. London: FDI, 1990, p. 24.

[5]Based on information received from Marius Andruska, Lithuania.

[6]Darby, M. L., and M. M. Walsh. *Dental Hygiene Theory and Practice.* Philadelphia: W. B. Saunders, 1995, pp. 15–17.

[7]Lennon, M. L. Dental health in Europe: A problem for disadvantaged groups: A discussion document. Department of Clinical Dental Sciences. University of Liverpool, England. October 1998.

[8]TSI, Hauptstraase 63, 4102 Binnengen, Switzerland. http://www.toothfriendly.ch.

[9]International Federation of Dental Hygienists, 55 Kemble Road, Forest Hill, London, SE23 2DH, England.

[10]FDI, 7 Carlisle Street, London, W1V 5RG, England.

[11]Pakhomov G. N. Oral Health Unit, World Health Organisation, CH-121 1 Geneva 27, Switzerland.

[12]Sally J. Marshall, President IADR, University of California, San Francisco School of Dentistry, Department of Restorative Dentistry, Box 0758, San Francisco, CA 94143-0758.

Get Connected

Multimedia Extension Activities

 www.prenhall.com/nathe

Use the above address to access the free, interactive companion web site created specifically to accompany this textbook. Here you will find an array of self study material to help you gain a richer understanding of the concepts presented in this chapter.

Chapter 5

LEGISLATIVE INITIATIVES AFFECTING DENTAL HYGIENE PRACTICE

OBJECTIVES

After studying this chapter, the dental hygiene student will be able to:

- define the legislative process.
- define the major bodies of law.
- describe the regulation of the dental hygienist.
- advocate the utilization of a dental hygienist without restrictive barriers.
- describe the responsibilities of dental hygienists in the United States.

COMPETENCIES

After reading this chapter and participating in the accompanying class activities, the dental hygiene student should be competent in the following:

- promote the values of oral and general health and wellness to the public and organizations within and outside of the profession.
- be able to influence consumer groups, businesses, and government agencies to support health care issues.

KEY WORDS

Bodies of Law
    Administrative
    Common
    Constitutional
    Statutory
Government Branches
    Executive
    Judicial
    Legislative

Legislature
Practice Act
Regulation
Rules
Statute
Supervision

INTRODUCTION

Many legislative initiatives affect the practice of dental hygiene. In fact, most states have bills introduced or changes to rules and regulations annually. Frequently legal changes to practice regulations may allow dental hygienists to more effectively treat the public. Certain changes can prohibit dental hygienists from providing care to the public. Further, many state dental organizations work to expand the scope of dental hygiene practice to on-the-job-trained personnel. Recent resolutions passed by the American Dental Association (ADA) support the alternative pathway model of dental hygiene education such as on-the-job (preceptorship) training of personnel.[1] Simply, the challenge dental hygiene faces today may well be professional survival.

Most recently, a statute was passed giving dental hygienists in New Mexico the freedom to provide dental hygiene in any setting without the supervision of dentists.[2] Interestingly, the state health policy commission, not the dental hygiene association, brought about the impetus for the change. The reason for the change, which is termed collaborative practice, was to increase access to care for the underserved population. In contrast, Kansas recently passed a change initiated by the dental association to the dental hygiene practice act, which allows dental assistants to provide supragingival scaling. Further, the American Dental Association had recently adopted the position to define oral prophylaxis as a dental prophylaxis performed on transitional or permanent dentition that includes scaling and/or polishing procedures to remove coronal plaque, calculus, and stains. In other words, if a patient goes to the dental office for a routine "cleaning," the patient probably will not realize that a dental assistant legally may provide just a polishing and bill it as a cleaning. Fortunately, the ADA unanimously rescinded this decision after the American Dental Hygienists' Association was able to explain the significance of this wording change to the dental insurance industry.

In 2003, the Federal Trade Commission issued a complaint against the South Carolina State Board of Dentistry alleging that it violated federal laws by illegally restricting the ability of dental hygienists to provide preventive dental services, including cleanings, sealants, and fluoride treatments, on-site to children in South Carolina schools. The Board of Dentistry had a passed an emergency regulation that contradicted the law that stated that all patients had to have an examination by a dentist before receiving dental hygiene treatment in schools. This issue is another prime example of an organized body of dentistry working diligently to hinder access to dental hygiene care.

STATE GOVERNMENT OVERVIEW

Even though the federal laws that are discussed in Chapter 11 affect dental hygiene *science*, the laws that affect dental hygiene *practice* are enacted and enforced by individual states. The federal government has no responsibility or authority for the reg-

Table 5–1. Comparison of State and Federal Government

Branches of Government	Federal Government	State Government
Legislative	Congress	State Legislature
Executive	President	Governor
Judicial	Federal Court	State Court

ulation of dental hygiene in states. Although the federal government does not play a major role in the governing of dental hygiene practice, it provides the model after which each state's system of government is fashioned. Table 5–1 compares the branches of government for state and for federal government.

State government has three **branches,** including the **legislative, executive, and judicial** branch. Each branch of government has a specific function and limited areas of authority, which is exclusive to that branch, as indicated in Table 5–2.

The legislative branch makes laws for the state, which would include laws affecting the licensing and practice of the dental hygienist. The executive branch carries out the laws passed by the legislature. This branch has the power to enforce laws made by the state legislators. An example of this branch is a police officer. Lastly, the judicial branch interprets the laws the legislature passes. Judges do not make laws, they simply interpret existing laws.

The major **bodies of law** include the **common** law, **statutory** law, **constitutional** law, and the **administrative** law, which are listed in Table 5–3. Common law is created by the courts via judicial decision and can be changed by the courts. It contains notions of common sense and precedent. Statutory law is written law, which is enacted by the **legislature,** helps promote justice, and can be changed by the legislature. Dental hygiene practice acts are statutory law. Constitutional law was developed after common law and statutory law. The people created it and the people have the power to change the law. It is the most powerful law; in fact, it

Table 5–2. Branches of State Government

Branch of Government	Function
Legislative	Create laws
Executive	Enforce laws
Judicial	Interpret laws

Table 5–3. Major Bodies of Law	
Type of Law	**Definition**
Common	Created and changed only by courts
Statutory	Created and changed by legislature
Constitutional	Created and changed by the people
Administrative	Delegation of legislative power to an administrative agency

takes precedence over both common law and statutory law. The fourth body of law is administrative law and is the result of the legislative branches voluntarily delegating some of its lawmaking authority to the executive branch. Administrative agencies such as state dental boards fall within this law. The legislature has the authority to say when and if they can develop rules and regulations.

Generally, state legislative process includes two legislative bodies, the Senate and the House of Representatives, sometimes referred to as the Assembly or House of Delegates. In most states, the legislature meets for up to six months once a year.

LAWS PERTAINING TO DENTAL HYGIENE

Laws pertaining to dental hygiene are generally found in the state dental hygiene **practice act.** However, federal laws do have the ability to affect dental hygiene practice. Policies enacted at the federal level pertaining to dental insurance and Medicaid may be able to affect dental hygiene practice. If a **rule** in the Medicaid law stated that dental hygienists could be reimbursed for oral examinations, oral prophylaxis, and other procedures, states may be inclined to ensure that their state laws and rules did not conflict federal law. In essence, state legislators may push for a change in the **statute** so that dental hygienists can deliver care without the direct **supervision** of a dentist. Then their state would have the benefit of federal money directed at dental hygiene care delivered in schools or practice settings other than the private dental offices.

For the most part, laws pertaining to dental hygiene practice are found in state laws. These statutory laws describe the allowable scope of practice, necessary dental supervision requirements, requirements necessary to obtain a dental hygiene license process, and suspension and revocation of licensure procedures. Many states have rules and **regulations** developed by the state dental board to aid in interpreting the laws of the practice act.

In order to make any statutory changes (changes to the practice of dental hygiene) it is necessary, in essence, for a thought (bill) to become a law. Figure 5–1 depicts the basic method in which a bill may become in fact a law. Both houses must pass a bill after it has spent time in specific committees, which may amend or change the bill, within each house. Many times a bill will "die" in a committee only to have the most vital ideas added to a totally different bill. Such a process acts as a

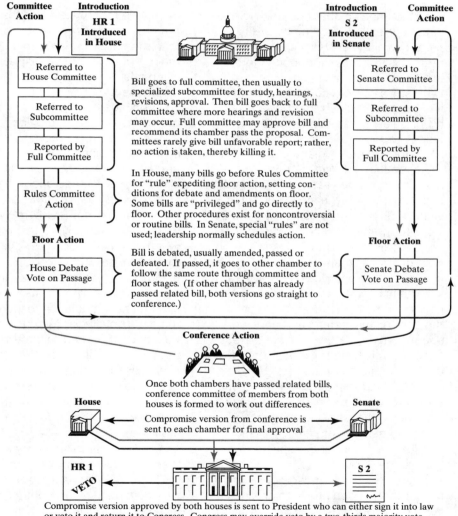

Figure 5–1.   How a Bill Becomes a Law

DENTAL HYGIENIST'S SPOTLIGHT
A Day in the Life of Wendy Bachman, RDH, BS

I started thinking about dental hygiene in the correctional setting before I started hygiene school. While taking my prerequisites, I was introduced to the health services administrator at the Western New Mexico Correctional Facility. When I explained that I was taking his class as a prerequisite for dental hygiene school, he encouraged me to apply for a dental hygiene position with the corrections department when I had my license. Three years later I called him and I have been working in corrections since 1996. I provide dental hygiene services for both male and female inmates.

Initially the dental hygiene position with the department of corrections was only ten hours per week so I also worked in private practice. I didn't anticipate how much I would enjoy working in the correctional setting and now work about thirty hours per week in corrections and still keep my foot in the private door six hours per week.

Working as a dental hygienist in the correctional setting is rewarding for me. The relationship I have with my supervising dentist is that of a colleague. He trusts my skills and respects my knowledge. I didn't know it could be so enjoyable working with someone and not for them. I don't have to produce a certain amount of money per day and he doesn't write my paycheck. This arrangement does not mean that I am unac-countable for my time, but that I have the time each patient requires rather than the obligatory sixty-minute appointment. We have mutual respect for our given talents, which allows the patient to receive the best level of care.

Because of the way the dental and medical services are provided to inmates, dental and medical staff work as an interdisciplinary team to help the patient/inmate achieve health. In hygiene school we all learned about the relationship between the patients' oral health and overall health. However, when you work in an interdisciplinary setting where you have access to the patients' medical history, physical, and complete blood count, you begin to appreciate the connection between systemic disease and oral health. It is my responsibility as the dental hygienist to educate the patient and other medical providers about periodontal health and how it relates to overall health. I find that most of my patients are extremely appreciative of the time I spend in patient education. In fact my patients in the correctional setting are much more appreciative of my time and willingness to share my knowledge than my private practice patients.

The level of appreciation I receive may be because I attempt to treat those incarcerated patients just as I would patients in private practice. I strive to pro-
(continued)

Dental Hygienist's Spotlight   *(continued)*

vide each patient with the best care that I can deliver regardless of the practice setting. I believe that my success in corrections has come from the fact that I treat those incarcerated patients as human beings first. It doesn't mean that I extend favors to them, but that I treat them within the standard of care for corrections and I do it in a respectful manner. Mom was right, treat people how you would like them to treat you.

As with any career you take the good with some bad. The bad in corrections is that the medical department still receives the lion's share of the budget. When money is tight, dental is asked to do more with less. More advanced medical procedures are considered the standard of care, while scaling and root planing or extraction (and oral irrigation with antimicrobials when I can fit it in the budget) are the only dental treatments for periodontal disease. As it is in many other areas, dental is still walking in medical's shadow. Often policies and procedures are written that base dental and periodontal treatment on the inmates' classification level (minimum, medium, or maximum security). Those inmates who are classified minimum security have access to fewer services than those at the medium or maximum security level regardless of the length of time that they will be incarcerated. Unfortunately, an inmate's need for dental treatment rarely follows the level of classification or the policy and procedure manual.

political compromise between legislators. If both houses fail to pass the bill, the bill will not become a law. If both houses pass the bill, it is necessary for the governor to sign it into law, or if the governor vetoes the bill, both houses may override the veto by a two-thirds majority vote.

STATE DENTAL BOARDS

State dental boards generally govern dental hygienists, although New Mexico and Iowa have dental hygiene committees that work with the board to effectively govern dental hygienists, and several other states have dental hygiene advisory committees. Interestingly, not all states have state dental boards. State dental boards generally consist of several dentists, one or two dental hygienists, and one or two public members. Because of the fact that no state dental boards have an equal number of dentists and dental hygienists on the board, the dentists on the board are basically governing dental hygienists in the state with no chance for a true voice for dental hygienists. The board is usually responsible for developing rules and regulations to interpret or further define the practice act, as well as granting and suspending or revoking licenses. This can become very limiting for dental hygienists, because the majority board members are dentists who can literally interpret the law to limit the practice of dental hygiene while increasing the functions that other on-the-job trained dental personnel can provide. Unfortunately, in many instances, the profession of dental hygiene has no power to affect their own practice, while dentists who have limited education in dental hygiene science make decisions regarding the practice of this science.

Table 5–4 includes states with individual dental hygiene committees. State dental boards are composed primarily of dentists, who are responsible for regulating dentistry and dental hygiene. Self-regulation of dental hygienists means that state governments turn to members of the dental hygiene profession for advice and assistance in carrying out the practice act. The basic guides for regulation for each profession are found in its practice act.

A rule is a statement of general applicability that implements, interprets law, or defines the practice and procedure requirements of an agency of a state government. Thus, a rule establishes a requirement, sets a standard, establishes a fee or rate, provides a set procedure, sets forth how a law will be implemented, gives guidance for

Table 5–4.   State Dental Hygiene Committees

Arizona	Advisory committee to the dental board
California	Administrative committee of the dental board
Delaware	Advisory committee to the dental board
Florida	Advisory committee to the dental board
Iowa	Self-regulating committee
Maryland	Committee of the dental board
Missouri	Advisory Committee to the dental board
New Mexico	Self-regulating committee
Oregon	Advisory Committee to the dental board. Appointed by the board president.
Texas	Advisory committee to the dental board
Washington	Committee to advise director of health department on dental hygiene rules and discipline

Note: In most instances, dental hygiene committees are advisory in nature and do not have rule-making powers. Committee members are usually not members of the regulatory (dental) board. Maryland, where committee members are also members of the dental board; New Mexico, where the committee has complete authority for the regulation of dental hygiene; and Washington, whose examination committee is separate from the dental board are the exceptions to state dental hygiene committees.
Source: www.adha.org.

compliance with law, describes the structure of an organization, or instructs members of the public how they must deal with or practice before any agency. Further, mandatory rules are those required by statute to promulgate. The rule-making process is ongoing, and state dental boards may promulgate rules at any time provided that they follow the provision of the law regulating that process found in the state's administrative procedures. A rule can be changed by the board initiating the rule-making process or by a person petitioning the board to promulgate, amend, or repeal a rule.

SUPERVISION OF DENTAL HYGIENISTS

All states have supervision requirements, meaning that dentists supervise dental hygienists. In fourteen states, dental hygienists may provide services in certain settings under various forms of unsupervised practice. Moreover, in nine states dental hygienists may enroll as Medicaid providers, thus billing and collecting for services rendered.

Table 5–5 defines the different types of supervisions of dental hygienists. Supervision is a major problem with respect to the utilization of the dental hygienists.

Table 5–5. Supervision of Dental Hygienists	
Type of Supervision	**Generally Accepted Definitions**
Unsupervised, Independent, Collaborative Practice	Dental hygiene practice without any supervision required from a dentist. Dental referral is necessary. In many states, a dental hygienist may practice only in certain public health settings.
General Supervision	The practice of dental hygiene without the "physically present" supervision of a dentist. The patients must be a patient of record of a dentist. Many states have additional stipulations such as the patient must have had an exam 30 days prior to or 30 days after dental hygiene treatment.
Indirect Supervision	During dental hygiene treatment, the dentist must be in the facility.
Direct Supervision	During dental hygiene treatment, the dentist must be in the facility. Sometimes, this is further prohibitive by requiring the dentist to be in the treatment operatory.

Supervision restricts the practice of dental hygiene usually to dental offices, and decreases the effectiveness of public health efforts.[3]

SUMMARY

Power is responsibility; it is service, not privilege. Its exercise is morally justifiable when it is used for the good of all, when it is sensitive to the needs of the poor and defenseless.[4] The organizations of dental hygiene continually strive to increase access to dental hygiene care. In fact, in order to effectively prevent dental diseases it is necessary for dental hygienists to become empowered in the political process and to be the voice for the underserved populations who currently face barriers to care.

REFERENCES

[1]American Dental Association House of Delegates Resolutions, 139th Annual Session, 1998.

[2]Nathe, C., and B. Posler. Collaborative practice: A form of independence. *RDH* 20 (1999): 16–19.

[3]Much of the information on government and laws was taken from and can be found in a curriculum module, *The Dental Hygienist as Change Agent.* Chicago: American Dental Hygienists' Association, 1992.

[4]Pope John Paul II. *An Invitation to Joy.* New York: Simon & Schuster, 1999.

Get Connected

Multimedia Extension Activities

www.prenhall.com/nathe

Use the above address to access the free, interactive companion web site created specifically to accompany this textbook. Here you will find an array of self study material to help you gain a richer understanding of the concepts presented in this chapter.

Unit II

DENTAL HYGIENE PUBLIC HEALTH PROGRAMS

Dental hygienists practicing in public health settings strive to attain oral health within a given population. As in private practice, one of the most important roles of the dental hygienist is to motivate patients to change values and to influence behaviors aimed at attaining oral health. When dental hygienists treat a target population, the most effective vehicle to improve health is through group education.

As previously discussed, it is vital for the dental hygienist to be able to educate patients in an individualized manner in private practice and to be able to provide that same education in a group presentation style. For example, dental hygienists practicing in a prison strive to improve the oral health of the inmates they treat. Dental hygienists consulting for a head start program would focus on attaining oral health of the children in this setting. Therefore, it is important for dental hygienists to understand the differences between various populations and how to effectively promote oral health.

Chapter 6

DENTAL HEALTH EDUCATION
AND PROMOTION

OBJECTIVES

After studying this chapter, the dental hygiene student will be able to:

- define dental health education and promotion.
- describe health education and promotion principles.
- outline the different learning and motivation theories.
- describe how a dental hygienist could best educate a population.

COMPETENCIES

After studying this chapter and participating in accompanying course activities, the dental hygiene student should be competent in the following:

- provide health education and preventive counseling.
- promote the values of oral and general health and wellness to the public and organization within and outside the profession.
- be able to include consumer groups, businesses, and government agencies to support health care issues.
- use screening, referral, and education to bring consumers into the health care delivery systems.

KEY WORDS

Behavior change	Health promotion
Habit	Values
Health education	

www.prenhall.com/nathe

INTRODUCTION

Dental hygienists frequently are asked to present information to groups of individuals regarding dental health education (Figure 6–1). Generally, these groups have underlying similarities and are referred to as target groups, which are discussed in Chapter 8. Although fundamental differences come into play when educating a group of individuals as opposed to an individual patient, many of the concepts are similar.

Dental health education provided to groups of individuals can be a more effective, productive, and inexpensive way to provide preventive dental care to the population. For these reasons, all dental hygienists need to be skilled in providing presentations to the community. This chapter focuses on dental health education and learning principles.

HEALTH EDUCATION

Principles

Historically, theorists postulated that health is a quality of life that includes physical, mental and emotional, and family and social health. The wellness scale defines a state of illness and death leading to completely healthy functioning individual

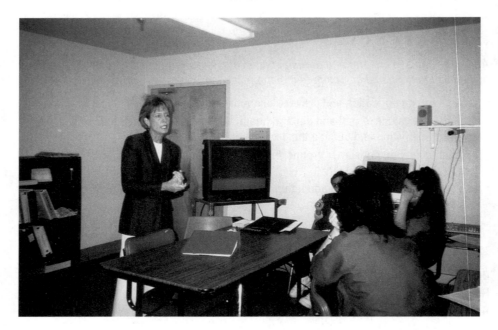

Figure 6–1. A Dental Hygienist Providing a Dental Health Presentation to School Nurses

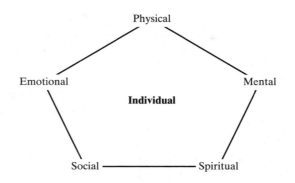

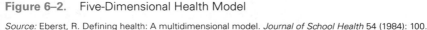

Figure 6–2.   Five-Dimensional Health Model

Source: Eberst, R. Defining health: A multidimensional model. *Journal of School Health* 54 (1984): 100.

with areas in between for quality of life indicators. Further, it has been accepted that the individual is a multidimensional being that consists of five dimensions. In this model the dimensions of health include physical, mental, and social, and adds spiritual and emotional aspects to the past model (Figure 6–2). It is helpful to look at the five dimensions as need systems, each needing specific input from the environment for complete development of the total individual. Listed in Table 6–1 are the five dimensions with corresponding input. Those specific characteristics of input refer to phenomena that feed each dimension in positive terms. Basically, if a

Table 6–1. Five-Dimensional Health Model		
Dimensions	**Positive Input**	**Negative Input**
Physical	Food, Toothbrush, Floss	Poor Nutrition, Inadequate Dental Care
Emotional	Trust	Mistrust, Fear of Dental Provider
Mental	Knowledge	Ignorance
Social	Interaction with People	Withdrawn, Inadequate Communication Skills
Spiritual	Values, Morality	No Morality, No Value Given to Dental Health

Source: Eberst, R. Defining health: A multidimensional model. *Journal of School Health* 54 (1984): 100.

given dimension receives an adequate amount of the necessary input, that dimension will theoretically have maximum potential for efficient function; conversely, if negative input is given, a detriment to health may develop.

Fortunately society has placed a never-before-seen emphasis on wellness and prevention, two concepts synonymous with contemporary dental hygiene practice. Because of these self-help trends, the dental hygienist's role in dental disease prevention and education is assuming more value to the public than ever before. Self-wellness is a concept that is extremely popular in the United States and focuses on living a healthy lifestyle and taking responsibility for one's health. A health behavior can be defined as an action that helps prevent illness and promotes health for the individual or population.

Health education can be defined as the teaching of health behaviors that bring an individual to a state of health awareness. **Health promotion** is the informing and motivating of people to adopt health behaviors.[1] Health promotion is similar to health education, but is more useful in making people aware of healthy ideas and concepts. In contrast, the intention of health education is to actually have the learner gain accurate knowledge about health behaviors and lifestyles. Both promotion and education are methods utilized to modify detrimental behaviors and promote self-wellness concepts. Although it is important to realize that the dental hygienist may provide an effective dental health presentation and the individuals may understand the presented health information, it does not necessarily mean that dental health behaviors will be practiced.

One example of a dental health promotional activity would be for the local dental hygiene association to work on banning sugary snacks and beverages from the vending machines in all elementary schools, middle schools, and high schools in the district. This promotional activity is not designed to be measurable by decreasing caries. However, it is designed to promote awareness for the need to decrease consumption of sugary snacks. If the local dental hygiene association actually held classes for the middle school teachers on dental health prevention modalities and the teachers passed a test that qualified them to teach dental health to students, the dental hygiene association would have accomplished a dental health educational activity.

DENTAL HEALTH EDUCATION PRINCIPLES

The primary goal of dental health education is the prevention of disease utilizing appropriate dental health interventions. Dental health education is a planned activity that utilizes the populations' knowledge, attitudes, culture, and values to promote oral health practices.[2]

Moreover, dental health education as a theory suggests that although a person may be educated on a particular health behavior, it is not until that person changes the behavior that it will impact dental health. Therefore, it is necessary to

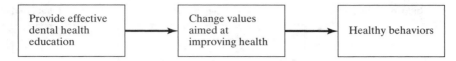

Figure 6–3. Goals of Dental Health Education

change the person's values regarding the behavior before behavior is changed. **Values** are the aspects that give meaning to our lives. They may have been derived early in life from our parents, grandparents, older siblings, teachers, or other influential people from whom we seek love and acceptance.[3] Figure 6–3 displays the steps necessary in changing behavior. Many students would now want to know how to change values of a patient with poor oral hygiene practices, which is the more difficult area. Obviously, if dental hygienists could change values that the population holds toward dental health, the population's suffering from dental diseases would dramatically decrease or possibly cease to exist. Unfortunately, changing values is a bit of a challenge. The following proposed theories will lend ideas on possible methods to utilize when changing values.

Psychology and education are related in terms of dental health. The successful use of any of these measures requires the interaction of dental hygienists and patients to achieve and maintain a maximum level of dental health. Three major factors are necessary for both parties to achieve this rapport: information, motivation, and psychomotor skills. It is necessary to consider the interrelationships of education, motivation, human values, socioeconomic needs, and behavioral modification to effectively change oral health behaviors.[4]

The dental hygiene student is aware that education is the basis for any dental hygiene treatment. In particular, dental health education is based largely on the scientific principles of psychology and sociology that facilitate learning and behavioral change in the individual.[5] In fact, the Health Belief Model found in Figure 6–4 suggests that for an individual to display a readiness to take action to avoid a disease or act in preventive manner, that individual would need to believe that he or she was susceptible or vulnerable, that the disease has serious consequences, that the behavior was beneficial, and lastly that it was important.[6] Basically, this theory is based on the premise that when individuals have accurate information they will make better health choices. In fact, the health belief model is used by the U.S. Public Health Service as a model for health interventions.

Table 6–2 depicts the Health Belief Model in relation to dental hygiene.

STAGES OF LEARNING

It is important to understand the increments in which a person actually learns information that is presented. The learning ladder in Figure 6–5 depicts an individual's natural progression from knowledge absorption to value adoption. This ladder

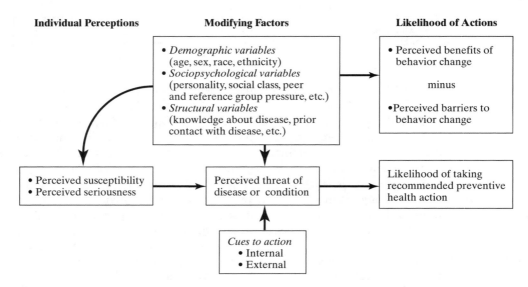

Figure 6–4. Health Belief Model

Source: Adapted with permission from Becker, M. H. *The Health Belief Model and Personal Health Behavior.* Thorofare, NJ: Charles B. Slack, 1974.

Table 6–2. Example of Health Belief Model in Dental Hygiene Practice	
1. Susceptibility	Individual believes that they are susceptible to oral cancer because they chew tobacco
2. Serious Consequences	Individual believes that oral cancer can be disfiguring and fatal
3. Beneficial	Individual believes that in order to decrease the risk of disfigurement, illness, and possibly death it would be beneficial to stop chewing
4. Salience	Individual makes the cessation of chewing tobacco top priority in life, and stops the practice

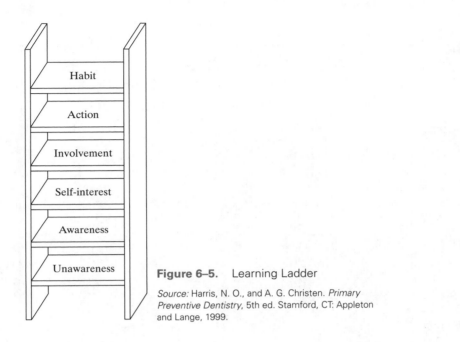

Figure 6–5. Learning Ladder

Source: Harris, N. O., and A. G. Christen. *Primary Preventive Dentistry*, 5th ed. Stamford, CT: Appleton and Lange, 1999.

has six rungs that begin with total lack of awareness of the topic and extend up to habit formation. The bottom increment is unawareness and is followed by awareness, which is the education provided by the health care worker. The person then enters the self-interest stage, which is characterized by a recognition of desire and involvement. The next stage is involvement in which the patient becomes involved in the learning process and that is followed by action and **habit.**

TRANSTHEORETICAL MODEL

The transtheorectical model is similar to the stages of learning and includes five stages of change that an individual must process. These changes are precontemplation, contemplation, preparation, maintenance, and action. The precontemplation stage has no intention to take action within the next six months, where preparation intends to take action within the next thirty days. When an individual takes action, it is followed by maintenance and can be thought of as termination when the overt behavior never relapses. An example of this theory could be as simple as an individual precontemplating daily flossing, starting to contemplate flossing every day, and finally taking action and flossing daily.

DENTAL HYGIENIST'S SPOTLIGHT
A Day in the Life of Mary Webb,
Student Dental Hygienist, United Kingdom

During the education of a dental hygienist, the students not only study all aspects of dental hygiene but are also required to study for the Certificate in Oral Health Promotion (OHP), which is an additional qualification to that of the diploma in dental hygiene.

Emphasis is placed on social psychology and behavior patterns of the individuals, as well as inequalities in health and barriers to dental health care.

As a senior student, I visit a day care center for people with disabilities. Many of the clients have arthritis or have suffered strokes or were born with disabilities. Clients have problems managing their own dental care and need a lot of support and custom-designed programs.

Part of my Certificate in OHP was to gain teaching practice, both in the practical aspects and also in presentation for my target group. Following discussion with the Community Dental Services in the area, I contacted the day care center. (The CDS are responsible for OHP in an area known as the Local Health Authority.)

I researched my clients' needs and made appropriate visual aids so that it would not only make my presentation interesting, but it would also help clients find the most suitable way of maintaining their own oral health.

A number of clients had problems using their hands and I made acrylic handles to insert standard toothbrushes and made use of soft rubber balls in which the toothbrush handles were pushed. I took along enlarged photographs of healthy and unhealthy

(continued)

Dental Hygienist's Spotlight   *(continued)*

mouths to show clients how plaque forms on teeth and the consequences of not removing it. For the elderly clients attending the day center, I made a photo montage to stimulate discussion about their dental needs.

A demonstration of toothbrushing techniques, using a volunteer, to the caretakers of the center was followed by a question-and-answer session with both clients and caretakers.

The CDS will continue to monitor and support the center, and I shall return to reinforce the dental health message that I left with them.

THEORY OF REASONED ACTION

The theory of reasoned action focuses on the belief that people make rational decisions based on intent. A person's behavior intent is a combination of knowledge, values, and attitudes. Therefore, a person's intent to perform a certain action is the most immediate and relevant predictor that the person will indeed carryout that action. The following excerpt is an example of the theory of reasoned action.

Example: Behavior/Cessation

Attitude toward the Behavior: "You know what? I think, smoking is dangerous for my health."

Subjective Norms: "I wonder if my wife would like me to quit smoking."

Perceived Behavioral Control: "I can quit smoking, even if I'm hooked on cigarettes!"

Intention: "I want to quit smoking right now!"

Behavior: "As you can see, I am not smoking anymore. Instead of taking a cigarette, when I get the cravings, I crumble paper now."[7]

SOCIAL COGNITIVE THEORY

The social cognitive theory—also known as the self-efficacy theory—postulates that knowledge, behavior, and environment act in a reciprocal manner to continually affect each other.[8] See Figure 6–6. The sources of self-efficacy include enactive attainment, vicarious learning, verbal persuasion, and affective status. This theory reinforces the belief that social pressure is the most powerful factor in influencing

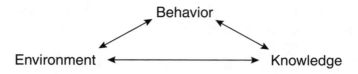

Figure 6–6.　Social Cognitive Theory

social norms. Basically, this theory emphasizes the power social leaders have in influencing our values and behaviors. One example of an application of this model would be the celebrity "Got Milk?" promotional advertisements.

EMPOWERMENT MODELS

The empowerment models are participant oriented, and social environments are considered to be important prerequisites for health education. Empowerment models have become more common in recent years and are practiced routinely by dental hygienists when instructing patients on brushing and flossing as patients become active learners during demonstration of skills. Empowerment models emphasize provider and patient working collaboratively toward treatment.

MOTIVATION

Motivation is definitely an important factor in learning. Motivation defined is the will of the individual to act. It is actually a drive that propels the individual to satisfy a need.[9] Remember the individual must be aware of the needs before motivation can occur.

Motivational models generally pinpoint the following considerations that need to be present for values to change. Individuals initiating a change need to be aware of their own values and must understand and know the patient's values and needs. It is important not to push the provider's values upon the patient, and it is important to determine what motivates the patient and understand the prior knowledge of dental care.

In fact, it is necessary to motivate a population in order to effectively promote value adoption and **behavior change.** Major factors that substantially impact the learner are listed in Table 6–3. Obviously a need must exist, or education and behavior changes would not be mandated. Attitudes are powerful influences on human behavior and learning because they help people make sense of life. Stimulation is an experience that makes us active, where affect is a major motivational fact pertaining to the emotion of the learner. Competence occurs when an individual gains control over his or her environment.[10]

Table 6–3.   Factors Influencing Motivation
Need
Attitude
Stimulation
Competence

Source: Chopoorian, K. How adults learn: The dental hygienist as an educator. *Dental Hygienist News* 9 (1996): 3–6.

The self-determination theory is a macrotheory of human motivation concerned with the functioning of personality within social contexts. This theory emphasizes the degree to which human behaviors are self-determined. Basically, this theory is based on the assumption that an individual makes his or her own choice when determining when to adopt dental healthy behaviors.

Maslow's Hierarchy of Needs

Many dental hygiene students are familiar with Maslow's Hierarchy of Needs—presented in Figure 6–7—and it is one theory that is advantageous for the dental hygienist to keep in mind. These levels are arranged in lower to higher level needs to represent the levels one must attain before full potential has been reached. Maslow theorized that when the needs at one level are met, then needs of higher levels can be addressed subsequently, in a linear, stairstep approach. In this hierarchy, the more advanced needs will not appear until lower needs have been acknowledged and addressed. In addition, when lower needs such as hunger reappear, all higher needs momentarily vanish.[11] Adapting this theory to dental

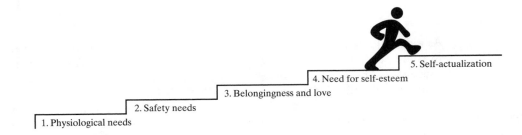

5. Self-actualization
4. Need for self-esteem
3. Belongingness and love
2. Safety needs
1. Physiological needs

Figure 6–7.   Maslow's Hierarchy of Needs

Source: Maslow, A. H. *Motivation and Personality*, 3d ed. New York: Harper and Row, 1987.

health, one can assume that when an individual has not met basic needs (such as living with a toothache), the next level of the need's hierarchy cannot be attained.

BEHAVIOR MODIFICATION

In order to change behaviors, it takes more than education; therefore, it is important to discuss behavior modification. In fact, most of us at one time or another have considered some form of action for change, usually for self-wellness. Many may have started exercising or dieting at the beginning of the year or before an important event, and many may have promised themselves to get more sleep or stop smoking, but all of us at some time or another have thought about changing for the betterment of our health.

Psychologists have theorized that behavior modification is accomplished by classical conditioning, operant conditioning, or modeling. Classical conditioning, described by Ivan Pavlov in the late 1920s, suggests that animals become conditioned to specific stimuli to act in a specific way. Theoretically, if a patient receives commendation for good oral hygiene at an appointment, that patient will be more likely to maintain good home care so that the dental hygienist will provide praise at subsequent appointments. Operant conditioning, described by Skinner, is based on the concepts of rewards and punishments in which good behavior is reinforced and bad behavior is disciplined. This concept suggests that if a pediatric patient receives dental treats following good behavior at the dental hygienist's office, good behavior is being reinforced, whereas if a pediatric patient exhibits bad behavior at the dental hygienist's office and is disciplined by the parents, bad behavior may not continue at subsequent appointments. Modeling behavior can facilitate learning through imitation. For example, if a child is present when the older sibling, who after exhibiting good behavior is being treated, that child may show good behavior through imitation. The behavior modification model suggests that it is necessary to travel through different stages in order to have behavior changed. It is important to note that all of these theories suggest that behaviors can indeed be changed.[11]

SUMMARY

As a dental hygienist, it is necessary to be able to conduct an effective presentation to successfully transform knowledge into positive behaviors. The key word here is successful. The goal of a presentation should be ultimately to instill the value of dental health and thus change the individual's behavior.

Remember, as a dental health educator, it is important to realize that education involves much more than simply relaying information. Effective dental health education should ultimately provide positive values toward dental health and affect behavior changes. Therefore, it is necessary to fully understand the knowledge level of the population and have some background in order to be aware of the values of the population and the individuals within the population. In addition, the educator must be aware of personal values and make sure to work in a positive manner to improve the dental health of the population.

REFERENCES

[1]Meeks-Mitchell, L., and P. Heit. *Health: A Wellness Approach.* Columbus, OH: Merrill Publishing, 1987, p. 6.

[2]DeBiase, C. B. *Dental Health Education Theory and Practice.* Philadelphia: Lea & Febiger, 1991, pp. 9–11.

[3]Seaward, B. L. *Managing Stress Principles and Strategies for Health and Well-Being.* Sudbury, MA: Jones and Barlett, 1999, pp. 83–90, 181–90.

[4]Becker, M. H. *The Health Belief Model and Personal Health Behavior.* Thorofare, NJ: Charles B. Slack, 1974.

[5]DeBiase, C. B. *Dental Health Education Theory and Practice.* Philadelphia: Lea & Febriger, 1991.

[6]Harris, N. O., and F. Garcia-Godoy. *Primary Preventive Dentistry,* 5th ed. Stamford, CT: Appleton and Lange, 1999.

[7]DeBiase, C. B. *Dental Health Education Theory and Practice.* Philadelphia: Lea & Febriger, 1991.

[8]http://hsc.usf.edu/~kmbrown/TRA_TPB.htm.

[9]Chopoorian, K. How adults learn: The dental hygienist as an educator. *Dental Hygienist News* 9 (1996): 3–6.

[10]Maslow, A. H. *Motivation and Personality,* 3d ed. New York: Harper & Row, 1987.

[11]Seaward, B. L. *Managing Stress Principles and Strategies for Health and Well-Being.* Sudbury, MA: Jones and Bartlett, 1999, pp. 83–90, 181–90.

Get Connected

Multimedia Extension Activities

 www.prenhall.com/nathe

Use the above address to access the free, interactive companion web site created specifically to accompany this textbook. Here you will find an array of self study material to help you gain a richer understanding of the concepts presented in this chapter.

Chapter 7

LESSON PLAN DEVELOPMENT

OBJECTIVES

After studying this chapter, the dental hygiene student will be able to:

- describe the process of lesson plan development.
- list and describe teaching strategies.
- list the characteristics of an effective teacher.
- develop a lesson plan.

COMPETENCIES

After studying this chapter and participating in accompanying course activities, the dental hygiene student should be competent in the following:

- provide health education and preventive counseling.
- promote the values of oral and general health and wellness to the public and organization within and outside the profession.
- be able to include consumer groups, businesses, and government agencies to support health care issues.

KEY WORDS

Dental hygiene process of care
Lesson plan
Organization

Preparation
Teaching strategies

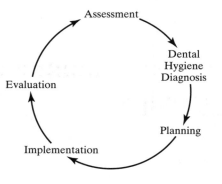

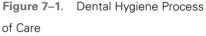

Figure 7–1. Dental Hygiene Process of Care

INTRODUCTION

Planning an effective presentation of dental hygiene principles to a target group involves the **dental hygiene process of care.** Utilizing this process, depicted in Figure 7–1, will enable the dental hygienist to follow logical steps in the development of an effective lesson. Figure 7–2 shows a dental hygienist who was asked to present dental health information to a parents' advisory board from a local Early Head Start Program. Notice the importance placed on planning the presentation. Although this dental hygienist (Figure 7–3) frequently educates her patients on the importance of infant oral health care, it is necessary to actually spend time planning when presenting to a group of individuals.

The best way to make sure that the presentation will be effective and successful is for the dental hygienist to be prepared. Moreover, **preparation** and **organization** decreases the initial nervousness some dental hygienists feel when being asked to present to a group. Use of the steps involved in the dental hygiene process of care, as outlined in Table 7–1, can assure an effective lesson plan and aid in an effective presentation.

ASSESSMENT PHASE

During the assessment phase, the target population's needs, interests, and resources should be defined. Many times a long-term care facility will contact dental hygienists to present dental health information to their nurse's aides. Before the planning phase begins, it is necessary for the dental hygienist to assess the population. If this stage is skipped, the presentation may not be pertinent to the target population. Remember, it is important to never assume things about a target population. In fact, for example, the dental hygienist does not effectively assess this population and decides to discuss periodontal diseases based on a population where

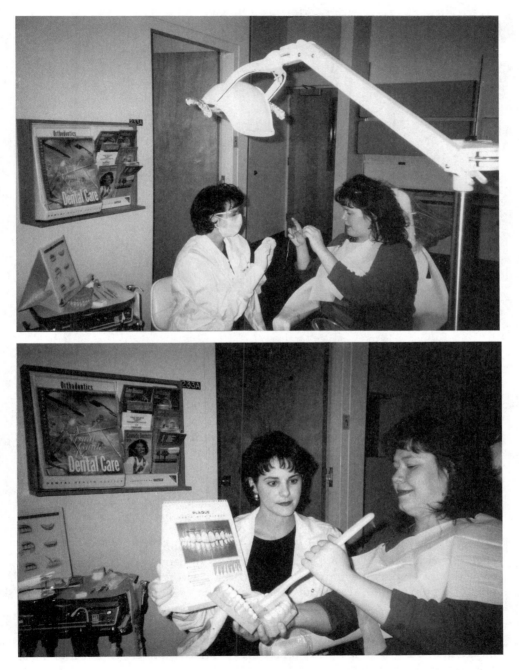

Figure 7–2. Dental hygienist providing patient education to a mother concerning her infant's home care regimen during a routine dental hygiene appointment.

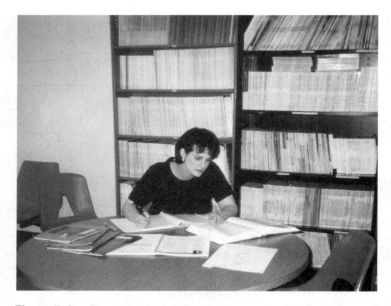

Figure 7–3. Dental hygienist planning a presentation for a group of 20 women with infants ranging from 2 to 8 months. The women are enrolled in the local WIC program.

more than 90 percent of this population has a periodontal disease. However, this facility is having difficulties with dentures. In particular, they are losing many dentures and have trouble keeping them clean. So actually, what they are interested in is information on denture identification and denture care. The target group may leave the presentation feeling disappointed that their specific needs were addressed only when they were able to ask questions during the last three minutes. How could this situation have been avoided? The dental hygienist could have avoided it by talking with a nurse's aide on the group's particular needs, interests, and abilities. Further, the dental hygienist would have been better prepared to answer questions.

Moreover, assessment includes defining the group's level of dental knowledge. Many target populations have similar levels of dental health knowledge, but some do not. And although many times dental knowledge is assessed at the beginning of a presentation, researching before the presentation is an excellent way to plan a knowledge-level appropriate presentation. Discussing the topics with the contact person is one way to assess the population and providing a brief survey to the group prior to the presentation would be one other assessment method. Also questioning the group about the topics they would be interested in learning can help in narrowing the topics.

Table 7–1.   Lesson Plan Development

Assessment
• Assess target populations' needs, interests, and abilities
• Assess resources

Dental Hygiene Diagnosis
• Formulate findings from assessment
• Prioritize goals

Planning
• Broad goal formulation
• Specific objectives
• Select teaching method(s)

Implementation
• Be prepared
• Effective teacher characteristics

Evaluation
• Qualitative measurement
• Quantitative measurement
• Information provided to appropriate parties

DENTAL HYGIENE DIAGNOSIS

Formulating a dental hygiene diagnosis cannot be accomplished unless a thorough assessment of the population has been conducted. When diagnosing a group, it is not important that the dental hygienist talk with each member of the group, but that a consensus is drawn after speaking to one or two contacts about the group's particular needs, interests, and capabilities. Specifically, dental hygiene diagnosis requires analysis of the data to identify dental needs that can be fulfilled through dental hygiene education.

One example of a dental hygiene case with corresponding diagnosis is as follows. Before giving a presentation to a support group for patients with diabetes, the dental hygienist contacted the group leader and staff nurse regarding the needs, interests, and capabilities of this group. The dental hygienist was told that many members complained of bleeding and sore gums and the desire to learn more about gum disease associated with diabetes. The dental hygiene diagnosis could be described as periodontal diseases associated with diabetes.

PLANNING

During the planning stages, it is necessary to develop a presentation goal and several objectives. This activity will help the hygienist define the actual information that needs to be presented to the group and how to effectively present this information.

After assessing and developing a dental hygiene diagnosis regarding a group, it is necessary to prioritize the groups' particular needs. One example may be that a parent teacher association (PTA) has asked the dental hygienist to come to their meeting to discuss dental care for fifteen minutes. After further questioning it was noted that the primary difficulties that the PTA group had were access to dental care for families with Medicaid insurance, motivating their children to brush, and helping parents with quick and easy nutritional food choices. In addition, some parents were interested in learning more about periodontal surgery, implants, and bleaching. When prioritizing, it is important to realize that in fifteen minutes an instructor would be unable to deliver comprehensive dental health education on all of the preceding topics. Therefore, it is necessary to prioritize the most beneficial and important topics for inclusion in the **lesson plan.**

Goals

The first step in planning a lesson would be to write the goal. A goal is a broad statement that reflects the final outcome that the instructor expects from the target group by the time the presentation is finished.[1] It is important to write only one or two broad goals that you expect the group to accomplish. After setting the overall goal, the instructor must remember that the more specific objectives will be defined in a more detailed manner.

Objectives

Writing objectives allows the dental hygienist to plan in detail the information that will be presented and discussed. An objective always includes a specific, observable action/behavior that the learner is to perform or exhibit.[2] Many times objectives include an audience, condition, and measurement. The audience to whom the objective is intended is defined. The condition, which entails relevant factors affecting the actual performance, is defined. An example of a condition would be following the presentation. The level of achievement is referred to as the measurement. The measurement describes acceptable performance. An example of an objective is as follows. Following the presentation, the physician's assistants will be able to describe the dental caries process in compliance with the presented information.

When writing an objective, it is important to be aware of three learning domains.[3] These domains are presented in Table 7–2. The first domain is the psychomotor domain, which describes actions. The behaviors in the psychomotor domain are the easiest to label with precise verbs when writing objectives. An example of an objective written for the psychomotor domain would be following the dental health presentation, the nurse's aides will be able to clean dentures effectively. These behaviors are concrete and observable, and the verbs that refer to them directly denote a neurophysical activity. Please see Table 7–3 for the verbs in the psychomotor domain.

The cognitive domain represents intellectual skills. Although the verbs used to describe behavior in this domain (presented in Table 7–4) may be slightly more abstract than verbs used in the psychomotor domain, the skills in this domain are not really difficult to translate into relatively precise verbs. An example of an objective in this domain is as follows: following the presentation, the first-grade school-children will identify three healthy snacks from the chart.

Finally, the domain that includes feelings, attitudes, values, and interests is referred to as the affective domain. See Table 7–5 for verbs used in this domain. Although this domain can be measured by qualitative assessment, the affective domain is not directly observable and not as easily measured as the behaviors in the other two domains. Yet, for those in the dental hygiene profession, the affective domain is extremely important. An example for this domain would be following completion of the current issues course, the dental hygienist will be able to defend,

Table 7–2.   Domains of Learning

Psychomotor	To describe actions
Cognitive	To describe behavior
Affective	To describe feelings

Levels of Learning

Knowledge	To know
Application	To apply
Problem solving	To problem solve

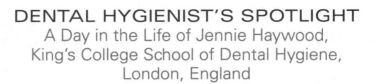

DENTAL HYGIENIST'S SPOTLIGHT
A Day in the Life of Jennie Haywood, King's College School of Dental Hygiene, London, England

After being asked to visit an infant/junior school and talk to young children between six and eight years of age, I planned how I was going to approach the session. I love working with children and making things, and I devised two papier-mâché heads; one showing "good" teeth and the other showing "bad" teeth. Basi- cally, they were two hollow balls and after talking about healthy foods the children were invited to "post" a selection of food pictures in their heads. The children had to decide which was a healthy food and which was an unhealthy snack. It was great fun and we all enjoyed the game. It also prompted a lot of questions from the children.

Display boards explained about sugars and tooth decay. We had a detective game on the boards. It consisted of a label from a selection of foods and a magnifying glass to look at the tiny list of ingredients printed on the empty packet of snacks and drinks. The children were surprised at the high levels of sugars found even in savory snacks.

A colleague also took another

(continued)

Dental Hygienist's Spotlight   (continued)

class, and we combined the classes and their teachers at the end of our sessions. We talked to the children and answered any questions they might have. The teachers chipped in too and were amazed at the ways in which sugar gets added to processed foods and drinks without them knowing. The teachers' evaluations of the sessions were positive and I hope to return in six months to evaluate the retention of the dental health messages I gave.

in writing, the dental hygienist's role in consumer advocacy with a passing grade. Table 7–6 includes verbs that are open to interpretation; therefore, these verbs are not a good choice when writing objectives.

Moreover, different levels of learning would include the knowledge level, application level, and problem-solving level (refer to Table 7–2). The knowledge level is the lowest level and simply implies that knowledge is gained. Applying the knowledge that was gained is the definition of the application level, and actually being able to solve a problem implies that the learner has mastered the problem-solving level. Understanding the domains and levels of learning will enable the dental hygienist to adequately define and plan the lesson.

Teaching Methods

Another important planning step is deciding which **teaching strategies** to use. In order to decide which method is most appropriate, or if more than one method is appropriate, the instructor will need to decide which method will promote the

Table 7–3. Verbs of the Psychomotor Domain	
brush	floss
clean	identify
detect	irrigate
disinfect	measure
demonstrate	probe
eat	screen
exercise	sterilize
experiment	

desired outcome. Further, is the method adaptable to the activities involved, and are the required resources present and feasible? Most important, the method should be interesting and motivating to the audience.

Lecture is probably the most well known and traditional method of teaching. Lecture is effective if a formal presentation of information is needed and the information is appropriate for the knowledge level. Lecturing is also effective when the intention is to create awareness of various ideas, issues, and beliefs. The drawback to using the lecture method is that the audience is not involved, thus decreasing

Table 7–4. Verbs from the Cognitive Domain	
collect	indicate
contrast	label
classify	list
compare	show
describe	recognize
diagnose	record
design	solve
explain	

Table 7–5.	Verbs from the Affective Domain
advocate	evaluate
assess	judge
believe	lead
challenge	live out
debate	persuade
defend	suggest
discuss	value
deduct	

motivation and learning. The lecture method is best used in conjunction with other methods.

Discussion involves interaction between the students and the instructor and more easily arouses interest, which helps students with reasoning abilities. Presentation is defined as employing the lecture and discussion methods in conjunction. Demonstration can be used with lecture or presentation methods when the desired outcome is learning a behavior such as brushing.

The inquiry method, sometimes referred to as problem-based learning, makes use of unfinished case studies in which the teacher acts as a facilitator and the student is responsible for gaining the correct information.[4] Group or individualized games and activities usually increase motivation and learning. Examples of games and activities

Table 7–6.	Verbs Open to Misinterpretation
appreciate	interpret
comprehend	know
empathize	like
familiarize	realize
grasp	think
have faith	understand

are CD-ROM interactive activities or puzzles, including playing dental health jeopardy as a group. Role-play and simulation activities can be utilized as a group. These methods can increase student comprehension and problem-solving skills when presenting information by affording everyone an opportunity to participate.

Educational Materials

Educational materials can add a great deal to a presentation. Visual aids help elicit excitement from the learners and contribute an organizing aspect to the lesson. Visual aids can include slides, videotapes, overhead transparencies, tooth model demos, oral hygiene aids, CD-ROMs, classroom games, puzzles, activity sheets, gloves, labcoats, masks, flipcharts, posters and books, to name a few (see Figure 7–4). On the other hand, educational materials, such as tooth models, can be a distraction if utilized improperly. Many times teachers will "pass around" the tooth model during a presentation, which can be disruptive to the learning process because the students are trying to listen to the teacher and practice the correct brushing method all at once. By planning the presentation well, effective integration of a tooth model can be accomplished.

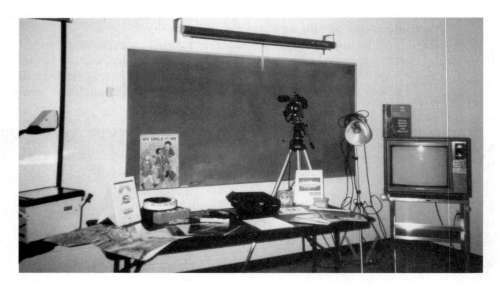

Figure 7–4. Dental health educational materials utilized in an elementary school. These materials can be used effectively as specific strategies to increase awareness of dental health basics.

An example of a lesson plan is provided in Figure 7–5. This lesson plan was prepared to teach eighth-grade students about the career of dental hygiene during a career month at school. During this month, students are preparing to register for classes in high school. More than fifty different individuals will take part during the month in providing students information about possible careers. This example can be helpful when developing a presentation.

IMPLEMENTATION

The most important criterion for implementation is to be prepared. By completing the first two phases, the dental hygienist should be well organized and feel confident regarding the presentation.

Classroom Management

An instructor who feels prepared and confident can effectively manage many different situations that may arise during the presentation (Figure 7–6). Surprisingly, managing a classroom of adults can be as important as managing children. In fact, methods involved in managing a class include being direct, enthusiastic, and organized. Notice any signals that the class is becoming uncontrolled, such as frequent talking, shuffling, or sleeping. By staying calm and conveying your enthusiasm, knowledge, and expectations, these signals can be stopped. Moreover, being well organized will increase instructor confidence and decrease the likelihood that the instructor may lose control of the class.

Characteristics of an Effective Teacher

Providing an effective presentation entails more than an effective assessment and planning phase, it actually includes motivating the students to learn and apply the information. Characteristics of an effective teacher provide light on the reasons why some teachers are more successful at initiating change than others. Communication skills are vital for an educator. Characteristics related to communication skills and most commonly associated with effective teachers are enthusiasm, flexibility, patience, and a personable manner. See Table 7–7 for a complete listing of characteristics of an effective teacher.

Being prepared is definitely the best way to increase the likelihood that the presentation will be effective. By carefully preparing the lesson, the instructor will be organized in the thinking process and should be confident in the material. Careful preparation includes gathering and organizing the information and

Figure 7–5.   Example Lesson Plan

Dental Hygiene Presentation

Audience: **24 eighth-grade schoolchildren**

Time: **15 minutes**

Goal: The goal of this presentation is to promote the career of the dental hygienist.

Objectives:

Following this presentation, the eighth-grade schoolchildren will be able to:
1. Describe the career of a dental hygienist.
2. Describe the settings in which dental hygienists work.
3. List the careers available in the dental field.

Teaching Methods:

Lecture
Discussion
Role playing

Audiovisual Aids:

Videotape on the Dental Hygiene Career (5 minutes)
Overhead transparencies
Dental Hygiene Career pamphlets

Introduction: Today we will be discussing the career of dental hygienists, their functions in dental care delivery, and other careers available in the dental field.

Rationale: It is important for eighth graders to be aware of career opportunities available, so that next year you can begin taking classes in high school that will help prepare you for college course work pertaining to the career you are interested in.

Transparencies utilized throughout underlined areas.

Dental Hygienists Defined: A dental hygienist is . . .

Educational Preparation: The University of New Mexico in Albuquerque offers a dental hygiene program in our state. All neighboring states offer dental hygiene programs in university and community college settings. Dental hygienists can receive associate, bachelor's and master's degrees in dental hygiene.

(continued)

Figure 7–5.   *(continued)*

When preparing for a dental hygiene career in high school it is good to remember that dental hygienists possess a strong background in the basic health and social sciences. Subjects that are recommended include biology, chemistry, physics, and anatomy and physiology as well as algebra, geometry, and calculus, and English and other social science courses.

Roles of the Dental Hygienists: Dental hygienists have six roles defined including manager, clinician, educator/health promotor, researcher, consumer advocate, and change agent. (Provide examples).

Practice Settings: Dental hygienists work in private dental offices, public schools, nursing homes and hospitals, military, state, and federal public health programs, dental industry, and business and research facilities. They provide oral health services through preventive, educational, diagnostic, and therapeutic sciences. In addition, many dental hygienists work as consultants.

View videotapes and answer questions concerning the videotape.

Careers Available in the Dental Field: Additional roles in the dental field include dentist, dental assistant, dental technician, and dental office manager/receptionist. (Provide examples of these careers.)

Conclusion: Today we discussed the dental hygiene career, education preparation of the dental hygienists, and other careers available in the dental field.

developing the presentation of this information. Further, effective planning should include practicing the presentation that has been developed.

Fear of Public Speaking

Many dental hygienists initially may be nervous when facing an audience. The best way to prevent this nervousness, or at least be able to make it through the presentation, is to be prepared. Practice in front of an audience, even if it is only one other person, until feeling completely confident. In addition, encourage questions from audience members; this opportunity will increase their participation and help the nervous instructor feel more confident that the audience is learning and listening.

EVALUATION

Evaluation is an ongoing process and actually is thought about in the planning phase when objectives and goals are being developed. Writing effective objectives will ensure that the dental hygienist can measure what is intended to be measured

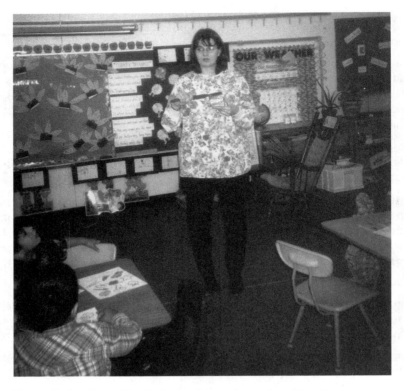

Figure 7–6. Dental hygienist implementing a dental health presentation to a group of schoolchildren.

Table 7–7.   Characteristics of Effective Teachers

Ability to interact

Enthusiastic

Flexible

Knowledgeable

Organized

Patience

Personable

Willingness to learn

and that the objective is measurable. Evaluation can also be determined by the smoothness of the presentation and audience interest and participation. Teachers should be well aware of the motivation level of the class. Remember, the more interested the students are and the more they participate, the more likely the objective will be met. Students that are motivated are more likely to adapt these effective dental health behaviors dental hygienists strive to promote.

Figure 7–7 is an example of a pretest/posttest examination for seventh-grade schoolchildren. A dental hygienist is presenting a lesson plan on the prevention of oral cancer and is planning to evaluate her lesson by utilizing a pretest/posttest evaluation. Other methods of evaluation can include games, activities, computer games and quizzes, or simply group questioning.

Moreover, it is imperative to evaluate the dental hygienist's effectiveness as an information conveyor. Figures 7–8 and 7–9 are examples of evaluation criteria for lesson plans and presentations. By working on meeting all of these evaluation criteria, the dental hygienist is increasing the chance that criteria for effective planning and presenting will be met.

Figure 7–7. Self-Evaluation Example

Oral Cancer Prevention Strategies Pretest
1. Smokeless tobacco products do less harm to oral tissues than smoking cigarettes.
   True
   False
2. Alcohol use increases the risk of oral cancer.
   True
   False
3. Regular dental hygiene examinations include oral cancer examinations.
   True
   False

Oral Cancer Prevention Strategies Posttest
1. Smokeless tobacco products do less harm to oral tissues than smoking cigarettes.
   True
   False
2. Alcohol use increases the risk of oral cancer.
   True
   False
3. Regular dental hygiene examinations include oral cancer examinations.
   True
   False

Figure 7–8. Lesson Plan Evaluation Checklist

1. Displays organized lesson plan
2. Demonstrates evidence of research of topic
3. Presents effective introduction
4. Presents lessons on level of target population's understanding
5. Presents expected behavioral objectives
6. Presents appropriate questions
7. Utilizes time efficiently
8. Develops and utilizes appropriate visual aids
9. Presents effective conclusion
10. Implements self-evaluation strategies

SUMMARY

Planning an effective lesson involves the dental hygiene process of care. The dental hygienist should thoroughly assess the target population's needs to develop an appropriate lesson. Goals and objectives should be developed to aid in presentation development with an emphasis on identifying measurable outcomes. Being prepared is the most important step in providing effective dental health education to groups.

Figure 7–9. Class Presentation Evaluation Checklist

1. Gives evidence of research of topic
2. Presents instruction on level of target audience's understanding
3. Selects appropriate teaching methods
4. Selects effective visual aids
5. Uses helpful visual aids
6. Adheres to time frame
7. Asks appropriate probing questions
8. Presents professional appearance
9. Maintains proper eye contact
10. Projects voice accordingly
11. Demonstrates a prepared, organized manner

REFERENCES

[1]Fodor, J. T., and G. T. Dalis. *Health Instruction: Theory and Application,* 4th ed. Philadelphia: Lea and Febiger, 1989; DeBiase, C. B. *Dental Health Education: Theory and Practice.* Philadelphia: Lea and Febiger, 1995; Dignan, M. B., and P. A. Carr. *Program Planning for Health Education and Health Promotion.* Philadelphia: Lea and Febiger, 1987; Smith, T. C. *Making Successful Presentations: A Self-Teaching Guide.* New York: Wiley and Sons, 1984.

[2]Gagliardi, L. *Dental Health Education: Lesson Plan and Implementation.* Stamford, CT: Appleton and Lange, 1999.

[3]Tolle, L. Dental Hygiene 400/500 Oral Health Promotion Course-Pak. Copytron, 1988.

[4]Smith, T. C. *Making Successful Presentations: A Self-Teaching Guide.* New York: Wiley and Sons, 1984.

Get Connected

Multimedia Extension Activities

 www.prenhall.com/nathe

Use the above address to access the free, interactive companion web site created specifically to accompany this textbook. Here you will find an array of self study material to help you gain a richer understanding of the concepts presented in this chapter.

Chapter 8

∙∙

TARGET POPULATIONS

OBJECTIVES

After studying this chapter, the dental hygiene student will be able to:

- define target populations to whom dental hygienists may provide services.
- describe cultural diversity.
- describe the effect culture has on dental hygiene care.
- list barriers to dental hygiene care.

COMPETENCIES

After studying this chapter and participating in accompanying course activities, the dental hygiene student should be competent in the following:

- promote the values of oral and general health and wellness to the public and organizations within and outside the profession.
- identify services that promote oral health and prevent oral disease and related conditions.
- be able to influence consumer groups, businesses, and government agencies to support health care issues.
- use screening, referral, and education to bring consumers into the health care delivery system.

KEY WORDS

Barriers to care	Faith-based initiatives
Cultural diversity	Target populations

INTRODUCTION

Target population is a term used to represent a certain segment of the population. The term is broad and can represent three-year-old children or a group of youths involved in a local church group or even elderly living in an assisted living community. Basically, age can be a representative factor of a target group, but it usually has other commonalities as well. An example would be that although the children in the group are three years old, they may also share other characteristics in that they attend the same Head Start program, live in the same geographic area, come from families in similar income sectors, have one parent, and live with extended families. In addition, many of the children have the same ethnic background. So although we know that these children are three years old, many factors are helpful when planning a dental hygiene in-service for this group. This chapter discusses target populations, cultural diversity, and **barriers to dental care** that may be encountered.

SPECIFIC TARGET POPULATIONS

Dental hygienists provide service and education to many different groups and frequently are asked to present dental health information to these groups. These groups are referred to many times as **target populations.** Target population, as mentioned already, is a group of individuals with similarities of some sort whether it be age, race, educational background, life situation, and/or health conditions.

This section contains brief discussions of some of the groups to whom dental hygienists may speak.

Family Caregivers: Family caregivers can be defined as the population in society that currently provides daily care to family members. These caregivers may be parents, grandparents, children, other relatives, or close friends. This care may be as comprehensive as dispensing medicine, both orally and intravenously to a family member, to helping the member with hygiene and sanitary functions, cooking, and feeding. This group usually assumes some responsibility specifically pertaining to oral hygiene care. In fact, many hospitals and health care organizations provide health education and caregiving classes to this group, which should include oral hygiene care.

Health Care Workers: This target group provides direct patient care and/or treatment and can include nurses, physicians, physician assistants, physical and occupational therapists, speech pathologists, and nurses aides. This group has considerable knowledge about the diseases of the target population, but may need additional information on the impact the disease or condition has in relation to oral health. The dental hygienist should be knowledgeable about the disease and ask health care workers about their experiences treating and caring for individuals with the disease.

Hospice Workers: This group of workers may include a variety of professionals all working together to make terminal illness more tolerable and comfortable for the patient and his/her families. Dental hygienists definitely can alleviate oral pain through education of caregivers and/or patients, dental hygiene treatment, and by referral to a dentist if needed. Dental hygienists may be the coordinator of dental care for the hospice program.

School Teachers: School teachers can influence students a great deal; therefore, this group can be particularly important to the dental hygienist. Theorists suggest that school teachers' discussion on dental health is more influential on students than a dental hygienist providing information once a year during dental health month. For this reason it is necessary that the teachers be equipped with proper dental knowledge and motivated to instill positive dental health behaviors to students. It is important that the teacher be able to recognize noticeable dental disease and have a dental hygienist to contact within the community. The dental hygienist can be effective in changing dental behavior by working with this group and collaborating with teachers.

Social Workers: Social work is the professional activity of helping individuals, groups, or communities to enhance or restore their capacity for social functioning and to create societal conditions favorable to the goals.[3] Social workers are a group who have a definitive influence on target populations. Depending on the populations that the social worker treats, the dental hygienist can work with the social worker in providing access to dental care and education for many groups in need. The dental hygienist should provide the social worker with proper oral hygiene knowledge and serve as a liaison between the social worker and patient.

Persons with Medical Conditions/Diseases: Most important to remember with this population is the relationship oral health has with overall health. If the patient is afflicted with a medically compromising disease such as cardiovascular disease, respiratory disease, metabolic and endocrine disease, immune compromising diseases, liver and kidney disorder, arthritis, physical disabilities, joint prostheses, and/or cancer, many symptoms, conditions, and diseases may be seen in the oral cavity. Dental education for the patient with a systemic disease is complicated but can help in alleviating many infections and may improve not only dental health but also overall health. When presenting to groups of this nature, remember to have information available on specific drugs that are commonly taken and the effects of these drugs on dental health, premedication coverage information if necessary, and oral manifestations of the disease.

Developmentally Disabled: Developmental disability is either present at birth or occurs during the developmental period. In fact, some defects are not present at birth and may appear years later. The major disorders in this category are mental retardation, cerebral palsy, epilepsy, and autism.[1] Education directed toward this

DENTAL HYGIENIST'S SPOTLIGHT
A Day in the Life of Sheryl Magnuson
Veteran's Affairs Dental Hygienist

As the senior dental hygienist at Veteran's Affairs Medical Center in Albuquerque, New Mexico, my primary responsibility is direct patient care, followed by a secondary responsibility of planning and administering various dental health programs.

I provide comprehensive dental hygiene treatment on ambulatory and nonambulatory patients. I routinely instruct patients at chairside, demonstrating the proper home treatment techniques and tailoring them to their individual needs. Bedside dental hygiene treatment is provided using specialized procedures for comatose patients, neurosurgical patients, and other types of nonambulatory patients.

On an independent basis, I plan, coordinate, and conduct programs for target populations such as diabetic, geriatric, and psychiatric patients. My training responsibilities also include instructing the nursing staff in the proper techniques of oral care. These techniques are applied to the bedridden, handicapped, disabled, and chronically ill patients.

For many years, I have routinely trained dental hygiene students here at the Veteran's Affairs Medical Center. Those responsibilities include conducting orientation classes and providing a meaningful academic and clinical instruction during their rotation.

group may consist of interventions aimed at reducing higher rates of periodontal disease and caries, as well as care of teeth that may be rotated and/or crowded. Specific drug interactions and appointment scheduling issues common to this group should be assessed.

Hearing Impaired: Hearing impairment can be described as functional but not effective hearing. Hearing aids may be utilized. On the other hand, deafness refers to an inability to understand speech even with the use of a hearing device. Figures 8–1 and 8–2, available on the website, depict sign language that can be utilized when educating this population. Visual aids are helpful when addressing the hearing impaired, as well as hands-on learning in which the entire group participates.

Visual Impairments: Limitations in sight range from a slight impairment in vision to complete blindness with no perception of light.[2] Education for blind individuals should focus on descriptions. It is recommended that audio and manual aids be utilized, allowing the individuals within the group to feel the teeth, brush, and floss while the dental hygienist demonstrates proper oral hygiene care. In addition, audiotapes can be useful. Few resources are available for blind individuals regarding dental health. Therefore, it may be helpful to work with an individual who is blind when creating teaching aids for a presentation.

Individuals Living in Poverty: In the United States, poverty affects over 10 percent of the population and consistently ranks children as the age group most afflicted by poverty.[4] In fact, the United States spends about 12 percent of its gross national product on public assistance and social insurance programs such as Social Security, Medicare, Aid to Families with Dependent Children (AFDC), food stamps, and Medicaid.[5] Some researchers believe that the growth of an urban underclass locked in a cycle of welfare dependency, joblessness, crime, and out-of-wedlock pregnancy has also contributed to the persistence of poverty.[6] However, some researchers propose that the culture of poverty, which can be explained as individuals living in poverty taking on their own culture, has not developed in the United States.[7] For the dental hygienist, accessing dental care for these individuals by working at finding dental providers who will accept Medicaid insurance is necessary. The dental hygienist may need to work with a social worker or case manager on locating funding for dental care if the individual or group is not enrolled or eligible for Medicaid insurance. Moreover, transportation issues may need to be resolved and language barriers may exist. As with all groups, education is needed to make individuals aware of dental diseases and promote dental disease prevention.

Inmates: This group can be defined as individuals living in a state or federal prison. In the United States, inmates have a right to health care, thus the demand for dental hygiene services. Preventive health care has proven practical and economical in all facets of health care delivery and this definitely is seen in dental care. Basically, by working in a correctional institution, dental hygienists can help decrease dental diseases and restorative and emergency dental conditions and subsequently decrease dental care costs within this group. Many inmates have had minimal or no prior dental hygiene treatment and so dental hygienists working with this population need to focus on the etiology of dental disease and oral health behaviors designed to prevent or control disease.

Ages: These individuals may be addressed at different age levels. Table 8–1, available on the student website, describes age specific competencies seen in different stages of life. During the time they spend in prison, many inmates live a healthier lifestyle, free from substance abuse and unhealthy behaviors. This is the ideal time to emphasize the value of optimum oral health on the body.

* *Prenatal:* Women who are pregnant present with a variety of oral health needs, including changes in their oral health because of pregnancy and the care of their infants' oral health needs. Pregnant women may suffer periodontal conditions exacerbated from hormonal fluctuations. Pyogenic granulomas are occasionally present during pregnancy as is pregnancy-induced gingivitis. Further, preterm births have been associated with periodontal disease in the mother. Remember

that these conditions can be prevented by meticulous oral hygiene and professional dental hygiene care, which is the message of the dental health educator.

- *Infancy:* Early childhood caries is a preventable disease. Many infants are fed a bottle in bed or sugary drinks from a bottle during the day, which end up causing early childhood caries, sometimes referred to as nursing (baby bottle) tooth decay. In addition many parents have questions about teething, the functions of the primary dentition, when to begin regular dental hygiene visits, and home care regimens. Dental hygienists may serve as a dental health educator, promoter, clinician, and refer infants/parents to dentists as needed.

- *Preschool:* Preschoolers are interested in learning and are busy striving for independence. Young children are impressionable, and, therefore, the education of this population is vital for a lifetime of good oral hygiene. In particular, in this stage of development a positive dental role model and education are absorbed rapidly. It is important to discuss the role of the dental hygienist and other dental care providers and to explain basic dental and nutrition knowledge. Interactive learning with the group is effective with coloring or other hands-on methods utilized.

- *Elementary Age Children:* This age group is interested in obtaining knowledge and continuing to strive for independence. It is important to discuss a more definitive concept of dental health care and preventive interventions such as fluoride and dental sealants. Children are attending school, and, therefore, the dental hygienist can easily schedule an educational presentation through their teacher. Teachers have influence in this age group, so dental educational materials aimed at integration into the math, reading, and social sciences curriculum is helpful for this age group.

- *Teenage Children:* This group strives for total independence and will enjoy a presentation on dental health without parental supervision. It is important to understand the issues in their lives. Moreover, many individuals in this age group are concerned with their looks or basic presentation. Discussing halitosis or tooth color may be effective at this age. In addition, teenagers look for positive reinforcements, which can take the form of rewards such as T-shirts and hats, for a job well done in oral home care. Also, many teenagers are involved in athletics, making a discussion of mouthguards critical with this population.

- *Adults:* Adults tend to be more cooperative in the learning process if they are aware of the benefits. They are focused on time constraints and only want to learn what is practical for them. Moreover, adults may have many issues concerning dental care, including fear and anxiety. Instructions about their children's oral health may also be provided. In addition, it is necessary to understand the individual's capabilities and values. If an individual has no value for oral care, then the education presented will be of little value. It is important to figure out how the dental hygienist can make oral health important in the individual's life and of real value to this person. Moreover, adults are interested in information about dental care delivery in general, and such discussion is appropriate with this group.

- *Older Adults:* Many older adults remain independent, whereas other older adults may have limited independence. Having background knowledge of this group's capabilities is necessary. Further, this group may be entitled to government funding of dental care; therefore, it is important for the hygienists to serve as a liaison between the elderly and the dental care delivery system. Moreover, dental caries, periodontal diseases, oral cancer, disease etiology and prevention, as well as nutrition, holistic health care, and specific dental services (tooth bleaching, cosmetic dentistry) may be addressed.

CULTURAL DIVERSITY

National Geographic described culture in the following excerpt.

No culture is static. Ideas, technologies, products, and people move from one place to another. When cultures come into contact through migration, trade, or the latest telecommunications devices, they influence each other. Sometimes cultures cross-pollinate, exchanging foods, music, sports. At other times, say critics of globalization, a culture swamps another like an invasive, fast-reproducing weed. Cultures have evolved in response to contact for thousands of years. But the pace has changed. In the past the influences of distant cultures came slowly, delayed by one journey. Today, because of the telephone, the television, the Internet, telecommunications satellites, world trade and long-distance travel, cultural influences can spread across the planet as fast as the click of a mouse.[7]

This definition stresses the fact that cultures involve a multitude of dimensions and rarely remain stagnate. The statement also suggests that the influence cultures have on each other and, hence, **cultural diversity,** are changing. Further, Pope John Paul II states, "At the heart of every culture lies the attitude man takes to the greatest mystery: the mystery of god. Different cultures are basically different ways of facing the question of the meaning of personal existence."[8] Dental hygienists must be aware of and show respect to different cultures' religious and ethnic differences and their influences within the culture, particularly in health care practices.

Cross-cultural dental hygiene is defined by Darby as the effective integration of the client's socioethnocultural background into the dental hygiene process of care (see Table 8–1). Culture is related to the dental hygiene process of care because often disease and health are culturally determined and because cultural factors can facilitate or impede health care goals and outcomes. Culture is the common set of beliefs, values, attitudes, and perceptions shared by a group of people. Basically, it is a person's culture that pervades that person's experiences,

Table 8–1.   Guidelines for Cross-Cultural Dental Hygiene

- Approach each client (individual, family, community) as an individual with unique characteristics and life experiences
- Try to get in touch with your own unique characteristics and life experiences. Sensitize yourself on how cultural factors have influenced your personal beliefs, attitudes, behaviors, practices, and values
- Try to identify biases and prejudices in your own life; their origins; their impact on interpersonal communication; their impact on your effectiveness as a health care provider, educator, manager, researcher, consumer advocate, and agent of change
- Become a lifelong student of other cultures, particularly the cultures unique to your community
- Assess the culturally related practices, attitudes, values, and beliefs of your clients as part of the dental hygiene process
- Display an accepting, nonjudgmental demeanor when presented with cultural diversity
- Reflect knowledge and recognition of the client's various cultural practices throughout the interaction
- Incorporate culturally relevant variables into the dental hygiene services that will be provided to the client
- Encourage the client to continue cultural health practices that can bring no harm; provide support, understanding, and time when trying to change a potentially harmful oral health practice that is culturally determined
- Determine whether the dental hygiene plan of care is in harmony with the client's cultural values; modify dental hygiene plan of care that conflicts with the client's culture
- Recognize special dietary practices of the client; provide nutritional counseling within the framework of the client's culture
- Develop collegial relationships with health professionals from various ethnic and minority groups as a way of promoting cultural exchange that ultimately improves dental hygiene care

Source: Darby, M. L., and M. M. Walsh. *Dental Hygiene Theory and Practice,* 2d edition. Philadelphia: W. B. Saunders, 2003.

relationships, and interactions. Table 8–2 is a guide to working with people of various cultural groups.[9]

Dental hygienists, regardless of their cultural origins, cannot afford to function under the ignorance of ethnocentrism. Ethnocentrism is the belief that the only culture of importance is the individual's culture and that others merely do not matter. Cross-cultural competence can be gained via self-analysis and awareness, travel, reading about and observing people from other cultures, validated verbal and nonverbal messages that are delivered and/or received, avoiding stereotypical thinking, considering cultural determinants of health and disease, and demonstrating culturally sensitive behavior throughout the dental hygiene process of care.[10]

FAITH-BASED INITIATIVES

Many religious groups play a significant role in health care. In fact, religious leaders tend to have a great influence on health care delivery and work diligently at helping those in need of health care. Religious leaders play a significant role in social changes, while educating many on the moral obligation of health care. Recently, the federal government initiated the development of an agency that ensures collaboration of the government and religious groups working to improve life for those in need. The mission of the Center for Faith-Based and Community Initiatives (CFBCI) is to create an environment within the Department of Health and Human Services (HHS) that welcomes the participation of faith-based and community-based organizations as valued and essential partners assisting Americans in need. The CFBCI's mission is part of the department's focus on improving human services for our country's neediest citizens.

BARRIERS TO DENTAL CARE

Many populations within a society face restrictive barriers to dental hygiene and dental care. The profession of dental hygiene strives to alleviate these barriers and improve access to care for these population strata. Barriers that individuals and populations may encounter are listed in Table 8–3.

Barriers to dental care can be defined as any limitation an individual may have to receiving dental services. Barriers can include age, cultural variances, language difficulties, disabilities, transportation issues, or financial limitations. Barriers may be easily overcome such as transportation problems that can be alleviated by a state program offering transportation to medical and dental appointments or

Table 8–2. Cultural Phenomena Affecting Health Care*

	African (Black) Americans	Asian/Pacific Islander Americans	American Indians, Aleuts, and Eskimos	Hispanic Americans	European (White) Origin Americans
NATIONS OF ORIGIN	West coast (as slaves) of Africa Many African countries West Indian islands Dominican Republic Haiti Jamaica	China, Japan, Hawaii, the Philippines, Vietnam, Asian India, Korea, Samoa, Guam, and the remaining Asian/Pacific islands	200 American Indian nations indigenous to North America Aleuts and Eskimos in Alaska	Hispanic countries Spain, Cuba, Mexico, Central and South America Puerto Rico	Germany, England, Italy, Ireland, former Soviet Union, and all other European countries
ENVIRONMENTAL CONTROL	Traditional health and illness beliefs may continue to be observed by "traditional" people	Traditional health and illness beliefs may continue to be served by "traditional" people	Traditional health and illness beliefs may continue to be observed by "traditional" people Natural and magico-religious folk medicine tradition Traditional healer: medicine man or woman	Traditional health and illness beliefs may continue to be served by "traditional" people Folk medicine tradition Traditional healers: *curandero, espiritista, partera, señora*	Primary reliance on "modern, Western" healthcare delivery system Remaining traditional health and illness beliefs and practices may be observed Some remaining traditional folk medicine Homeopathic medicine resurgent
BIOLOGICAL VARIATIONS	Sickle cell anemia Hypertension Cancer of the esophagus Stomach cancer	Hypertension Liver cancer Stomach cancer Coccidioidomycosis	Accidents Heart disease Cirrhosis of the liver Diabetes mellitus	Diabetes mellitus Parasites Coccidioidomycosis Lactose intolerance	Breast cancer Heart disease Diabetes mellitus Thalassemia

152

	Coccidioidomycosis Lactose intolerance	Lactose intolerance Thalassemia			
SOCIAL ORGANIZATION	Family: many single-parent female-headed households Large, extended family networks Strong church affiliations within community Community social organizations	Family: hierarchical structure, loyalty Large, extended family networks Devotion to tradition Many religions, including Taoism, Buddhism, Islam, and Christianity Community social organizations	Extremely family-oriented to both biological and extended families Children are taught to respect traditions Community social organizations	Nuclear families Large, extended family networks *Compadrazzo* (godparents) Strong church affiliations within community Community social organizations	Nuclear families Extended families Judeo-Christian religions Community and social organizations
COMMUNICATION	National languages Dialect: Pidgin French, Spanish, Creole	National language preference Dialects, written characters Use of silence Nonverbal and contextual cueing	Tribal languages Use of silence and body language	Spanish or Portuguese are the primary languages	National languages Many learned English rapidly as immigrants Verbal, rather than nonverbal
SPACE	Close personal space	Noncontact people	Space very important and has no boundaries	Tactile relationships: touch, handshakes, embrace Value physical presence	Noncontact people: aloof, distant Southern countries: closer contact and touch
TIME ORIENTATION	Present over future	Present	Present	Present	Future over present

*Please remember that not all individuals from a given culture will act or think in the same manner. All individuals possess an inherent variability within cultural groups. This chart is not meant to generalize populations, but to serve as a beginning guide.

Adapted from: Spector, R. "Cultures, Ethnicity, and Nursing," in *Fundamentals of Nursing*, 3rd ed, eds. Potter, P. and Perry, A. (St. Louis: Mosby, 1992), p. 101.

Table 8–3.   Barriers to Dental Hygiene and Dental Care

- Age
- Language
- Habit
- Culture
- Poor Finances
- Lack of Faith in Treatment
- Education
- Misunderstanding
- Fear
- Transportation
- Values
- Safety of Treatment
- Illiteracy
- Attitudes
- Denial of Disease
- No Dental Providers
- Belief in Invulnerability
- Convenience
- Social Issues
- Education Levels
- Provider Conflicts
- Dental Hygienists' Supervision Requirements

may be more complicated such as statutes that do not allow a registered dental hygienist to provide dental hygiene care in a school setting.

Barriers to care can often be a compilation of factors. For instance, a two-year-old child with severe stages of early childhood caries with Medicaid insurance may face a barrier to care if no pediatric dentists or qualified general dentists in the immediate area are willing to provide treatment. Their reluctance may be due to the age of the child, the lack of qualified dental providers, the severity of the disease, or the type of insurance. One factor may limit access to care for this child or several factors may be involved.

Another example of a single barrier to care may be a teenager who believes that his teeth are invulnerable to the effects of periodontal disease. This teenager may not believe that keeping his teeth for a lifetime takes a commitment to home care as well as professional care. This individual may not respond to information presented about the periodontal condition of his mouth, which may be a limitation to the services offered by the dental hygienist. Hopefully, the dental hygienist can alleviate this barrier by gearing the educational therapy toward values the teenager possesses. For example, the dental hygienist may be able to discuss the effect of periodontal disease on halitosis, which may interest the teenager.

The professional dental hygienist assumes the responsibility for increasing access to quality dental hygiene and dental care. This responsibility requires an understanding of barriers and working to alleviate these barriers.

SUMMARY

It is important for the dental hygienist practicing in community settings to be aware of the barriers some populations face when trying to access dental hygiene care. Moreover, many populations have similarities in terms of cultural identity. The dental hygienist needs to be aware of the different cultural philosophies, ideas, and practices. Moreover, it is vital for the dental hygienist to learn about the population before providing treatment or education so these initiatives can be effective.

REFERENCES

[1] DeBiase, C. B. *Dental Health Education Theory and Practice.* Philadelphia: Lea and Febiger, 1991.

[2] Ibid.

[3] Zastrow, C. *Introduction to Social Welfare Institutions,* 3d ed. Chicago: Dorsey Press, 1986.

[4] Proctor, B. D., and J. Dalaker. US Census Bureau. Current Population Reports P60-219. *Poverty in the United States:* 2001. Washington, DC: U.S. Government Printing Office, 2002.

[5] Sawhill, Isabel V. Poverty in the United States. *Concise Encyclopedia of Economics.* Liberty Fund, Inc. Ed. David R. Henderson. Library of Economics and Liberty. 8 September 2003.

[6] http://www.poverty.smartlibrary.org.

[7] Millennium supplement: Culture. *National Geographic* 196 (1999): 1.

[8] Pope John Paul II. *An Invitation to Joy.* New York: Simon & Schuster, 1999.

[9] Darby, M. L., and M. M. Walsh. *Dental Hygiene Theory and Practice,* 2d edition. Philadelphia: W. B. Saunders, 2003.

[10] Ibid.

Get Connected

Multimedia Extension Activities

 www.prenhall.com/nathe

Use the above address to access the free, interactive companion web site created specifically to accompany this textbook. Here you will find an array of self study material to help you gain a richer understanding of the concepts presented in this chapter.

Chapter *9*

PROGRAM PLANNING

OBJECTIVES

After studying this chapter, the dental hygiene student will be able to:

- describe the various program planning paradigms.
- define the dental hygiene program planning paradigm.
- describe various dental public health programs.
- develop a dental public health program plan.

COMPETENCIES

After studying this chapter and participating in accompanying course activities, the dental hygiene student should be competent in the following:

- identify services that promote oral health to prevent oral disease and related conditions.
- assess, plan, implement, and evaluate community-based oral health programs.
- use screening, referral, and education to bring consumers into the health care delivery system.

KEY WORDS

Dental hygiene process of care
Paradigm

Prevention programs
Program planning

www.prenhall.com/nathe

INTRODUCTION

Dental hygienists frequently provide dental health presentations to target populations as discussed in the preceding chapters. Actually planning a dental health program entails more than just providing dental health education to a group. It generally consists of providing dental hygiene and dental treatment geared toward a population's needs.

Program planning is much more than just planning a program; it encompasses the assessment, diagnosis, implementation, and evaluation stages in addition to the planning stage. Few would argue that before a program can be planned, one must review past programs and identify a paradigm to follow when constructing programs. Applying ideas to programs should be less complicated within the framework of a paradigm and then completing it with a specific group's needs and resources.

Program planning and implementation are quite possibly the most exciting areas of public health. It is motivating and intriguing to look deeply into a population's needs and create dental programs to meet those needs. Existing paradigms and programs will be presented and a new dental hygiene program planning paradigm is discussed in this chapter.

DENTAL HYGIENE PUBLIC HEALTH PROGRAMS

The following section is devoted to the presentation of current dental public health programs. The first section describes generic programs that are implemented throughout various regions of the United States, and the later section describes specific private and publicly funded programs.

Prevention Programs

Historically, localities fluoridated the school water supply, but now many local areas across the country implement a school fluoride mouthrinse program. This program is employed in the local schools, and students take time out to "swish and spit" as it is sometimes called. Dental hygienists coordinate the program and teach school teachers how to administer the program.

Dental sealant programs are also common. Dental hygienists and dentists (where it is required for supervision) travel to schools placing sealants and provide oral hygiene instruction. This type of program enables students who may not visit the dental office to have the preventive benefits of dental interventions. It is an inexpensive method to prevent dental caries, especially in the 50 percent of the population that does not receive dental care via private dental offices.

A dental hygienist in a school program may implement a program to fabricate athletic mouthguards for all sports teams. This program would be designed to prevent oral trauma and concussions and may be more frequently seen in a middle school or high school.

Dental health educational programs are abundant throughout the world and strive to provide preventive dental health tools to large populations. Many are instituted in schools, but can also be seen in long-term care facilities, health care support groups, and day care facilities. However, many educational programs are sporadic and have no measurable outcomes assessment. The program may consist of a dental hygienist visiting a third-grade class to present twenty minutes of dental health education.

Many large dental supply companies have materials developed for the sole purpose of mass education. When using these materials, it is necessary that the dental hygienists make sure the information presented is helpful and scientifically valid. The materials should not be just an advertisement with little gain to the consumer. If carefully critiqued by the dental hygienists, these materials can be valuable in dental health promotional activities. Appendix B provides a listing of companies that have educational materials available for the dental hygienist.

Dental hygienists may also develop and implement health promotion programs such as programs designed to promote dental health. The dental hygiene association may sponsor a poster designing contest during children's dental health month. The students may be asked to design a poster that depicts a dental health message. The winners may receive a prize, and the dental hygiene association may utilize the poster on a billboard during the next legislative session. Another example of a promotional project would be the addition of a dental operatory to the local children's museum. This would help send a message of exploration and applied science to children in the area. This message would be an example of a health promotional activity. Many tobacco prevention programs are promotional in nature.

Healthy Smile Program: School-Based Dental Health Program

The University of New Mexico, Division of Dental Hygiene, and the Albuquerque Public Schools collaborated to develop a school-based dental program. This program, which is coined the Healthy Smile Program, was developed to provide urgent treatment to children and prevent dental diseases through education, screenings, referrals, and follow-up.[1] The screenings include dental caries and plaque indexes before and after the educational and treatment interventions are provided to effectively evaluate the program (Figure 9–1).

This program differs from many dental health programs because it is interdisciplinary in nature. Dental hygienists, school nurses, schoolteachers, social workers, and parents collaborated to develop, implement, and evaluate this program. The dental hygienists educate the students, parents, and teachers and provide screenings; the school nurses coordinate the health care needs of the students; the

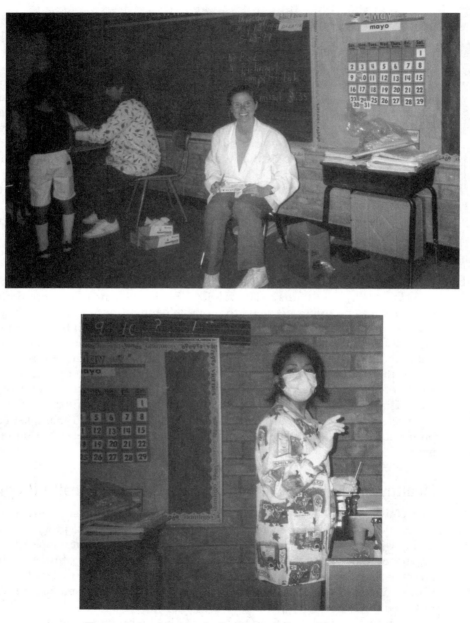

Figure 9–1. Healthy Smile Program Dental Screening

teachers educate their students; and the social workers assist the parents in accessing care by helping meet the transportation, social, and funding needs for students. Most important, the parents become involved in obtaining dental care for their children. The involvement of a social worker in this dental health program increased the children's chances of actually obtaining dental care.

Moreover, the New Mexico Dental Hygienists' Association became a collaborating participant in this program with the development of Free Cleaning and Sealant Clinics on the weekends for students in these schools. The greatest benefit from this program was the number of families that were linked up with Medicaid insurance and the New Mexico Healthy Kids Funds by the program's social worker. These clinics provided yet another opportunity to obtain much needed services and enroll more of the population in these government-funded programs.

Dental Program at Inner City Health Center: Volunteer Dental Treatment Program

The Inner City Health Center (ICHC), established in 1983, is a private, nonprofit, volunteer-based health care facility committed to providing medical and dental care and counseling services to the medically uninsured and low-income families living in the Denver metropolitan area.[2] The Dental Program primarily serves adults and children in emergency situations. Because Medicaid insures these children, the clinic refers most of the pediatric population to specialized dental facilities, which serve children, allowing ICHC to help those low-income adults who have no dental insurance. Patients pay on a sliding fee scale, according to their ability to pay.

In conjunction with ICHC's medical clinics, the dental clinic provides dental screenings to adults and children, dental education in prevention and maintenance, hypertension screening, oral cancer detection and referral for treatment, evaluation for child and spousal abuse, smoking and tobacco cessation programs, and complete dental care, including all aspects of restorative dentistry. New clients must take a preventive oral hygiene course, which is offered one day a month. The preventive program of ICHC's Dental Program, including its highly effective Pediatric Dental Caries Prevention Program (a joint venture between the Dental Program and the Pediatric Department at ICHC), is an essential component to the overall program, which strives to assure the oral health of one of the highest risk and most dental needy populations in America.

ICHC networks with dozens of local dental professionals, community organizations, businesses, and other medical and dental organizations. In addition, ICHC and its dental program also provide structured job training to students training to be dentists, dental hygienists, dental assistants, and dental receptionists. ICHC receives no government funding except Medicare/Medicaid reimbursements; patient fees, foundations, corporate gifts and grants, fund-raisers, and general donations from churches and individuals generate its income.

Soroptimist Dental Project: Mobile Dental Treatment Program

Established in 1942, the Soroptimist Dental Project is a comprehensive program that provides dental health education in school classrooms and free dental care in a mobile dental unit to indigent students (K–12) in Zanesville, Ohio.[3] The program's mission is to provide students with a lifelong understanding and personal acceptance of healthy nutritional habits and the value of dental care. With prevention as a goal, students learn that their teeth can, and should, last a lifetime.

Dental health education is the cornerstone of the program. All 4,900 public school students receive dental health education as part of their school curriculum. A dental hygienist visits each classroom in the eight elementary schools, GRADS programs (students who are expectant mothers), and special education classes. Middle school and high school students receive dental health education as part of their health education classes.

During the school year, a mobile dental unit travels to all eleven Zanesville public schools to provide a wide range of dental services, including dental screenings, cleanings, fluorides treatments, sealants, restorations, extractions, and emergency services to qualified students. Each year approximately 450 students without other resources for dental care receive dental treatment through the program.

The Soropitimist Club of Zanesville refunds the cost of the program supplies and equipment. The staff expense of the dental hygienist and dentist's contracted services are covered by the Zanesville Board of Education.

Matthew 25: Faith-Based Dental Treatment Program

Almost twenty years ago, a dream of helping the needy became a reality for a group of people from St. Mary's Catholic Church who wanted to bring alive the verses from Matthew 25 . . . a biblical call to care for the poor.[4] This program is an example of a faith-based initiative. A medical clinic opened in 1976, and within two years, a dental clinic opened. Matthew 25 provides dental care for the low-income non-Medicaid individuals. Dental cleanings, examinations, simple extractions, and restorations are available, and dentures are also made in the clinic with lab work done by Indiana University Dental Lab Students. A children's dental sealant clinic is also offered. The goals of Matthew 25 are to provide direct health and dental care or access for those individuals unable to receive care elsewhere, promote health and safety though education and health screenings, and to strive to reduce complications of chronic disease through education, health monitoring, medical evaluation, and maintenance with medication. Since its inception, Matthew 25 has continued to expand over the years. Now more than 360 volunteers and six part-time staff members and numerous agencies and organizations work directly with Matthew 25. The organization does not rely on governmental grants.

DENTAL HYGIENIST'S SPOTLIGHT
A Day in the Life of Christine Murphy, RDH, BS

Christine Murphy is the dental clinic director for the Pueblo of Isleta in New Mexico. Beginning in 1979, she has worked as a dental assistant and office manager for many years. In 1991 she attended the University of New Mexico (UNM) and graduated from the UNM Division of Dental Hygiene in 1996. She filled in for several dental offices and taught clinically at UNM while she searched for the "perfect job." She is past-president of Sigma Phi Alpha and currently in her second term as president of the High Desert Dental Hygiene Society, the local component of the American Dental Hygiene Association. In January 1998 she found her place in the dental field.

She was hired part time as the dental hygienist for the Pueblo of Isleta just south of Albuquerque, New Mexico. Christine worked two days a week when first hired because she was not sure she would like public health. She continued to teach at the university and worked one day a week for a temporary service. Soon after she began to work with the people of Isleta, she knew it was the place she wanted to be. Soon she was working three days on the Pueblo while she finished the semester at UNM.

In April 1999 she was named interim director for the Pueblo's dental clinic while a search was made to hire a dentist. Christine was instrumental in assisting the tribal council to select a dentist. During such time she kept the dental clinic operational. She developed a budget, staffed the clinic, and scheduled part-time dentists to provide dental care for the community. As a result in October 1999 she was named permanent director of the clinic by the Isleta Tribal Council.

The dental clinic is an interdisciplinary functioning unit. They work with the diabetic program, the Head Start

(continued)

Dental Hygienist's Spotlight   *(continued)*

program, the elderly center, WIC, and work closely with the health clinic staff. Southwest Indian Polytechnic Institute and the staff of the dental clinic at Isleta work together to provide more extensive dental services such as oral surgery, orthodontics, periodontal surgery, and endodontic therapy. Christine helps coordinate all these programs.

She enjoys working for the tribe primarily because of the lack of restrictions in patient care. Financial or time constraints are not a factor when planning treatment. The people are so appreciative of the work done at the dental clinic that it is a pleasure for Christine to get up and go to work in the morning.

Operation Smile Dental Hygiene Program: International Dental Health Educational Program

Operation Smile was founded in 1982 by Dr. William Magee, a plastic surgeon and dentist, and his wife, Kathy, a nurse and clinical social worker.[5] The Magees traveled to the Philippines with a group of American physicians and nurses in 1981, where they provided surgery to children with cleft lip and palate deformities. They became frustrated by the realization that more children needed treatment than could be seen during one visit, which led to the beginning of Operation Smile. Operation Smile (OS) is a private nonprofit, volunteer medical service organization providing reconstructive surgery and related health care to indigent children and adults in developing countries and the United States (Figure 9–2).

Volunteer health care teams travel to various locations and provide surgeries for disfigurements such as cleft lip and palate deformities, tumors, orthopedic problem cancrum oris, and burn scars. Specifically, one commonly seen disease is referred to as cancrum oris or noma. Cancrum oris is an acute, necrotizing process involving the mucous membrane of the mouth. The condition is most commonly seen in children with poor oral hygiene, malnutrition, and debilitating disease. It is characterized by rapidly spreading and painless destruction of bone and soft tissues. Healing frequently occurs, but often with disfiguring effects. OS physicians are able to perform reconstructive surgeries to patients with cancrum oris. Dental hygienists have an important role in the prevention and control of this disease.

American children in need of reconstructive surgery and dental work were treated free of charge as well. The organization has grown to provide education and training to health care workers to achieve long-term self-sufficiency.

The Operation Smile Dental Hygiene program focuses on training teachers and health care workers to prevent and control oral disease and to promote dental

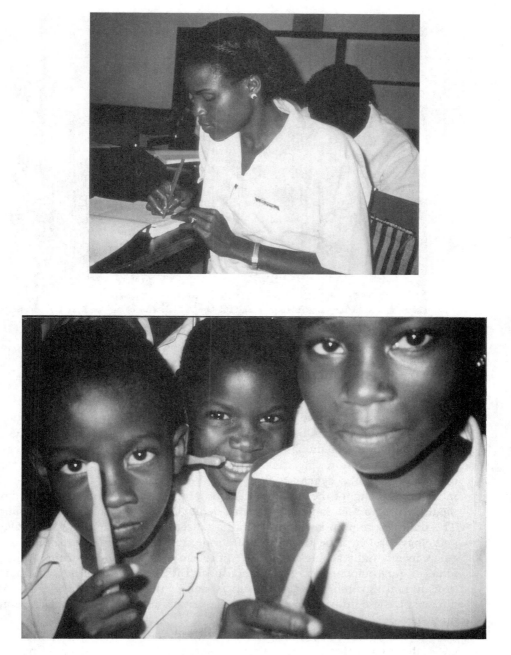

Figure 9–2. Operation Smile International Dental Hygiene Program Training

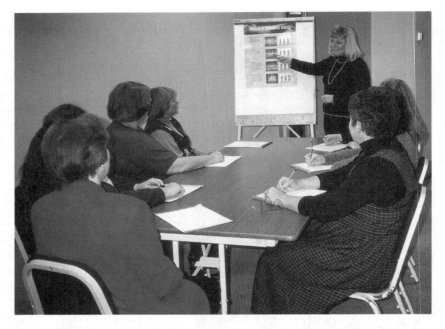

Figure 9–3. A dental hygienist meets with several administrators and health care workers during a planning meeting for school-based dental hygiene program.

health though an organized effort (Figure 9–3). The dental hygienists are crucial in facilitating dental care in the countries OS serves. The primary role of the OS dental hygienist is the planning and implementation of two-week training programs designed to educate teachers and health care providers on dental hygiene fundamentals. The dental hygienists first secure dental care, educational supplies, and monetary funding for the dental hygiene program. The OS dental hygienists implement the program in conjunction with a dental counterpart from the host country. The training program is composed of basic lectures, including oral anatomy, oral pathology, oral hygiene techniques, fluoride, nutrition, dental screenings, dental emergencies, and teaching strategies. At the end of the didactic portion of the program, the participants present the oral health lesson to local schoolchildren and provide oral screenings under the supervision of the OS dental hygienists. More important, these individuals may serve the community as a dental hygiene consultant when dental health concerns arise.

In many developing countries, dental conditions are often a low priority because these countries are faced with such tremendous health issues. One way to improve the quality of life and challenge the exhausting health issues is through prevention. For this reason dental hygiene plays a critical role in these countries.

DENTAL HYGIENE PROCESS OF CARE

Comparison between the dental hygienist in private practice and public health is an interesting way to analyze the inherent differences between providing dental hygiene care and education on an individualized basis versus on a population basis. By delving into the intricacies involved in the **dental hygiene process of care,** it helps in understanding how private practice programs differ from public health programs.

EXISTING PROGRAM PLANNING PARADIGMS

Many postulate that one of the reasons dental public health seems difficult to grasp for students is the fact that so many **paradigms** exist for the development of a public health program. The following paradigms have been utilized in the past to describe planning a public health program.

The first truly **prevention program** planning model was developed by Dr. Fones (see Figure 9–4) in 1927. The model depicted the present-day efforts to prevent and cure disease. Fones depicted the main efforts for disease prevention above the health line and the tube used to represent the path of those who became ill, chiefly from preventable disease. The bottom of the tube represents mortality; the other end of the tube, passing through the convalescent stage to emerge again into the health area. Fones was a staunch believer in prevention and when presenting this model emphasized the fact that very few schools had a well-defined health program.[6]

Figure 9–5 displays the Planning and Implementation Strategy Flowchart. This model emphasizes the need for ongoing revisions and needs assessments, while noting the importance of assessment and planning. DeBiase suggests that the steps involved in planning a dental health educational program include identifying the target population, conducting a needs assessment, designing the program, then implementing and evaluating the program.[7] Of course, this model describes a process for developing an educational program rather than a program equipped with dental treatment objectives.

Harris and Garcia-Godoy define the steps of this process as survey, analysis, program planning, program operation, finance, and evaluation.[8] The emphasis of this paradigm lies within the business aspects of a dental public health program. The Association of State Territorial Dental directors proposed a seven-step model for assessing oral health needs and developing community plans as shown in Figure 9–6. The plan is comprehensive and addresses existing state infrastructure and policies. Moreover, quality assurance plays an important role in this model.

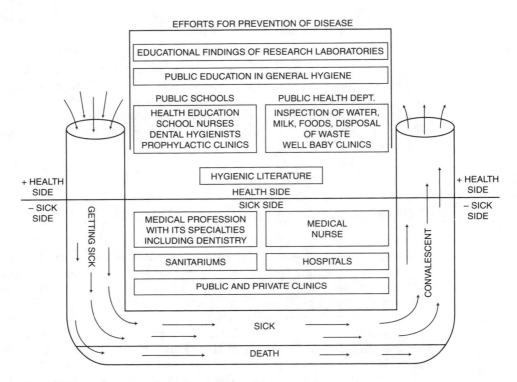

EFFORTS FOR PREVENTION OF DISEASE

| EDUCATIONAL FINDINGS OF RESEARCH LABORATORIES |
| PUBLIC EDUCATION IN GENERAL HYGIENE |

PUBLIC SCHOOLS | PUBLIC HEALTH DEPT.

HEALTH EDUCATION
SCHOOL NURSES
DENTAL HYGIENISTS
PROPHYLACTIC CLINICS

INSPECTION OF WATER,
MILK, FOODS, DISPOSAL
OF WASTE
WELL BABY CLINICS

HYGIENIC LITERATURE

+ HEALTH
SIDE

− SICK
SIDE

HEALTH SIDE
SICK SIDE

+ HEALTH
SIDE

− SICK
SIDE

GETTING SICK

MEDICAL PROFESSION
WITH ITS SPECIALTIES
INCLUDING DENTISTRY

MEDICAL
NURSE

CONVALESCENT

SANITARIUMS | HOSPITALS

PUBLIC AND PRIVATE CLINICS

SICK

DEATH

Figure 9–4. Prevention Program Planning Model

Source: Fones, A. C. *Mouth Hygiene,* 3d ed. Philadelphia: Lea & Febiger, 1927. ©Lippincott Williams & Wilkins.

Although many different paradigms are available, all possess common threads, aspects that are necessary during program development of all natures. These common threads are described in the dental hygiene program planning paradigm.

DENTAL HYGIENE PROGRAM PLANNING PARADIGM

The dental hygiene program planning paradigm shown in Table 9–1 utilizes the dental hygiene process of care model when describing the steps in program planning.[9] Assessment, dental hygiene diagnosis, planning, implementation, and evaluation are the basic increments of program development.

Assessment

During the assessment phase, the dental hygienist assesses the population's needs, facility needs, resources, and funding. Population needs can be assessed through surveys or dental screenings utilizing specific dental indexes. Dental indexes will

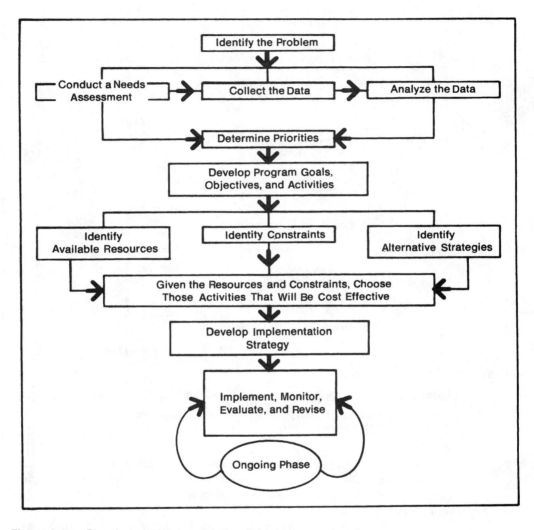

Figure 9–5. Planning and Implementation Flowchart

Source: Gluck, G. M., and W. M. Morganstein. *Jong's Community Dental Health,* 4th ed. St. Louis: Mosby-Yearbook, Inc., 1998.

provide the planner with objective information about the population's dental needs. Surveys or personal interviews will aid in gathering information about demand, perceived needs, approximate knowledge-level of the population, and existing problems and issues.

Information about the demographics (age, socioeconomic status, educational level, cultural diversity, and other important details) of the population should be

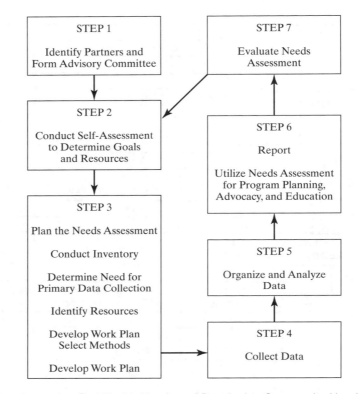

Figure 9–6. Assessing Oral Health Needs and Developing Community Needs

Source: Seven-Step Model for Assessing Oral Health Needs and Developing Community Plans. Guidelines for State and Territorial Oral Health Programs. July 1997.

gathered, and specific dental needs should be identified. Many times it does not take additional efforts to gather information about population demographics. This information can be found in documentation from the facility, community, or existing grant applications.

Moreover, it is necessary to identify facilities that may be involved, whether it be a public school, nursing home, or other organization. Specific information on available space, equipment, and dental and educational materials for the program is necessary. In addition, resources and funding identification are important for planning the program.

Personnel needs, sometimes referred to as labor force planning, are important. When assessing personnel issues, it is important to understand the state practice act, which may allow for dental hygienists to work without supervision of dentists, thus decreasing personnel needs. Moreover, it is necessary to assess for the ultimate coordination of the program. It makes the program operation run more smoothly if a dental professional coordinates. Many times if a different health

Table 9–1.   Dental Hygiene Program Planning Paradigm

Assessment

Assessment via surveys, existing data, or dental screenings:

- Population's dental needs
- Demographics
- Facility
- Personnel (manpower)
- Existing resources
- Funding

↓

Dental Hygiene Diagnosis

- Prioritization of needs
- Formulation of diagnosis to provide goals and objectives for blueprint

↓

Planning

- Identify methods to measure goals
- Develop blueprint
- Address constraints and possible alternatives

↓

Implementation

- Program will begin operation
- Revision and changes identified and employed

↓

Evaluation

- Measuring of goals via surveys and dental indexes
- Qualitative and quantitative evaluation
- Ongoing revisions employed

care worker coordinates the program they are unaware of appointment scheduling and other issues inherent in dental care. If the program is combined with a larger public health program, dental coordination should be addressed.

Dental Hygiene Diagnosis

The dental hygiene diagnosis is the natural conclusion to the assessment phase and focuses on those needs that can be fulfilled through dental hygiene care. Dental hygiene diagnoses must be prioritized to provide direction for the dental hygiene actions that follow.[9]

The diagnoses will basically address the needs and be prioritized depending on importance. The following case is one example of a dental hygiene diagnosis. The assessment uncovered the following. In the prison's population it was determined via two dental indexes that moderate to advance periodontal diseases and heavy calculus were present in the majority of inmates. After analyzing the survey, it was reported that most inmates had not had their teeth cleaned for more than fifteen years. The dental public health planner developed the following dental hygiene diagnosis: periodontal disease associated with no regular dental hygiene care. After providing the dental hygiene diagnoses for the population needs, the next phase can commence.

Planning

After prioritizing the goals and deciding which direction the program will follow, it is necessary to draw up a dental program blueprint. This blueprint is created during the planning stage, along with the methods to measure the program's effectiveness. The effectiveness of a program can be measured both quantitatively and qualitatively. In essence, pretest/posttest exams and dental indexes should be developed and/or chosen to measure the goals quantitatively. Surveys, interviews, and personal statements contribute to the qualitative measure of a program.

The target population should be assessed during the planning stage. Information regarding this population provides the basis for formulation of program operations. The blueprint identifies possible constraints that might be encountered and details strategies to overcome difficulties. In addition, alternative areas to develop resources should be addressed. See Figure 9–7 for an example of an operational blueprint for a dental program. Practice management should be developed to set a standard for management issues inherent to programs. Strategies for setting standards are discussed in Chapter 16.

Implementation

At this stage the program will actually begin operations. Revising the program and employing changes as necessary also come into play at this point. A program planner should not be discouraged by difficulties evidenced at this stage. Most

Figure 9–7.   Example of an Operational Program Planning Paradigm

BLUEPRINT FOR THE
1998–1999 HEALTHY SMILE PROGRAM

The goal of this project is to utilize school and community resources in the development of a program that would favorably impact the dental health of first-grade students in the Rio Grande cluster.

Funding, Materials, and Personnel Needs were met by a grant from APS Medicaid-in-the-Schools Funding.

Education

Parents

Objective: To educate patients on dental health and improve referral system.

Methods: Presentations by dental hygienists, newsletter advertisements, PTA meetings, Parent Partner Association meetings, and interaction with social workers.

Evaluation: Increase in dental care utilization, report from social worker.

Alternative: Meet with principals if not seeing an increase in dental care utilization.

Children

Education

Objective: To improve the level of dental health knowledge.

Methods: Presentations by dental hygienists, coverage by teachers, parent involvement.

Evaluation: Passing grade (75%) on the worksheet completed by students at the end of the curriculum.

Alternative: Revise educational portion.

Plaque

Objective: To decrease the level of plaque detected during screening.

Methods: Screenings.

Evaluation: Pretest and Post-Test Plaque Index (PlI).

(continued)

Figure 9–7.   *(continued)*

Caries

Objective: To decrease the number of caries and to increase the number of restorations and extractions in the children screened.

Methods: Screenings.

Evaluation: Pretest and Post-Test Decayed Extracted Filled Teeth Index (DEFT).

Referrals

Objective: To increase the utilization of dental services.

Methods: Referrals given by school and follow-ups by social worker.

Evaluation: Follow-up with parents via social worker, report from social worker on number of parents contacted and number of the children treated.

Alternatives: Find out why it has not worked in each case and work on the additional needs, such as transportation, funding, etc.

Teachers

Objective: To increase the coverage of dental health education in the curriculum.

Methods: Donate dental health educational material and meet with APS administration about school dental health curriculum.

Evaluation: Pretest and Post-test survey to teachers.

Alternatives: Meet with teachers when program is not working.

programs require revisions, due to difficulties not forecasted or to additional needs originally not assessed.

Evaluation

Evaluation of the program is important and must be addressed to determine the program's success. Moreover, it aids in the ongoing revisions necessary to keep the program functioning at the optimum level. Program evaluation is discussed in Chapter 10.

SUMMARY

Effectively planning and implementing a dental public health program can be challenging and exhausting. It is important to remember the dental hygiene process of care at all stages; with careful assessment and planning, most difficulties can be avoided.

REFERENCES

[1]Nathe, C. N. et al. A group effort for the kids. *RDH* 10 (1999): 36–40.

[2]*Community Preventive Dentistry Awards, Highest Awards Publication.* Chicago: American Dental Association, 1999.

[3]*Community Preventive Dentistry Awards, Highest Awards Publication.* Chicago: American Dental Association, 1999.

[4]Matthew 25 Health/Dental Clinic. Suzy Beard, Dental Director. Fort Wayne, Indiana, October 1999.

[5]Nathe, C. Operation Smile: Dental Hygiene Program. *Dental Hygienist News* 7 (1994): 9–10.

[6]Fones, A. C. *Mouth Hygiene,* 3d ed. Philadelphia: Lea and Febiger, 1927.

[7]DeBiase, C. B. *Dental Health Education Theory and Practice.* Malvern, PA: Lea & Febiger, 1991.

[8]Harris, N. O., and Garcia-Godoy, F. *Primary Preventive Dentistry,* 5th ed. Stamford, CT: Appleton and Lange, 1999.

[9]Darby, M. L. The dental hygiene process. *Dental Hygiene* 55 (1981): 6, 10.

Get Connected

Multimedia Extension Activities

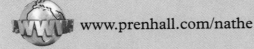 www.prenhall.com/nathe

Use the above address to access the free, interactive companion web site created specifically to accompany this textbook. Here you will find an array of self study material to help you gain a richer understanding of the concepts presented in this chapter.

Chapter 10

PROGRAM EVALUATION

OBJECTIVES

After studying this chapter, the dental hygiene student will be able to:

- describe the mechanisms of program evaluation.
- compare qualitative and quantitative evaluation.
- list and define the goals of various dental indexes.

COMPETENCIES

After studying this chapter and participating in accompanying course activities, the dental hygiene student should be able to:

- utilize, interpret, and analyze appropriate indices for patient assessment.
- determine outcomes of dental hygiene interventions (reevaluation) using indices, instruments, exam techniques, and patient self-report.
- assess, plan, implement and evaluate community-based oral health programs.
- use screening, referral and education to bring consumers into the health care delivery system.

KEY WORDS

Clinical evaluation
Dental index
Formative evaluation

Nonclinical evaluation
Summative evaluation
Measurement

www.prenhall.com/nathe

INTRODUCTION

The evaluation of programs is focused on finding out how well programs work by using scientific techniques. It is concerned with basically ascertaining how effective a program was. Ultimately, without program evaluation dental health programs cannot be promoted as an effective tool in preventing and/or treating dental diseases.

The focus of evaluation is started at the beginning during the program planning phase. Particular focus is placed on assessing and determining the health needs of a target population and determining the content of the program to make sure that it will be meaningful to the population. In addition, evaluation is used to determine the strengths and weakness of teaching personnel, strategies, and organization and to assess the desired outcomes of the program.

Measuring the goals by survey and dental index comparisons should commence, and revisions should be developed to improve the outcomes. Evaluation of the program is an ongoing process. Moreover, it is important to provide qualitative and quantitative documentation of the program to the target population, administrators, funding agency, and public on an ongoing basis. Table 10–1 illustrates the questions to ask when planning the program. Qualitative evaluation answers the question, "How well did we do?" whereas quantitative evaluation answers the question, "How much did we do?"

Program evaluation should focus on the measurement of the goals and objectives of the program being implemented. **Formative evaluation** of a program refers to the internal evaluation of program. It is an examination of the process and is usually conducted in program planning. **Summative evaluation** judges the merit of a program after it has been implemented.

The process of obtaining program evaluation and utilizing the **measurements** to evaluate the operation of a program is often referred to as performance management. Similarly, the process of utilizing such measures to enhance the pro-

Table 10–1. Questions to Ask When Planning the Program
What should be evaluated?
Who should be evaluated?
Who should administer the evaluation?
When should the evaluation be conducted?
How should the evaluation be conducted?

duction of desired outputs and the achievement of desired outcomes has become known as performance management.

Basically, the focus of evaluation should occur during all phases of program planning and should include a formal and informal systematic and regular evaluation of goals and objectives by using specific measurement instruments and outcome assessments.

Moreover, the quality of the program and personnel should be assessed, as well as the progress and effectiveness of activities and identification of problems and solutions to assist in revision and modifications to meet goals and objectives. Evaluations of the perceptions and attitudes of the population should additionally be evaluated.

EVALUATION TECHNIQUES

There are many ways to evaluate a dental public health program. Basic standards exist to monitor program effectiveness. The methods utilized are grouped into two areas: traditional nonclinical measurements and clinical methods (see Table 10–2). **Nonclinical evaluation** methods included face-to-face personal interviews, telephone interviews, and surveys. **Clinical evaluation** methods includes basic screenings and epidemiological examinations that utilize dental indices. Further, basic screenings can consist of the use of a tongue blade and dental mirror. Epidemiological exams consist of detailed visual-tactile assessment of the oral cavity with dental instruments, a dental mirror, and a dental light. However, both screenings and examinations do not constitute a comprehensive diagnosis and are charted according to the dental index used. Many different areas can be evaluated as depicted in Table 10–3.

Table 10–2. Methods of Evaluation	
Nonclinical Methods	**Clinical Methods**
Face-to-Face Personal Interviews	Basic Screenings
Telephone Interviews	Epidemiological Examinations
Surveys	
Document Analysis	

Table 10–3.   Areas of Evaluation
Access to Care
Dental Caries
Dental Care Delivery
Dental Hygiene Treatment
Dental Fluorosis
Dental Treatment Need
Dental Sealants
Occlusion
Oral Cancer
Oral and Craniofacial Diseases and Conditions
Oral Disease Disparities
Oral Health and Quality of Life
Oral Trauma
Periodontal Diseases
Social Impact of Oral Health
Tooth Loss
Water Fluoridation

DENTAL INDEXES

Although the **dental indexes** to be utilized in the program were developed during the planning stage, it is during implementation that the specific index will be employed. A dental index is actually a numerical value describing the status of a given population. It is designed to compare diseases or conditions before and after treatment or program implementation. Dental indexes can serve as a legal record, can be used for comparison, and may also motivate patients to maintain good oral hygiene. They actually help evaluate the effectiveness of a program or specific treatment. Characteristics of a dental index include clarity, simplicity, objectivity, validity, and reliability that it is quantifiable, sensitive, and relatively easy. Table 10–4 further describes these desirable characteristics.

DENTAL HYGIENIST'S SPOTLIGHT
Nina Flores, RDH, BS

I got involved in dental public health during my military service. I worked as a dental specialist/dental lab technician in Albuquerque, New Mexico, at Kirtland Air Force Base. I knew then that I was interested in becoming a dental hygienist. I trained in many public health settings during my education at the University of New Mexico and upon graduation participated as a member of the National Health Service Corps. I was able to work as a dental hygienist in Louisiana in a community health center. Upon returning to Albuquerque, I worked as a dental hygienists in a civil service position with the Indian Health Service. I had the opportunity to coordinate patient outreach programs and participated in grant writing. And although I was based in a city clinic, I also was able to travel to multiple clinics in the rural areas providing dental hygiene services. Then the opportunity of a lifetime presented itself to me. The First Nations Community HealthSource was adding a dental component to service Native Americans in New Mexico. First Nations Community HealthSource is a primary-care clinic located in Albuquerque's Southeast Heights that principally serves a significant Native American population with culturally appropriate care. First Nations offers a full range of health care to its Indian and non-Indian clients, including primary care, behavioral health, and substance abuse services. For adults, there is family planning, prenatal and postpartum care, and preventive diabetic programs. For children, there are immunizations, WIC services, and nutritional programs. In the behavioral health area, First Nations offers crisis intervention, psychological testing, and family therapy. A recent congressional appropriation allowed the clinic to start dental services.

I have been the Dental Program Manager since October 2001 and have been able to create and coordinate the dental clinic from the inception. I have been able to successfully obtain grants and work in an administrative arena daily. I was able to take my dental hygiene skills and reach many by working every day as a dental public health administrator.

Different categories of indexes exist, including the simple index, cumulative index, irreversible index, and the reversible. A simple index measures the presence or absence of a condition, whereas a cumulative index measures all the evidence of a condition past and present. An irreversible index measures conditions that will not change, such as dental caries, whereas a reversible index measures conditions that can be changed such as plaque.

Table 10–4. Characteristics of a Dental Index	
Characteristic	**Defined**
Clarity	Criteria are understandable
Simplicity	Easily memorized
Objectivity	Not subject to individual interpretation
Validity	Measures what is intended
Reliability	Reproducible, examiner consistency and calibration
Quantifiable	Statistics can be applied
Sensitivity	Ability to detect small degrees of difference
Acceptability	No pain to subjects, minimal expense

Please see the student website for more information on labeling of tooth surfaces and teeth numbers. In many types of indexes, only a few teeth or tooth surfaces are screened. Usually these teeth are the six teeth that include numbers 3, 9, 12, 19, 25, and 28 as shown in Figure 10–1. These teeth are referred to as Ramjford teeth. There are many types of frequently utilized dental indexes. A few of the many frequently used indexes are briefly described in Table 10–5.[1]

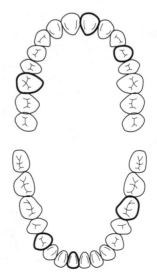

Figure 10–1.   Ramjford Teeth

Table 10–5. Common Dental Indexes

Plaque, Debris, and/or Calculus

PHP: Patient Hygiene Performance
- To assess the extent of plaque and debris over a tooth surface

PHP-M: Patient Hygiene Performance Modified
- A modification of the PHP index

Plaque Control Record
- To record the presence of bacterial plaque on individual tooth surfaces

Plaque-Free Score
- To determine the location, number, and percent of plaque-free surfaces of individual motivation and instruction

Pl1: Plaque Index
- To assess the thickness of plaque at the gingival area

OHI: Oral Hygiene Index
- To measure existing plaque and calculus as an indication of oral cleanliness
- The OHI has two components, the debris index and the calculus index; the practitioner can evaluate both or just one

OHI-S: Simplified Oral Hygiene Index
- The same as the OHI, but only used six specific teeth

VMI: Vope-Manhold Index
- To assess the supragingival calculus after a dental cleaning

Gingival Bleeding

GBI: Gingival Bleeding Index
- To record the presence or absence of gingival inflammation as determined by bleeding from interproximal gingival sulci

SBI: Sulcus Bleeding Index
- To locate areas of the gingival sulcus bleeding upon gentle probing

Eastman Interdental Bleeding Index
- Measures papillary bleeding

(continued)

Table 10–5. *(continued)*

Gingival Changes/Gingivitis

GI: Gingival Index
• To assess the severity of gingivitis based on color, consistency, and bleeding on probing

MGI: Modified Gingival Index
• A modified GI, does not utilize bleeding upon probing

P-M-A: Papillary Marginal Attached Index
• To assess the extent of gingival changes including papillary, gingival margin and attached gingiva in large studies

Periodontal Diseases

PI: Periodontal Index
• To assess and score the periodontal disease status of populations in large studies

PDI: Periodontal Disease Index
• To assess the prevalence and severity of gingivitis and periodontitis and to show the periodontal status of an individual or a group

CPITN: Community Periodontal Index of Treatment Needs
• To screen and monitor individual or group periodontal treatment needs

PSR: Periodontal Screening and Recording
• A modified version of the CPITN to screen and monitor individuals or group periodontal needs

LPA: Loss of Periodontal Attachment
• Assesses the loss of periodontal attachment

ESI Extent and Severity Index
• Measures the extent and severity of loss of periodontal attachment

GPI: Gingival Periodontal Index
• Assesses the gingivitis and pocket depth in the dentition

Dental Caries

DEFT or S: Decayed Extracted, Filled Primary Teeth, or Tooth Surfaces
• To calculate the status of decay, extractions, and filled primary teeth or tooth surfaces

(continued)

Table 10–5. *(continued)*

DMFT or S: Decayed Missing Filled Permanent Teeth
- To calculate the status of decay, missing, and filled teeth or surfaces within the dentition, an indicator of dental caries activity

RI: Root Caries Index
- To calculate the status of root caries, usually recommended for adult surveys

Malocclusion

Malignment Index
- Assesses the rotations and tooth displacements

Occlusal Feature Index
- Assesses the crowding and interdigitation and vertical and horizontal overbites

Treatment Priority Index
- Assesses orthodontic treatment needs

Occlusal Index
- Assesses the various characteristics of occlusion including dental age, molar relation, overbite, overjet, posterior crossbite, posterior open bite, tooth displacement, midline relations, and missing permanent maxillary incisors

Dental Aesthetic Index
- Assesses esthetics of occlusion based on the impact it has on the social and psychological well-being of the individual

Dental Fluorosis

Developmental Defects of Dental Enamel
- Scores enamel opacities, regardless of origin to avoid any bias

Fluorosis Index
- Rate of fluorosis within a population, sensitive to mild through severe cases

Fluorosis Risk Index
- To assess fluorosis, particularly the specific time of enamel formation

Tooth Surface Index of Fluorosis
- Rate of fluorosis within a population; more sensitive than the fluorosis index

(continued)

Table 10–5. *(continued)*

Others

Cleft/Lip Palate
• Calculated as the terms of rate in the number of births in a population

Oral Cancer
• Calculated as the terms of rate in a population, sometimes broken down into strata

GOVERNMENTAL EVALUATION OF ORAL HEALTH

Healthy People 2010 have specific focus areas for oral health.[2] The oral health goal of Healthy People 2010 is to prevent and control oral and craniofacial diseases, conditions, and injuries and to improve access to related services. In fact, all of the oral health objectives in Healthy People 2010 include a way to measure the objective. Please see Table 10–6 for specific objectives and evaluation mechanisms.

A National Oral Health Surveillance System (NOHSS) has been developed based upon a set of oral health indicators from *Healthy People 2010*.[3] NOHSS is a collaborative effort between the Centers for Disease Control and Preventive and The Association of State and Territorial Dental Directors and is designed to help public health programs monitor the burden of oral diseases, the dental care delivery system, and fluoridation. (See Figure 10–2.) The oral health indicators include the list depicted in Table 10–7.

SUMMARY

Evaluation is a mandatory phase of any type of dental hygiene treatment, including public health. There are a variety of evaluation mechanisms that can be utilized in program planning. Program evaluation should be conducted during all phases of program planning. Dental indexes are frequently used to determine effectiveness of program planning at the prevention and treatment of dental diseases.

Table 10–6. Healthy People 2010: Oral Health Objectives and Evaluation

Objectives	Measurement Mechanism
Decrease deaths from oral and pharyngeal cancer	Number of oral cancer deaths per 100,000 population
Increase early detection of oral and pharyngeal cancer	Percentage of individuals with recent oral and pharyngeal examination within the past year
Increase annual examinations for oral and pharyngeal cancer	Percentage of persons with recent oral and pharyngeal cancer diagnosed at earliest stage
Decrease dental caries experience	Percentage of persons with ≥ 1 dft or DMFT
Decrease untreated dental decay	Percentage of persons with ≥ 1 dt or DT
Decrease permanent tooth loss	Percentage of persons with 28 teeth, no teeth extracted
Decrease complete tooth loss	Percentage of persons with all teeth extracted, edentulous
Reduce periodontal diseases	Percentage of persons with ≥ 1 bleeding site. Percentage of persons with ≥ 4 mm LOA in at least 1 site
Increase use of dental sealants	Percentage of persons with ≥ 1 sealant on permanent molars
Increase community water fluoridation	Percentage of people served by community water systems with optimal fluoride levels
Increase use of oral health care system	Percentage of individuals with annual dental visits
Increase use of oral health care system by residents using long-term care facilities	Percentage of nursing home residents with dental service within last year
Increase dental services for low-income children	Percentage of low-income children and adolescents with preventive dental service within last year
Increase school-based health centers with oral health component	Percentage of school-based health centers with an oral health component
Increase health centers with oral health component	Percentage of local health departments and community-based health centers with oral health component
Increase referral for cleft lip or palate	Percentage of states with system for recording and referring orofacial clefts

For more information, see http://www.healthypeople.gov.

Figure 10–2. National Oral Health Surveillance System

Analytic considerations for the surveys
(BRFSS, NHANES, NHIS, YRBSS) Estimates for certain population subgroups may be based on small numbers and be subject to relatively large sampling error. When the number of events is small and the probability of such an event is small, considerable caution must be observed in interpreting the conditions (cell size < 50). Data from multiple years may be pooled to obtain adequate sample size.

BRFSS
The Behavioral Risk Factor Surveillance System is a state-based, ongoing data collection program designed to measure behavioral risk factors in the adult, non-institutionalized population 18 years of age or older. Every month, states select a random sample of adults for a telephone interview. This selection process results in a representative sample for each state so that statistical inferences can be made from the information collected.

BSS
The Basic Screening Survey is a standardized set of surveys designed to collect information on the observed oral health of participants, self-report or observed information on age, gender, race and Hispanic ethnicity, and self-report information on access to care for preschool, school-age, and adult populations. The surveys are cross-sectional and descriptive. Observations of gross dental or oral lesions are made by dentists, dental hygienists, or other appropriate health care workers in accordance with state law. The examiner records presence of untreated cavities and urgency of need for treatment for all age groups. For preschool children, presence of early childhood caries and caries experience are also recorded. For school-age children, presence of sealants on permanent molars and caries experience are also recorded. Presence of edentulism (no natural teeth) is recorded for adults. States may use one or more of the surveys in the BSS to conduct screenings to obtain oral health status and dental care access data at a level consistent with monitoring Healthy People objectives. Training materials are provided with the surveys and technical assistance on sampling and analysis are available to states undertaking these surveys using the standard protocol. BSS was developed by the Association of State and Territorial Dental Directors with technical assistance from the Division of Oral Health, National Center for Chronic Disease Prevention and Health Promotion, Centers for Disease Control and Prevention.

1992 Fluoridation Census
The 1992 Fluoridation Census provides the fluoridation status for each state. States reported each fluoridated water system and the communities each system served; the status of fluoridation—adjusted, consecutive, or natural; the system from which water

(continued)

Figure 10–2.   *(continued)*

was purchased, if consecutive; the population receiving fluoridated water; the date on which fluoridation started; and the chemical used for fluoridation, if adjusted.

2000 Water Fluoridation Reporting System

Populations Receiving Optimally Fluoridated Public Drinking Water—United States, 2000 (*MMWR* Vol. 51, No. 7; 144–147.) provides the most recent information on the status of water fluoridation by state.

NHANES

Oral health data were collected in the National Health and Nutrition Examination Survey (NHANES I, NHANES III, and NHANES IV).

NHANES I was conducted between 1971 and 1975. This survey was based on a national sample of about 28,000 persons between the ages of 1–74. Extensive data on health and nutrition were collected by interview, physical examination, and laboratory analyses. The sampling design of NHANES I did not include persons of Hispanic/Latin origin.

NHANES III, conducted between 1988 and 1994, included about 40,000 people selected from households in 81 counties across the United States. To obtain reliable estimates, infants and young children (aged 1 to 5 years), older persons (aged 60 years and older), Black Americans and Mexican Americans were sampled at a higher rate. NHANES III also placed an additional emphasis on the effects of the environment upon health. Data were gathered to measure the levels of pesticide exposure, the presence of certain trace elements in the blood, and the amounts of carbon monoxide present in the blood.

NHANES IV began in April 1999 and will be a continuous survey visiting 15 U.S. locations per year. Approximately 5,000 people will be surveyed annually. Oral health data from NHANES IV will be added to NOHSS when the survey is completed.

NHIS

The National Health Interview Survey is a cross-sectional household interview survey on the health of the civilian noninstitutionalized population of the United States. The sampling plan follows a multistage area probability design that permits the representative sampling of households. NHIS data are collected annually from approximately 43,000 households including about 106,000 persons.

PRAMS

The Pregnancy Risk Assessment Monitoring System collects state-specific, population-based data on maternal attitudes and experiences prior to, during, and immediately following pregnancy. The PRAMS sample of women who have had a recent live birth is drawn from the state's birth certificate file. Each participating state samples between

(continued)

Figure 10–2. *(continued)*

1,300 and 3,400 women per year. Women from some groups are sampled at a higher rate to ensure adequate data are available in smaller but higher risk populations. Selected women are first contacted by mail. If there is no response to repeated mailings, women are contacted and interviewed by telephone. Data collection procedures and instruments are standardized to allow comparisons between states. PRAMS provides data for state health officials to use to improve the health of mothers and infants. PRAMS allows CDC and the states to monitor changes in maternal and child health indicators (e.g., unintended pregnancy, prenatal care, breastfeeding, smoking, alcohol use, infant health).

State Synopses

The Synopses of State Dental Public Health Programs collects oral health program information provided to the Association of State and Territorial Dental Directors (ASTDD) annually by each state's dental director or oral health program manager. ASTDD, in conjunction with CDC's Division of Oral Health, presents that information with data from standard sources (U.S. Census, Department of Education, Bureau of Labor Statistics, etc.) on the State Synopses Web site. Each state has its own synopsis which contains state-specific information on demographics, oral health infrastructure, oral health program administration and oral health program activities. An interactive national trend table aggregates that information to track changes over time. Maps display which states conduct each of 12 types of oral health activities and which states have full-time dental directors.

YRBSS

The Youth Risk Factor Surveillance System is a school-based survey conducted biennially to assess the prevalence of health risk behaviors among high school students. YRBSS includes national, state, territorial and local school-based surveys of high school students. The school-based survey employed a cluster sample design to produce a representative sample of students in grades 9–12. Survey procedures were designed to protect the students' privacy by allowing for anonymous and voluntary participation.

Source: http://www.cdc.gov/nohss/DSMain.htm.

Table 10-7.   Specific Indicators
Caries Experience
Complete Tooth Loss
Dental Sealants
Dental Visits
Fluoridation Status
Oral and Pharyngeal Cancer
Teeth Cleaning
Untreated Caries

REFERENCES

[1] See Wilkins, E. *Clinical Practice of the Dental Hygienist,* 8th Edition. Malvern, PA: Williams and Wilkins, 1999, for a detailed description on how to calculate dental indexes.

[2] U.S. Department of Health and Human Services. *Healthy People 2010: Understanding and Improving Health,* 2nd ed. Washington, DC: U.S. Government Printing Office, November 2000.

[3] http://www.cdc.gov/nohss.

Get Connected

Multimedia Extension Activities

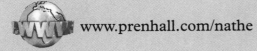 www.prenhall.com/nathe

Use the above address to access the free, interactive companion web site created specifically to accompany this textbook. Here you will find an array of self study material to help you gain a richer understanding of the concepts presented in this chapter.

Unit III

DENTAL HYGIENE RESEARCH

Dental hygiene practice is based upon published research, meaning that practitioner decisions are derived from documented evidence rather than anecdotal tradition. This is commonly referred to as evidence-based practice. Moreover, dental hygienists share the responsibility not only to practice science-based modalities, but also to increase the scientific body of knowledge that encompasses the dental hygiene sciences. It is imperative for the practitioner to be able to fully understand basic research principles. Additionally, dental hygienists must be able to critically evaluate scientific literature and dental care products and modalities. Most importantly, dental hygiene professionals must effectively communicate accurate information to the public, which it serves.

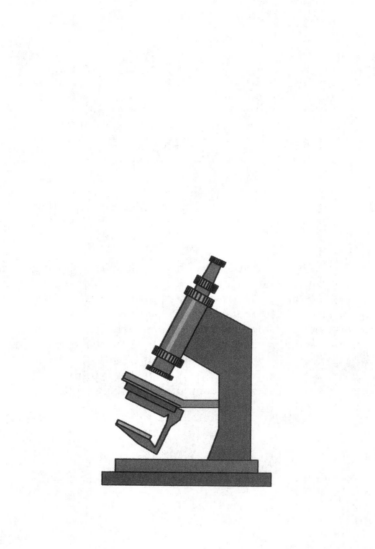

Chapter 11

THE ORAL EPIDEMIOLOGY
OF DENTAL DISEASES

OBJECTIVES

After studying this chapter, the dental hygiene student will be able to:

- define oral epidemiology and related terms.
- list and describe the publications reporting oral epidemiology.
- describe oral epidemiology and its relationship to dental hygiene.
- describe the current epidemiological issues of disease.

COMPETENCIES

After studying this chapter and participating in accompanying course activities, the dental hygiene student will be competent in the following:

- recognize and use written and electronic sources of information.
- evaluate published clinical and basic science research and integrate this information to improve the oral health of the patient.
- accept responsibility for solving problems and making decisions based on accepted scientific principles.
- recognize the responsibility and demonstrate the ability to communicate professional knowledge verbally and in writing.

KEY WORDS

Incidence	Oral epidemiology
Morbidity	Prevalence
Mortality	

INTRODUCTION

The study of disease in a target population is called epidemiology. The population can be as large as the entire globe or as small as a nursing home or elementary school. This science is concerned with many aspects of disease as it affects groups of people. Without the benefit of epidemiology and research, the dental hygienist in the private office would not understand how the patient acquired the disease or how to effectively offer treatment and suggest methods of prevention.[1] However, epidemiology includes more than the study of disease in a population. The science and tools of epidemiology are also used to study other trends related to health care, such as needle stick injuries among dental workers, the success of Hepatitis B immunization campaigns, and suicide rates among dentists, to name a few. As health care concerns become broader and more holistic, the science of epidemiology will expand to meet those research needs.

THE MULTIFACTORIAL NATURE OF DISEASE

Epidemiology attempts to understand the causes of disease in a population. At the turn of the century with the discovery of bacteria, the cause of acute disease was generally easy to establish. If a susceptible person was exposed to a particular bacterium in sufficient quantities, that person became ill with a disease. A simple cause-and-effect mechanism was understood to be at work. With the advent of antibiotics, life spans were extended, and the study of chronic disease became paramount. Within the last few decades, science and medicine have come to understand chronic disease (as well as many acute ones) as multifactorial processes. With cancer, for example, many factors interacted to cause the disease, including genetics, lifestyle, diet, occupational or recreational exposure to carcinogenic agents, and perhaps even a viral agent. No longer can a simple cause-and-effect mechanism be identified. Dental disease follows a similar multifactorial pattern (see Figure 11–1). Likewise, scientists are now exploring multifactoral approaches to the treatment of disease often referred to as holistic care. Designing such approaches makes research into the causes and treatments of disease much harder, but also much more necessary than ever.

EPIDEMIOLOGICAL TERMINOLOGY

Epidemiology also studies the trends or occurrence of disease in populations, commonly referred to as the incidence and prevalence of a disease. Although the terms may be unfamiliar, these examples will be familiar to most people. Incidence and prevalence are even occasionally reported in television commercials. **Incidence** is

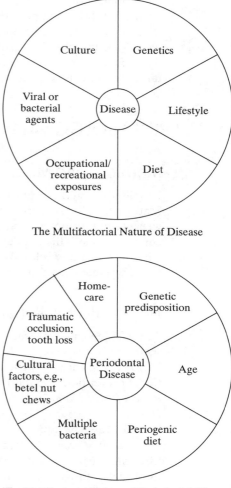

The Multifactorial Nature of Disease

The Multifactorial Nature of Periodontal Disease

Figure 11–1.   Multifactorial Nature
of Disease

simply the number of new cases of a disease during a certain period. For example, one hundred children at Knollwood Elementary School were diagnosed with caries in 1999. The **prevalence** of a disease is the number of people in a population with the disease at any given time. An example of prevalence would be that at the present time 95 percent of Americans have gingivitis. **Mortality** refers to the death rate in a population, and **morbidity** refers to the disease or sickness rate in a population.

Dental conditions readily lend themselves to the study of epidemiology. Specific tools have been developed to study dental disease more quickly and accurately. These tools are called dental indexes. They exist for a wide variety of dental conditions and diseases and are used to document the incidence, prevalence, and severity of disease in populations. For a thorough discussion of dental indexes, see Chapter 10. Because standard dental indexes have been in use for a long time and have been thoroughly tested to assure their validity, they make excellent tools for researchers who want to gather data on dental conditions. Please see Table 11–1 for commonly used terms and corresponding definitions in **oral epidemiology.**

ORAL EPIDEMIOLOGY REPORTS

Morbidity and Mortality Report

People interested in knowing current, relevant epidemiological facts in the United States typically subscribe to the Center for Disease Control and Prevention's weekly publication entitled the *Mortality and Morbidity Weekly Report* either in hard copy or online. This publication is a compilation of cogent issues currently studied. The data in the weekly *MMWR* are provisional, based on weekly reports to the CDC by state health departments.

Healthy People Reports

The U.S. federal government publishes reports that review the most current research in health care, including oral diseases. This report is entitled *Healthy People.* In 1979, the surgeon general's *Healthy People* Report laid the foundation for a national prevention agenda. Further, in 1980 *Promoting Health/Preventing Disease: Objectives for the Nation* and *Healthy People 2000: National Health Promotion and Disease Prevention Objectives* both established national health objective and served as the basis for the development of state and community plans.

    Healthy People 2010 sets the prevention agenda for the United States. It identifies the most significant preventable threats to health and establishes goals to reduce these threats. It builds upon health initiatives pursued over the past two decades. It contains a section on oral health, which sets the objectives outlined in Table 11–2.

Surgeon General's Reports

The first-ever comprehensive report on the status of the nation's oral health, released May 25, 2000, by Surgeon General David Satcher, MD, PhD, underscores the critical relationship between oral health and general health throughout life because the condition of the mouth directly mirrors the condition of the body.[2] In fact, the range of oral, dental, and craniofacial diseases and conditions that take a toll on the U.S. population is extensive. Specifically, there were eight major findings in the report included described in Table 11–2.

Table 11–1.	Terminology
Epidemiology:	The study of the amount, distribution, determinants and control of diseases and health conditions among given populations.
Epidemic:	A disease or condition occurring among many individuals in a community or region at the same time and usually spreading rapidly. Often called an "outbreak" of disease. Widespread outbreaks across a region or continent may be termed *pandemic* in extent.
Endemic:	A relatively low, but constant level of occurrence of a disease or health condition in a population.
Disease rates:	The number of cases or deaths among a population or target group during a given time period, expressed as a ratio. Rates are often statistically "adjusted" to make valid comparisons across different populations or to detect trends within the same population.
Mortality:	The ratio of the number of deaths from a given disease or health problem to the total number of cases reported.
Morbidity:	The ratio of "sick" (affected) individuals to well individuals in a community. It often measures the level of nonfatal health consequences (severity) of a disease or condition.
Prevalence:	A numerical expression of the number of all existing cases of a disease or problem in a population measured at a given point or period in time.
Incidence:	The number of new cases of a disease in a population over a given period of time.
Etiology:	The theory of causation for a disease or condition.
Risk factors:	Characteristics of an individual or population, which may increase the likelihood of experiencing a given health problem (e.g., age, gender, educational level, socioeconomic status).
Index:	A standardized method used to describe the status of an individual or group with respect to a given condition. Indexes usually involve a graduated scale for measuring the extent of the health problem.
Surveillance:	Methods or systems used to monitor disease and morbidity in a population periodically or on an ongoing basis. It is an important function of the Centers for Disease Control (CDC), National Center of Health Statistics (NCHS), and state health departments.

Table 11–2. Surgeon General's Major Findings

- Oral disease and disorders in and of themselves affect health and well-being throughout life.
- Safe and effective measures exist to prevent the most common dental disease—dental carries and periodontal diseases.
- Lifestyle behaviors that affect general health, such as tobacco use, excessive alcohol use, and poor dietary choices, affect oral and craniofacial health as well.
- There are profound and consequential oral health disparities within U.S. populations.
- More information is needed to improve Americans' oral health and eliminate health disparities.
- The mouth reflects general health and well-being.
- Oral diseases and conditions are associated with other health problems.
- Scientific research is the key to further reeducation in the burden of disease and disorders that affect the face, mouth, and teeth.

The report itself highlights the relationship between oral health and general health. Interestingly, the mouth and face are referred to as a mirror of health disease. Over twenty diseases and conditions that cause lesions of the oral mucosa were discussed. And associations among oral infections and diabetes, heart disease/stroke, respiratory ailments, and adverse pregnancy outcomes, such as premature births and low birth-weight babies, were addressed. The report also addressed the effects oral diseases have on well-being and quality of life. As hygienists are aware, tooth pain and oral disfigurement have impacts on eating, sleeping, cultural significance, social function, and economics.

And although the report does not mention the critical effect the dental hygiene profession has had in the past and can impact in the future on the prevention and treatment of dental diseases in America, it does highlight fluoridation, school water fluoridation, dietary fluoride supplements, fluoride mouthrinse programs, fluoride varnishes, dental sealants, and community programs as approaches to promote oral health and prevent oral disease. Fluoridated drinking water is reported to have made the single greatest impact on the prevention of oral diseases by providing fluoridated water to communities at a cost of 68 cents to $3.00 per person, depending on population size, which results in a 65 percent reduction in dental decay and cavities; yet only half of all U.S. water supplies are fluoridated.[3] This translates into 18,000 communities and 40 million children who go without fluoride in their drinking water.[4]

DENTAL HYGIENIST'S SPOTLIGHT
Beth McKinney, RDH, MS

I have been in public health most of my eighteen-year career as a dental hygienist. I received my bachelor of science degree in dental hygiene from the University of Maryland in Baltimore, Maryland, and my master of science degree in dental hygiene from Old Dominion University, in Norfolk, Virginia. I spent three years working in the dental insurance field doing quality assurance work. I then spent four years working for the Naval Dental Center in Norfolk, Virginia. It was exciting to treat a cohort of sailors and naval aviators along with twenty-two other dental hygienists in the command. I was employed by a dental contract agency in this position. I had the tremendous opportunity to spend two years at the National Institutes of Dental and Craniofacial Research, which is part of the National Institutes of Health in Bethesda, Maryland. I was able to work in a hospital setting treating patients and assisting with various research projects. I now work for Montgomery County in Maryland where I am responsible for maternity clients and quality assurance in the dental programs. In all these positions, I have enjoyed the mixture of clinical practice along with other skills such as administration, teaching, and research. Dental public health has allowed me to fully develop my skills as a health care professional.

A framework for action was discussed in the report, including the following recommendations:

- Change perceptions regarding oral heath and ideas so that oral health becomes an accepted component of general health.
- Accelerate the building of the science and evidence base, and apply science effectively to improve oral health.
- Build an effective health infrastructure that meets the oral health needs of all Americans and integrate oral health effectively into general health.
- Remove known barriers between people and oral health services.
- Use public-private partnerships to improve the oral health of those who still suffer disproportionately from oral disease.

In 2003, the U.S. Surgeon General published *A National Call to Action to Promote Oral Health (Call to Action)* which describes the ongoing effort to address the country's oral health needs in the twenty-first century. The *Call to Action* builds on *Oral Health in America: A Report of the Surgeon General* and the *Healthy People 2010* focus area on Oral Health. The *Call to Action* expands on these efforts by enlisting individuals from research, clinical care, and the community to work in collaboration for the oral health of society.

Global Oral Data Bank

The Global Oral Data Bank contains oral epidemiologic data from around the world. Data have been obtained from standard surveys assisted by the World Health Organization (WHO) or from published literature using comparable methods. In many cases they apply to large groups from the most populous parts of a country providing a working estimate rather than being fully representative. Sources/references are given under every data presented in the relevant country pages.

THE EPIDEMIOLOGY OF ORAL DISEASES

The range of oral, dental, and craniofacial ideas and conditions that affect the populations is extensive. Just as there is no single measure of overall health or overall disease, there is no single measure of oral health or the burden of oral diseases and conditions.[2] The following sections present epidemiological data of each specific oral disease or condition.

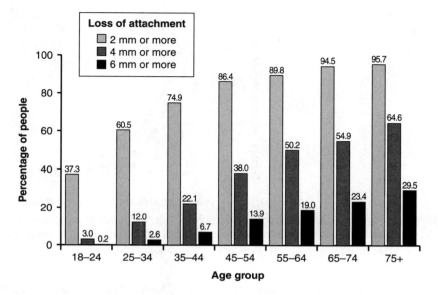

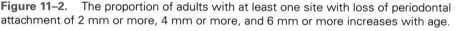

Figure 11–2.   The proportion of adults with at least one site with loss of periodontal attachment of 2 mm or more, 4 mm or more, and 6 mm or more increases with age.

Sources: Adapted from NCHS 1996; Burt and Eklund 1999.

Periodontal Diseases

As most dental hygienists could anecdotally predict, the majority of adults twenty-five years and older have at least 2 mm or more loss of attachment (see Figure 11–2).[5,6] In fact, the percentage of adults with 6 mm or more loss of attachment at one or more sites increases at older age groups with 19 percent of 55 to 64 year olds and 23.4 percent of 65 to 74 year olds have this amount of loss or more (see Figure 11–3).[5,6]

Men are more likely than women to have at least one tooth site with a 6 mm or more loss of attachment (see Figure 11–4).[5,6] Furthermore, at every age, a higher proportion of those at the lowest socioeconomic status (SES) have at least one site with attachment loss of 6 mm or more compared with those at higher SES level (see Figure 11–5).[5] Moreover, a higher percentage of non-Hispanic black persons at each age group have at least one tooth site with 6 mm or more of periodontal attachment losses compared with other groups.[5]

Tooth Loss

By the age of 50, most individuals in the United States have lost an average of 12.1 teeth, including third molars.[2] Overall, a higher percentage of individual living below the poverty level are edentulous than those who are living above (see Figure 11–6).[5,6]

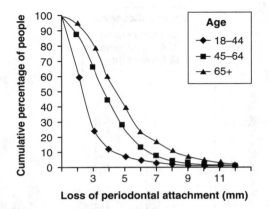

Figure 11–3. Although older adults have more periodontal attachment loss than younger adults, severe loss is seen among a small percentage of individuals at every age.

Sources: Adapted from NCHS 1996; But and Eklund 1999.

Although the overall rate of edentulism for adults 18 and older is approximately 10 percent, the rate increases with age, so that about a third of those 65 years and older are edentulous (see Figure 11–7).[7] In fact, of all population groups, Mexican Americans are the least likely to lose all of their teeth.[5]

Dental Caries

Dental caries is one of the most common childhood diseases. Among 5- to 17-year-olds, dental caries is more than 5 times as common as a reported history of asthma and 7 times as common as hay fever (see Figure 11–8).[5] The majority of

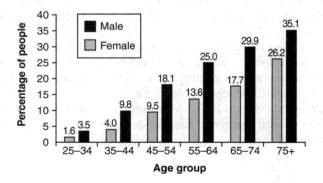

Figure 11–4. Males are more likely than females to have at least one tooth site with 6 mm or more of periodontal loss of attachment.

Sources: Adapted from NCHS 1996; Burt and Eklund 1999.

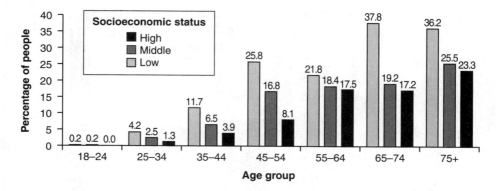

Figure 11–5. The percentage of adults with at least one tooth site with 6 mm or more of periodontal attachment loss is greater among persons of low socioeconomic status at all ages.

Sources: Adapted from NCHS 1996; Burt and Eklund 1999.

children aged 5 to 9 years had at least one carious lesion or filling in the coronal portion of either a primary or a permanent tooth.[5] This proportion increased in 77.9 percent for 17 year olds and 84.7 percent for adults 18 years or older.[5,7] Additionally, 49.7 percent of people 75 years or older had root caries affecting at least one tooth.[5]

Despite progress in reducing dental caries, individuals in families living below the poverty level experience more dental decay than those who are economically better off.[5] Furthermore, the caries seen in these individuals are more likely to be untreated than caries in those living above the poverty level.[5] See Figure 11–9. In addition to poverty level, the proportion of teeth affected by dental caries also varies by age and race/ethnicity.[5] Poor Mexican American children aged 2 to 9 have the highest number of primary teeth affected by dental caries compared with poor non-Hispanic blacks and non-Hispanic whites.[5] Among the nonpoor, Mexican American 2 to 9 year olds have the highest number of affected followed by non-Hispanic black and non-Hispanic whites.[5]

Adult populations (aged 18 and older) show a similar pattern.[5] The proportion of untreated decayed teeth is higher among the poor than the nonpoor (see Figure 11–10).[5] Regardless of poverty-level status, adult non-Hispanic blacks and Mexican Americans have higher proportions of untreated decayed teeth than their non-Hispanic white counterparts.[5]

Improvements have been noted over the past 25 years to 30 years with regard to dental caries.[5,7] Younger adults have experienced a decline in dental caries during this time period, as measured by the average number of teeth without decay or fillings (see Figure 11–11).[5,7] The number of untreated decayed teeth per person has also declined among all age groups.[5,7]

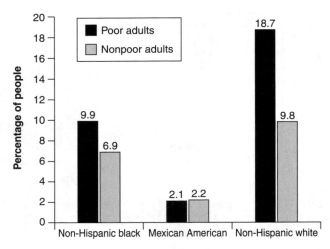

Figure 11–6. Complete tooth loss varies by race/ethnicity and poverty status: a higher percentage of poor and nonpoor non-Hispanic white adults (18 and older) have no teeth compared with non-Hispanic blacks and Mexican Americans.

Source: NCHS 1996.

Oral and Pharyngeal Cancer

Approximately 30,200 individuals develop oral and pharyngeal cancers every year in the United States, and, sadly, of these cases, about 7,800 Americans die each year.[8] The overall five-year survival rate for people with oral and pharyngeal cancer is about 52 percent.[9] Tobacco use has been estimated to account for over 90 percent of cancers of the oral cavity and pharynx.[10] Thus this represents the greatest single preventable risk factor for oral cancer (see Figure 11–12).

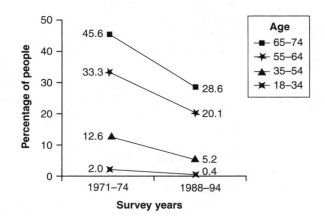

Figure 11–7. The percentage of people without any teeth has declined among adults over the past 20 years.

Sources: NCHS 1975, 1996.

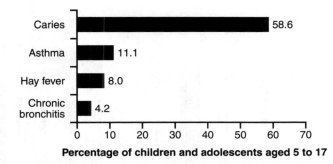

Figure 11–8.   Dental caries is one of the most common diseases among 5- to 17-year-olds.

Note: Data include decayed or filled primary and/or decayed, filled, or missing permanent teeth. Asthma, chronic bronchitis, and hay fever based on report of household respondent about the sampled 5- to 17-year-olds. *Source:* NCHS 1996.

Incidence rates for oral and pharyngeal cancers are higher for black individuals than for whites.[11] And in the United States, Asians and Pacific Islanders, American Indians and Alaska Natives, and Hispanics have lower incidence rates than whites and blacks (see Figure 11–13).[11]

Interestingly, the incidence rate for oral cavity and pharyngeal cancers is decreasing, with an estimated annual percentage decrease of .5 percent per year between 1973 and 1996.[9] Overall mortality rates for oral and pharyngeal cancers declined by 1.6 percent per year between 1973–96.[9]

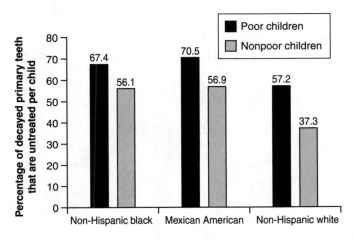

Figure 11–9.   Poor children aged 2 to 9 in each racial/ethnic group have a higher percentage of untreated decayed primary teeth than nonpoor children.

Source: NCHS 1996.

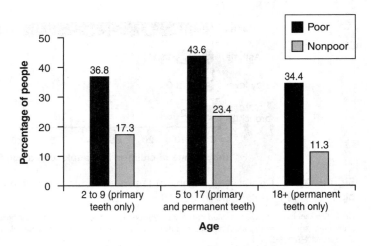

Figure 11–10. A higher percentage of poor people than nonpoor have at least one untreated decayed tooth.

Source: NCHS 1996.

Mucosal Infections and Diseases

The prevalence of recurrent herpes lesions is estimated to be between 15 and 40 percent.[12] Infection with the oral herpes simplex virus has been related to SES factors with 75–90 percent of individuals from lower socioeconomic populations developing antibodies by the end of the first decade of life.[13]

The prevalence of recurrent aphthous ulcers has indicated that the prevalence in the general population can vary from 5 to 25 percent.[14–17] The most frequently occurring lesions appear in the eighteen to twenty-four age group (see Figure 11–14).[7]

Figure 11–11. Since 1971–74, the average number of permanent teeth without decay or fillings has increased among 18- to 54-year-olds.

Sources: NCHS 1975, 1996.

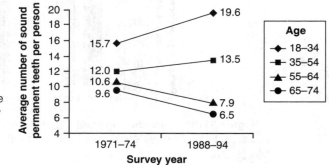

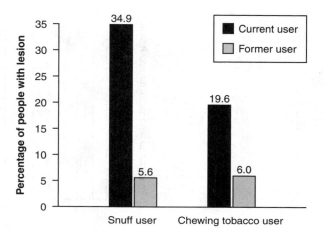

Figure 11–12.   Tobacco-related oral lesions are more common in 12- to 17-year-olds who currently use spit tobacco.

Source: Adapted from Tomar et al. 1997.

Oral candidiasis is found in individuals with impaired immune function, whereas oral human papillomavirus infections are common among individuals with HIV.[2] Denture stomatitis affects 26 percent of the people who have two full dentures.[2]

Cleft Lip/Palate

Cleft lip and palates are one of the most common classes of congenital malformation in the United States. The prevalence rates are 1.2 per 1,000 live births for cleft lip with or without cleft palate and .56 per 1,000 births for cleft palate alone.[18] Clefts lip/palates are more common in North American Indians (see Figure 11–15).[19]

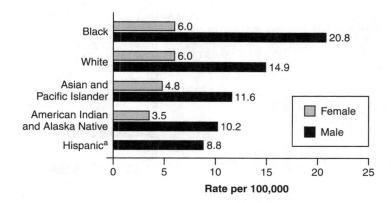

Figure 11–13.   Males have higher incidence rates of oral and pharyngeal cancers than females.

Note: Age adjusted to the 1970 U.S. standard.
[a]Data are unavailable for Hispanic females.
Sources: Adapted from Wingo et al. 1999; SEER Program, 1990–96; Ries et al. 1999.

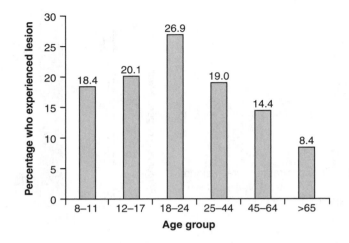

Figure 11–14.   A substantial percentage of the population, particularly among young adults, has experienced recurrent aphthous lesions (canker sores) in the past 12 months.

Source: Adapted from NCHS 1996.

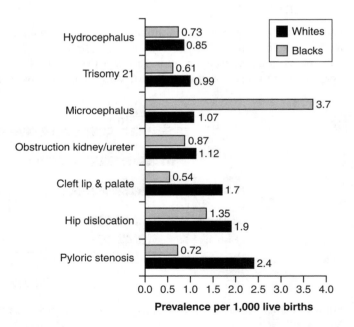

Figure 11–15.   Cleft lip and deft palate are among the most common congenital malformations, and prevalence varies by race.

Source: Schulman et al. 1993.

Injury

The leading causes of head and face injuries that result in emergency room visits include falls, assaults, sports injuries, and motor vehicle collision.[2] There were 20 million visits per year to emergency departments for craniofacial inures.[20] Less serious injuries that were treated by dentists in private office accounted for 5.9 million cases.[21]

Toothaches

Oral facial pain can greatly reduce quality of life.[2] Toothache pain can be caused by dental caries infections, periodontal infections, trauma, mucosal sores, and temporomandibular joint (TMJ) disorder. Twenty-two percent of adults experience at least one type of oral facial pain per six-month period.[22] In fact, adults living in poverty were more likely to report toothaches than adults living above the poverty level.[23]

SUMMARY

More information is needed in the field of oral epidemiology. In fact, many oral health disparities exist between gender, race/ethnicity, age, and SES. Periodontal diseases and dental caries are major issues in the nation's health and are widespread in the United States. These findings reflect the overall minor value society places on oral health care. Moreover, there are a variety of oral diseases and conditions that individuals in the United States experience. The dental hygienist must be aware of the epidimiology of all oral diseases, conditions and manifestations.

Author's Note

Most of the information on the epidemiology of oral diseases and conditions in the United States was derived from the following: U.S. Department of Health and Human Services. *Oral Health in America: A Report of the Surgeon General.* Rockville, MD: U.S. Department of Health and Human Services, National Institute of Dental and Craniofacial Research, National Institutes of Health, 2000.
For More Information on the Report: http://www.hhs.gov.

REFERENCES

[1]Darby, M. L. The missing link in professional validation. *RDH* 5 (1985): 10–15.
[2]U.S. Department of Health and Human Services. *Oral Health in America: A Report of the Surgeon General.* Rockville, MD: U.S. Department of Health and

Human Services, National Institute of Dental and Craniofacial research, National Institutes of Health, 2000.

[3]Ringlelberg, M. L., S. J. Allen, and L. J. Brown. Cost of fluoridation: 44 Florida communities *Journal of Public Health Dentistry* 52 no. 2, (1992): 75–80.

[4]U.S. Department of Health and Human Services (USDHHS). Fluoridation census, 992. Atlanta: U.S. Public Health Service, Centers for Disease Control and Prevention, Division of Oral Health, 1993.

[5]National Center for Health Statistics (NCHS). Third National Health and Nutrition Examination Survey (NHANES III) Reference Manuals and Reports, 1996.

[6]Burt, B. A. and S. A. Eklund. *Dentistry, Dental Practice, and the Community.* Philadelphia: W. B. Saunders, 1999.

[7]National Center for Health Statistics (NCHS) First National Health and Nutrition Examination Survey (NHANES I). Hyattsville, MD: NCHS U.S. Department of Health and Human Services, Public Health Services, Centers for Disease Control, 1975.

[8]American Cancer Society (ACS). *Cancer Facts and Figures.* Atlanta, GA: American Cancer Society, 1999.

[9]Ries, L. A. et al., eds. *SEER Cancer Statistics Review 1973–1996.* Bethesda, MD: National Cancer Institute, 1999.

[10]Tomar, S. L. et al. Oral mucosal smokeless tobacco lesions among adolescents in the United States. *Journal of Dental Research* 76 no. 6 (June 1997): 1277–86.

[11]Wingo P. A. et al. Annual report to the nation on the status of cancer, 1973–1996. With a special section on lung cancer and tobacco smoking. *Journal of the National Cancer Institute* 91 (1999): 675–90.

[12]Scully, C. Herpes simplex virus (HSV). In Millard H. D., and D. K. Mason, eds. *World Workshop on Oral Medicine, 1988 Jun 19–25.* Chicago: Year Book Medical Publishers, 1989, p. 160.

[13]Whitley, R. J. Prospects for vaccination against herpes simplex virus. *Pediatric Annals* 22 (1993): 726–32.

[14]Axell, T., H. Mornstad, and B. Sundstrom. The relation of the clinical picture to the histopathology of snuff dipper's lesions in Swedish population. *Journal of Oral Pathology* 5 no. 4 (July 1976): 229–36.

[15]Embil, J. A., R. G. Stephens, and F. R. Manuel. Prevalence of recurrent herpes labialis and aphthous ulcers among young adults on six continents. *Canadian Medical Association Journal* 113 no. 7 (October 4, 1975): 627–30.

[16]Ship, I. I. Epidimiologic aspects of recurrent aphthous ulcerations. *Oral Surgery Oral Medicine Oral Pathology* 33 no. 3 (March 1972): 400–406.

[17]Ship, I. I., V. J. Brightman, and L. L. Loaster. The patient with recurrent aphthous ulcers and the patient with recurrent herpes laibalis: a study of two population samples. *Journal of the American Dental Association* 75 no. 3 (September 1967): 645–54.

[18]Schulman, J. et al. Surveillance for and comparison of birth defect prevalence in two geographic areas—United States, 1983–88. *Morbidity and Mortality Weekly Report* 42 no. 1 (March 19, 1993): 1–7.

[19]Lowry, R. B., N. Y. Thunem, and S. H. Uh. Birth prevalence of cleft lip and palate in British Columbia between 1952 and 1986: Stability of rates. *Canadian Medical Association Journal* 140 no. 10 (May 15, 1989): 1167–70.

[20]Gift, H. C., and M. Bhat. Dental visits for orofacial injury: Defining the dentist's role. *Journal of the American Dental Association* 124 no. 11 (November 1993): 92–96, 98.

[21]Kaste, L. M., H. C. Gift, M. Bhat, and P. A. Swango. Prevalence of incisor trauma in persons 6–50 years of age: United States, 1988–1991. *Journal of Dental Research* 75 (Spec. No. February 1996a): 696–705.

[22]Lipton, J. A., J. A. Ship, and D. Larach-Robinson. Estimated prevalence and distribution of reported orofacial pain in the United States. *Journal of the American Dental Association* 124 no. 10 (October 1993): 113–21.

[23]Vargas, C. M., M. D. Macek, and S. E. Marcus. Sociodemographic correlates of tooth pain among adults: United States 1989. *Pain* 85 nos. 1–2 (March 2000): 87–92.

Get Connected

Multimedia Extension Activities

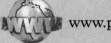 www.prenhall.com/nathe

Use the above address to access the free, interactive companion web site created specifically to accompany this textbook. Here you will find an array of self study material to help you gain a richer understanding of the concepts presented in this chapter.

Chapter 12

:::

RESEARCH IN DENTAL HYGIENE

OBJECTIVES

After studying this chapter, the dental hygiene student will be able to:

- describe the reasons for conducting research in dental hygiene.
- define the purpose of dental hygiene research.
- list and explain the various research approaches.
- compare research designs.

COMPETENCIES

After studying this chapter and participating in accompanying course activities, the dental hygiene students will be competent in the following:

- recognize and use written and electronic sources of information.
- recognize the responsibility and demonstrate the ability to communicate professional knowledge verbally and in writing.
- accept responsibility for solving problems and making decisions based on accepted scientific principles.
- expand and contribute to the knowledge base of dental hygiene.

KEY WORDS

Informed consent

Literature review

Research approaches

Sampling techniques

www.prenhall.com/nathe

INTRODUCTION

Dental public health is based upon programs that have demonstrated effectiveness in achieving health for the population. In order to develop programs that are measurable in terms of effectiveness, it is necessary for the dental hygienist to understand basic research principles.

In fact, most dental hygiene practice exists within the confines of a private clinical setting. The dental hygienist is concerned with a single patient at any given time; diagnosing that individual's condition and conducting both prevention programs and treatment are designed to put that patient in an optimal state of oral health. But the ability of that dental hygienist to do so is really predicated on a much larger sphere in which the study of dental disease and the creation of dental practices originate: the world of public health research.

RESEARCH AND DENTAL PUBLIC HEALTH

The study of disease in populations is accomplished by conducting research using the scientific method. The accuracy of the research determines the usefulness of the information obtained and the conclusions that can be drawn. Is this important to the private practitioner? If dental hygiene advice and treatment are to be based on known methods with predictable results rather than anecdotes, then it is crucial. Students in the early twenty-first century are likely to learn the practice of dental hygiene based on the research done by other practitioners and scientists as reported in medical and dental hygiene journals. For example, in a patient with condition x, the standard treatment modality is y. Z results can be expected in 85 percent of cases treated in this fashion. Dental hygienists who graduated from school several decades ago were more likely to base their practices on what their instructors learned from trial and error and anecdotal reports of other hygienists, the proverbial "what worked for them." Although this approach is frequently the mode for treatment, for medical science it is not the most scientific or the most reliable method.

How has dental hygiene practice changed as a result of research? For many years, instructors taught that fluoride treatments were done only after scaling and polishing. Likewise the patient at home was instructed to do brushing and flossing prior to rinsing with fluoride. Why? The prevailing argument was that the plaque needed to be removed for the fluoride to be effective. It remained the standard for many years. However, research has not born out the truth of this teaching. Research studies have revealed that fluoride can indeed penetrate plaque.[1]

The "truth" is that plaque removal is not necessary for fluoride treatments, either at home or in the office, to be effective. This type of practice is referred to as evidenced-based practice, implying that dental hygiene practice is based upon documented evidence from critically reviewed research.[2] How many dental hygienists still practice and teach to their patients the "old" way of thinking? Here, the anecdotal method and the method based on scientific research differ widely. The importance of conducting dental hygiene research is in its scientific basis for the practice of dental hygiene. The benefit of understanding something about research methods is that it allows any dental hygienist, whether directly involved in conducting research or only occasionally reading about it, to critically decide whether the research has scientific merit and should be applied in daily practice. If dental hygiene is to evolve as a specific, scientific discipline, a separate research base must be established. Dental hygienists need to conduct dental hygiene research in order to validate our current methods of practice and to investigate new ones. Because of what is now known about the multifactorial nature of disease, trying an anecdotal treatment on patient A with success does not guarantee that patient B will enjoy the same success.

TYPES OF RESEARCH

Dental hygiene research can be categorized in many ways. All have strengths and weaknesses. A pilot study is a small version of a proposed study, which is carried out on a small, sometimes intentionally chosen sample. It is a way of working out unforeseen errors in research design. After conducting a pilot study, revisions can be made in the research design to allow for better accuracy of results before the larger study is conducted.

Various approaches can be utilized for dental hygiene research; all involve observation, description, measurement, analysis, and interpretation of occurring phenomena.[3] Types of research can be classified as historical, descriptive, prospective (epidemiological), retrospective (ex post facto), and experimental. Please see Table 12–1 for examples of these studies.

Historical Approach

Natural history studies attempt to learn about and characterize a new disease and its process over time. It helps to establish the incidence and prevalence of a disease in a population. Various methods may be used to gather data, from questionnaires to clinical testing. No interventions are studied in this type of research.

Descriptive Approach

The descriptive approach includes a variety of types of studies. These include approaches that contain survey, observational, and correlation studies.

Table 12–1. Research Approaches

Approach	Definition/Purpose	Methods	Limitations	Example Applications
Historical	To determine the meaning of past events	Records review Interviews Literature review	Location of accurate data Gaps in the knowledge No replication Biased reports Distortion of events	The development of the American Dental Hygienists' Association Water fluoridation from 1945 to 1975
Descriptive	To describe and interpret current events or situations Types: **Survey** Gathers broad information about status quo. Usually involves a large sample size	Questionnaires Opinionnaires Interviews Indices	Lacks depth	Use of pit & fissure sealants by dental hygienists Caries experience of high school sophomores
	Case Study In-depth report on a single person, group, event, or situation	Interviews Observation Testing Records review	Unique Cannot be replicated Subject to bias	Orthodontic case report Water fluoridation in Meridian, Idaho

Type	Description	Disadvantages	Examples
Developmental	Studies growth, development, maturation, or change over a period of time		
Cross Sectional	Studies a cross-section of the population in a limited period of time	Obtaining representative population	Primary teeth exfoliation patterns
Longitudinal	Studies the same population over an extended period of time	Time consuming Longer financial commitment Loss of subjects	Changes in the periodontium over time
Document or Content Analysis	Analyzes the documents themselves Examination of records or documents for specific information or presentation style	Subjectivity in evaluation	Evaluation of dental journals for types of articles printed Sex biases in dental hygiene textbooks

(continued)

Table 12–1. (*continued*)

Trend Study	Combines descriptive and historical research to establish patterns from the past and present in order to predict future occurences	Records review Review of the Literature Interviews Observation Surveys	Long-range prediction is less valid and reliable than short-range prediction	Actions of the ADHA from 1960 to 1984 regarding expanding the duties of dental auxiliaries The use of sugar substitutes in carbonated beverages
Correlational Study	Measure the relationship between variables	Comparison of two sets of data	Correlation does not indicate a cause-effect relationship exists between variables (Post Hoc Fallacy) Plausible rival hypotheses	Frequency of flossing and periodontal disease Predental hygiene grades and clinical dental hygiene grades
Experimental	To investigate cause-and-effect relationships Involves manipulation of variables	Manipulation of one or more independent variables Control of extraneous variables	Artificiality due to amount of control Decreased external validity	Effect of intraoral sodium bicarbonate rinses on the periodontal ligament of laboratory rats. Life expectancy of dental restorative materials in vitro.

		Measurement of dependent variable(s) Use of a control group		
Quasi-experimental	Approximates true experimental approach but lacks control of true experimentation	Same as experimental except lacks the control of a true experimental design	Decreased internal validity Lack of control of extraneous variables	Effect of intraoral sodium bicarbonate rinses on the periodontal ligament of dental patients. Life expectancy of dental restorative materials in vivo
Ex Post Facto (Causal-Comparative)	To investigate existing differences to determine possible causes. (Reverse of experimental approach)	Reverse of experimental approach Independent variable is not manipulated	Cannot determine causal relationship Can only determine functional relationship Independent variable cannot be manipulated	Periodontal Disease (study adults over 40 with periodontal disease and adults over 40 without periodontal disease) Oral Cancer (similar methodology)

Source: Adapted from Darby, M. L., and Bowen, D. M. *Research Methods for Oral Health Professionals.* St. Louis: C. V. Mosby, 1980.

Survey research is that type of research done with data collecting techniques such as written or oral questionnaires or dental indexes. No interventions can be done in this kind of research.

Observational studies are those that simply observe events as they are. No intervention is done. Observational studies, like natural history studies, attempt to comprehensively describe a condition or situation.

In 1777, a Gloucestershire milkmaid told her physician, Dr. Edward Jenner, that contracting cowpox had been a fortunate event, since it conferred protection against smallpox. This bit of folk wisdom led Jenner to write his friend and mentor John Hunter about the possibility of preventing smallpox on a grand scale. Jenner's studies established the scientific principle that eventually resulted in driving smallpox from the face of the earth. The incentives and rewards for conducting clinical research from a simple case study were never clearer.[4] A case study is research about a specific incidence of the disease in one person. A case series is a report about a small group of people and cannot be generalized to the overall population. It often, however, makes for the most interesting reading and frequently is applicable to clinical practice.

Correlation research attempts to establish the cause and effect of a disease; however, this approach does not provide evidence for a cause-and-effect relationship between variables, rather than a correlation relationship. This approach is exploratory in nature and should then be followed up with an experimental study to determine whether a cause-and-effect relationship exists. Indexes and survey methodology as well as clinical testing may be used. Correlation research can look both forward and backward in time at a population, as well as study specific instances of the disease occurrence.

Epidemiological Approach

Epidemiological research follows a subpopulation, or cohort, of people with the disease over time. It may be a natural history study or the research may be investigating a treatment. Longitudinal studies are those that follow the study participants over long periods of time. Most research in breast cancer, for example, is done with longitudinal studies. Cross-sectional studies use many subjects from many subpopulations, but they are only looked at or investigated one time.

Thirty years ago in Claxton, Georgia, population 2,000, a rural physician became intrigued with the unusually high rates of cardiovascular morbidity and mortality in his region. His quest for a reason, aided by university-based researchers, the National Institutes of Health, and the Centers for Disease Control, led to more than 100 published reports and to a preventive-based medical model for disease.[5]

Retroactive (Ex Post Facto) Approach

A retrospective study looks at a group of people with the disease in the past. Usually this type of research is conducted via medical records. Obviously this type of research is not experimental in nature. An interesting example of this approach is a study of pregnant women that describes a mother's nutrition and fluoride uptake during gestation. An investigator may utilize past medical records to ascertain the nutritional habits and fluoride uptake of women during the forty weeks of gestation. Infant records of dental caries could be compared with the results. Obviously, a researcher would not wish to recommend that the control group does not ingest any fluoride or inadequate nutrition as an experimental group in this type of study; consequently, a retroactive study, although not controlled, can lend some valuable information.

Experimental (Prospective) Approach

Experimental research, or clinical trials, is probably the research most familiar to the lay person. In this type of research, an experimental treatment or intervention is studied in a group of people or animals. The treatment may be a new drug or surgical procedure. Most commonly, experimental research is conducted by double-blind studies, that is, a research project where neither the subjects nor the investigators know who is in the control (or placebo) group and who is in the group that received the experimental treatment. This type of study is considered to be highly reliable because it eliminates a great deal of bias on the part of the researcher. If the investigator does not know which treatment a subject received, then the researcher cannot make any suggestive comments to the participant, and the data collection can be done without any preconceived expectations. How is a double-blind study accomplished? Suppose a dental hygienist were providing services in a correctional facility and wanted to evaluate the relative merits of rinsing with chlorhexidine over a commercially available mouthrinse. A pharmacist could dispense two rinses: both blue and mint flavored in identical unmarked bottles. The pharmacist would keep a record of which subjects received which rinse but neither the hygienist nor the subjects would know. The hygienist, therefore, could not inadvertently suggest to the patients that one rinse is superior, and any indexes would be scored without the preconceived expectation that the subjects on chlorhexidine "should" be better than the control subjects. The dental hygienist, then, could not bias the results of the study.

A quasi-experimental study is actually designed as an experimental study but lacks inherent control. Results may be used when planning further studies.

THE RESEARCH QUESTION

Research is a time-consuming, tedious, and often expensive venture. It is carefully planned and executed. Often it is unrewarding when the null hypothesis proves to be correct and the experimental treatment had no benefit. Research design should be carefully planned. The first step in the planning process is the development of a hypothesis. Where do hypotheses come from? Hypotheses are the result of asking a question that can be researched.

> Question: Does brand X toothpaste really whiten teeth?
>
> Positive Hypothesis: Brand X does significantly whiten teeth.
>
> Null Hypothesis: There is no statistically significant difference between brand X and a placebo when comparing the whitening of teeth.

> Question: Which mechanical means of instrumentation is superior?
>
> Positive Hypothesis: Ultrasonic instrumentation is significantly better than hand scaling.
>
> Null Hypothesis: Ultrasonic instrumentation is not significantly better than hand scaling.

Often the questions arise from researcher observations and questions about observed occurrences. They can also come from questions arising out of previous research projects and from colleagues' experiences. In order for a hypothesis to be considered researchable, it must possess the characteristics in Table 12–2. Hypotheses are often stated in the null form, which actually provides a psychological advantage of sorts. If the researcher finds that a significant difference does exist, the null hypothesis can be rejected. By so doing the investigator is saying that a difference does exist.[6]

RESEARCH DESIGN

Once a valid hypothesis is stated, then the researcher must write a research proposal or protocol. Planning and conducting research is not for the faint of heart. It requires dedication and patience. The entire research process is summarized in Figure 12–1. Writing a research protocol involves several steps. The first of course is defining the problem by formulating a hypothesis. This step is followed by conducting a review of the literature to determine what is currently known about the issue. The researcher may find that the question has already been answered, or may find little information on the subject.

The second step is to design the research project. How will the question be answered? What method will be used to gather data? Will the project require any manipulation of subjects? Will human subjects be needed? Will additional collaborators be needed to conduct the research? How will they be calibrated? Will funds and/or supplies be needed? How will they be purchased? Will human subjects

Table 12–2.   Hypothesis Characteristics

Feasible
    Adequate number of subjects
    Adequate technical expertise
    Affordable in time and money
    Manageable in scope

Interesting to the investigator

Novel
    Confirms or refutes previous findings
    Extends previous findings
    Provides new findings

Ethical

Relevant
    To scientific knowledge
    To clinical and health policy
    To future research directions

Source: Hulley, S., and S. Cummings. *Designing Clinical Research.* Baltimore, MD: Williams & Wilkins, 1988.

be compensated? Have the data collection instruments been used before and are they valid? Can the resulting data be statistically analyzed? What statistical methods will be used? How many subjects are needed? Will a control group be used? How will the sample groups be selected? Does a pilot study need to be conducted first?

All these questions, and likely others as well, need to be carefully thought out and planned before the researcher recruits the first subject or sends out the first questionnaire. For this reason, research is often time-consuming and requires months or years to conduct. Teaching actual methodology of research is beyond the scope of this textbook; for more detailed information, the reader is referred to specific textbooks on research and/or a separate class on the subject.

RESEARCH METHODS

Developing the methods of a study depends on the **research approach** chosen. If a descriptive study is chosen, development of a survey may be indicated. Designing historical approaches and retroactive studies should be completed while choosing the statistical methods that will be utilized. It is necessary at this step to fully develop the design and statistical methods that will be employed.

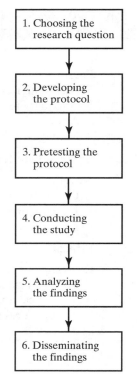

Figure 12–1.   Research Process

Experimental approaches are frequently clinical, laboratory, or epidemiological in nature and tend to employ specific designs. Designs employed may include a two-group pretest/posttest, time series, posttest only, Solomon three- and four-group designs, quasi-experimental and factorial designs. Figure 12–2 explains these frequently employed designs.

Experimental research frequently uses placebos and control groups. The control group is the matched group with the disease/condition not receiving the experimental treatment. The placebo is commonly thought of as the "sugar pill" but in fact the term placebo is more wide reaching. It may, in fact, be a sugar pill—a nontreatment. More likely though it is either the standard drug of choice for a disease or the standard treatment procedure against which the experimental one is being compared. The placebo effect is a term commonly used to refer to the real physical benefit that occurs when the subjects (patients) believe that they are taking something that will make them better. It speaks strongly to the multifactorial nature of disease and its treatment. Good experimental designs take this effect into account.

Is it ethical to use placebos when investigating life-threatening illnesses? The scientific method regarding the use of placebos underwent change during the era when many of the drugs now used to treat HIV were being developed. The study populations were understandably upset at possibly getting a placebo when they had

One-Group Time Series Design

Repeated Pretest Measures	Independent Variable	Repeated Post-Test Measures
Y_1 Y_2 Y_3	X	Y_4 Y_5 Y_6

Control Group Time Series Design

Group	Repeated Pretest Measures	Independent Variable	Repeated Post-Test Measures
E	Y_1 Y_2 Y_3	X	Y_4 Y_5 Y_6
C	Y_1 Y_2 Y_3	—	Y_4 Y_5 Y_6

Randomized Subjects Pretest/Post-Test Design

Groups	Pretest	Independent Variable	Post-Test
(R) E	Y_1	X	Y_2
(R) C	Y_1	—	Y_2

Randomized Subjects Post-Test Only Design

Group	Independent Variable	Post-Test
(R) E	X	Y_2
(R) C	—	Y_2

Randomized Matched Subjects Post-Test Only Design

Group	Independent Variable	Post-Test
(RM) E	X	Y_2
(RM) C	—	Y_2

Solomon Three-Group Design

Group	Pretest	Independent Variable	Post-Test
(R) E	Y_1	X	Y_2
(R) C_1	Y_2	—	Y_2
(R) C_2	—	X	Y_2

Figure 12–2.   Research Design

Source: Darby, M. L., and D. M. Bowen. *Research Methods for Oral Health Professionals: An Introduction.* St. Louis, MO: C. V. Mosby, 1980.

a fatal, incurable disease. The new standard in drug trials is now to do preliminary statistics after a period of a few months. If the new drug is unequivocably effective, all participants are offered the drug. If not, then those participants who received the placebo are offered the same trial period with the experimental drug after they complete the study if they so desire. Fortunately, dental hygiene research does not typically deal with such ethical dilemmas.

SAMPLING TECHNIQUES

Generally, it is impossible for a researcher to study an entire population that may be affected by a particular disease. The logistics and cost of such research would be prohibitive. Therefore, the researcher selects a sample population to study. To generalize research results to the whole population, the researcher must be sure that the sample is a representative subset. The best way of ensuring adequate representation is to take a random sample. Every possible subject is selected independently and has an equal chance of being selected. Selection can be done by lottery for a small sample or by

DENTAL HYGIENIST'S SPOTLIGHT
A Day in the Life of Ruth Nowjack-Raymer, RDH, MPH, PHD

Ruth Nowjack-Raymer was raised on a farm in the foothills of the Appalachian Mountains in eastern Ohio.

Oral disease prevention was virtually unheard of at that time, and many people assumed that they had "soft teeth" and that dental decay, periodontal disease, and tooth loss could not be prevented. In addition to lack of knowledge about oral disease prevention, this part of the country periodically had unemployment rates over 20 percent; thus, dental care was a luxury many could not afford.

Dr. Nowjack-Raymer had never heard of dental hygienists until she was looking at college catalogs and read about a profession whose goal it was to prevent dental disease. Prevent dental disease . . . how exciting! She imagined becoming a registered dental hygienist and returning to her home area to practice oral disease prevention in a mobile dental hygiene clinic going from town to town, to schools, work sites, and on home visits to people in need.

In 1969 Dr. Nowjack-Raymer entered The Ohio State University, Division of Dental Hygiene, and worked in the dental school's administrative office, cleaned houses, and was a nurse's aide in a nursing home at night.

A few weeks prior to completing the dental hygiene curriculum, Dr. Nowjack-Raymer learned that dental hygienists, even though they were licensed, were not permitted at that time to practice in public health settings without direct supervision. Her plans to provide prevention-oriented services from a mobile unit in rural Ohio were dashed. So, she continued her education and received a bachelor's degree in science with an emphasis on health education. Following graduation she worked in clinical practice for a decade and became involved with the component dental hygiene organization hoping to find a way to bring preventive care to under- and unserved people.

Dr. Nowjack-Raymer quickly rose through the ranks within her component (Columbus) and constituent (Ohio) dental hygiene organizations, serving as president of both. Involvement with the professional organizations gave her many opportunities to develop skills in management, project development and implementation, and lobbying within the state legislature.

Shortly thereafter the Ohio Department of Health vitalized its dental public health activities by hiring a progressive public health dentist who created numerous positions for baccalaureate-educated dental hygienists. The dental director had met Dr. Nowjack-Raymer through her role in the Ohio Dental Hygienists' Association and encouraged

(continued)

Dental Hygienist's Spotlight   *(continued)*

her to consider a career in public health.

In 1982 she joined the staff and was delighted to implement school-based fluoride programs in both rural and urban settings. Her long-held dream of preventing oral diseases amongst under- and unserved populations was finally being realized.

In 1984 Dr. Nowjack-Raymer received a master's of public health from the University of Michigan where she studied epidemiology, biostatistics, critical review of the literature, scientific writing, and public health administration. In addition she had the opportunity to do clinical dental examinations in accordance with epidemiological methods and analyze the data. All these new skills were essential to her public health career. One of the requirements for a master's in public health at the University of Michigan was the completion of an internship. Dr. Nowjack-Raymer was thrilled to have the opportunity to serve as an intern with the World Health Organization at its headquarters in Geneva, Switzerland. Her project was to evaluate health education approaches used by all of the varied WHO programs with respect to adults in developing nations. Through this internship Dr. Nowjack-Raymer had the opportunity to meet and interview leaders in international public health from many diverse areas, including typhoid, malaria, immunizations, and pharmaceutical distribution, and to hear the fascinating stories of their successes and frustrations. She

worked closely with the Oral Health Unit and learned of their tireless efforts globally, and she observed their expertise in the protocol of multicultural, international diplomacy.

Following the internship she returned to the Ohio Department of Health as the manager of the Family and Child Health component of the Division of Dental Health and was in charge of developing, implementing, and monitoring programs, policies, and grants for the state's Maternal and Child Health Clinics and Project Head Start.

In 1985 Dr. Nowjack-Raymer was asked to join the staff of what is now the National Institute of Dental and Craniofacial Research in Bethesda, Maryland, a part of the National Institutes of Health of the U.S. federal government. As a clinical trials specialist, Dr. Nowjack-Raymer coordinated and provided oversight of school-based clinical trials related to fluorides and dental sealants. During her fourteen years with the National Institute of Dental and Craniofacial Research, Dr. Nowjack-Raymer, who is now a public health research specialist, has served as a principal investigator, coproject officer, and coordinator of clinical trials and epidemiologic studies related to periodontal disease prevention, the oral manifestations of HIV infection, and a planned national survey of school-aged children. She completed a fellowship in oral clinical research methods at the University of Washington in Seattle as a

(continued)

computer selection for a large sample. Diseases that are more rare, such as juvenile periodontitis, may not lend themselves to such techniques. A researcher may desire to study an entire sample population that can be attained.

Systematic technique samples every nth subject; randomizing a sample would more likely create a sample more similar to the population than systematic sampling. Similarly if the researcher wants to study the prevalence of oral cancer at a nursing home, the research may be able to study the "whole" population. Results, however, could not be applied to other nursing homes because in essence a convenience sample was studied. For the study to be generalized, a sample of residents in multiple facilities would be needed.

A researcher has the ability to further stratify the sample during the study. By defining information such as age, gender, income level, or educational levels of subjects, the investigator can further generalize results to these strata within the population. For example, within a periodontal disease study an investigator may be able to suggest that males tended to have better oral hygiene during the study than females by stratifying the samples. This information can indeed be helpful when studying disease.

INFORMED CONSENT WHEN USING HUMAN SUBJECTS

Public health research often involves studying people. When research involves human subjects, an **informed consent** must be obtained with one exception. If the research is of the survey methodology, such as a questionnaire or an interview, the willing participation of the subject in answering the questions is their informed consent. The subject can decline to participate or can refuse to answer specific questions. However, all research that involves a clinical trial and human subjects must undergo a review process by one or more supervisory committees, commonly called review boards. These committees may be connected to the institution where the researcher works, the organization funding the research, or the facility where the research is being conducted.

If one is simply testing different types of toothpastes, writing a cumbersome document to protect the subjects may seem to be a bit of overkill. However, what if the new toothpaste causes demineralization of teeth? Never underestimate informed consent. Understandably, if an investigator is looking at a new drug to treat schizophrenia, getting informed consent becomes more problematic. In some instances, the experimental treatment is of a more serious nature, and the subject may be a small child or a person diagnosed with Alzheimer's or a mental illness. Obtaining an ethically and legally valid informed consent becomes extremely important.

Informed consent is part of examining the ethics of the research project as a whole. Federally established guidelines regulate research conducted on people. An outline for an informed consent is presented on the website with a sample informed consent document.

INTRODUCTION AND LITERATURE REVIEW

The first step in conducting research is to provide a thorough introduction that includes the purpose of the study. This is also the area that provides persuasive significance of the study. Providing significance to the study is an important step for any researcher. Obviously it is important to persuade the reader as to the importance and necessity of the research. This is the area that can really make a reader interested in the study.

The review of the literature provides detailed information from previous studies conducted and existing paradigms for treatments or product use. The **literature review** should cite many sources and should include studies published in peer-reviewed periodicals. By portraying an accurate account of the present knowledge in a subject, the dental hygienist is able to relate this information to evidence-based practice.

SUMMARY

Once completed, research needs to be disseminated to the professionals and the appropriate public if it is to be of any benefit. Without the distribution of the results to the target populations, the dental hygienist in private practice will not be able to incorporate new knowledge and techniques into daily practice that will benefit both clinician and patient. Oral health and hygienists' occupational health can and do suffer as a result. Quality research is published in peer-reviewed publications. Through this mechanism, the science of the laboratories becomes the art of patient care.

REFERENCES

[1]Ripa, L.W. Open questions and form. In S. Wei, ed. *Clinical Uses of Fluoride*. Conference in San Fransisco, 1984.

[2]Fourth national research conference agenda. Chicago: American Dental Hygienists' Association, 1999.

[3]Darby, M., and D. Bowen. *Research Methods for Oral Health Professionals: An Introduction*. St. Louis, MO: C.V. Mosby, 1980.

[4]Berg, A. O. et al. *Practice-Based Research in Medicine*. Kansas City, MO: American Academy of Family Physicians, 1986.

[5]Darby, M., and M. Walsh. *Dental Hygiene Theory and Practice,* 2d edition. Philadelphia: W. B. Saunders, 2003.

[6]Burns, N., and S. Grove. *The Practice of Nursing Research,* 2d ed. Philadelphia: W. B. Saunders, 1993.

Get Connected

Multimedia Extension Activities

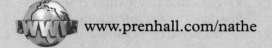 www.prenhall.com/nathe

Use the above address to access the free, interactive companion web site created specifically to accompany this textbook. Here you will find an array of self study material to help you gain a richer understanding of the concepts presented in this chapter.

Chapter 13

··

BIOSTATISTICS

by Chris French-Beatty, RDH, PhD

OBJECTIVES

After studying this chapter, the dental hygiene student will be able to:

- define and describe data analysis and interpretation.
- identify data by its type and scale of measurement.
- define and describe descriptive and inferential statistics.
- select and compute appropriate measures of central tendency and measures of dispersion.
- describe and construct frequency distributions and graphs.

COMPETENCIES

After studying the chapter and participating in accompanying course activities, the dental hygiene student should be competent in the following:

- recognize and use written and electronic sources of information.
- evaluate the credibility and potential hazards of dental products and techniques.
- evaluate published clinical and basic science research and integrate this information to improve the oral health of the patient.
- accept responsibility for solving problems and making decisions based on accepted scientific principles.
- expand and contribute to the knowledge base of dental hygiene.

KEY WORDS

Clinical significance
Correlation
Data analysis
Degrees of freedom
Interpretation

p values
Scales of measurement
Variables
   Continuous
   Discrete

www.prenhall.com/nathe

INTRODUCTION

The subject of biostatistics is a course unto itself, and fortunately for the twenty-first-century hygienist, computer programs are available to do all the computations. For the researcher who is not familiar with statistical analysis, consultation with a statistician experienced in this field is highly recommended when planning research projects. If the number of subjects is insufficient (less than thirty), not long enough in duration (typically, less than six months), or the wrong statistical tests are run on the data, the resulting conclusions are, of course, invalid. Repeating the research study due to statistical errors is frustrating for the principal investigator and highly aggravating to the financial sponsors.

Upon completion of a research project or program evaluation, data must be analyzed in preparation for interpretation of the results. **Data analysis** involves the application of statistical tests to the data in order to organize, describe, summarize, and analyze it to answer a research question or test a hypothesis.[1] Once the data have been analyzed, the researcher must interpret these results. **Interpretation** of results requires that critical thinking be used to explain the meaning and application of the findings and identify possible factors that could influence the results.[1] The procedures used to analyze the data are termed biostatistics. This chapter provides an overview of the topic.

Biostatistics are used to demonstrate response to dental hygiene therapy, to test products and treatment regimes used in dental hygiene therapy, to determine the needs of target populations, to evaluate dental health care and oral hygiene educational programs, and for a variety of other purposes in relation to oral health care.[2] Understanding the analysis of data is important for the dental hygienist to be able to practice therapies that are based upon scientific evidence.

Although not every dental hygienist will conduct research studies or evaluate community programs, each and every dental hygienist must understand the research process, including data analysis and interpretation, in order to critically apply the results of published studies to the practice of dental hygiene. Students of research often reflect a bias that statistics are undependable because they can be used to "say whatever you want them to say."[2] However, the appropriate application of sound principles of biostatistics will produce results that are valid. A foundation in biostatistics will help the dental hygienist understand the literature.

Commercial software packages, such as Statistical Package for the Social Sciences (SPSS) and Statistical Analyses System (SAS), are available for data analysis, and graphics programs, such as Microsoft Excel, are available for the presentation of data.[3] Even so, the dental hygienist must have a working knowledge of statistics to operate these programs. For the researcher who is not intimately familiar with statistical analysis, consultation with a statistician experienced in this field is highly recommended during the proposal stage when planning a research project or public health program.

CATEGORIZING DATA

Data are the information that are collected by a researcher.[4] Actually, data are the plural term; the singular term is datum. Data can be quantitative, meaning that numbers can represent the data, and statistics can be applied to them, or nonquantitative, sometimes referred to as qualitative. Each piece of information is called an item of data, and a group of all the data items collected is called a data set.

Data are classified as continuous or discrete. A **discrete** (sometimes called categorical) **variable** is made up of distinct and separate units or categories, also referred to as mutually exclusive, and is counted only in whole numbers. These are two terms that mean the same thing. Discrete, or categorical, variables are considered to be qualitative in nature. An example of this type of variable would be male/female or red/blue/yellow. The number of DMF teeth is discrete, as it is not possible to have a fraction of a tooth. So are religious preference and SES. However, sometimes the distinction in unimportant in application as many discrete variables, especially those that have a large number of possible scores, can be treated meaningfully as continuous for statistical analysis.[5] For example, it is meaningful to express a mean of 2.5 on a DMF, Plaque Index, Gingival Index, most other dental indices, and many rating scales, but an average religious preference of 1.8 has no meaning. A dichotomous variable is a categorical variable that places subjects into only two groups, such as male/female or pass/fail.[4]

On the other hand, a **continuous variable** is one that can be expressed by a large and infinite number of measures along a continuum. These variables can be expressed in fractions and are considered quantitative. For example, height, weight, and time are continuous because they fall on a continuum and have value when expressed as fractions. Data are also classified by **scale of measurement**. Four scales of measurement exist: nominal, ordinal, interval, and ratio. The higher the level of data, the more information it conveys about the differences among values.[4]

The nominal scale of measurement organizes data into mutually exclusive categories, but the categories have no rank order or value. Ethnic group membership is an example. Blacks may be placed in category A, Asian in category B, American Indian and Alaska native in category C, native Hawaiian and other Pacific Islanders in category D, and White in category E.

The ordinal scale of measurement organizes data into mutually exclusive categories which are rank ordered based on some criterion, but the difference between ranks is not necessarily equal. An example is classification of level of difficulty of patients in a dental hygiene clinic: Class 0, 1, 2, 3, and 4. The higher class reflects greater difficulty, but a class 4 is not necessarily twice as difficult as a class 2.

The interval scale of measurement has equal distance between any two adjacent units of measurement, but there is no meaningful zero point. In other words, the zero point is arbitrary, not determined by nature. An example is the Fahrenheit measurement scale. Scores on an interval scale can meaningfully be added and subtracted but not multiplied and divided. We can say that 90°F is 45° warmer than 45°F, but we cannot say that 90°F is twice as hot as 45°F.

The ratio scale of measurement contains all the characteristics of the preceding scales, but also has an absolute zero point determined by nature. Blood pressure, height, and weight are examples of ratio variables. We can say that a person who weighs 150 pounds is twice as heavy as a person who weighs 75 pounds.

In general, discrete data use the nominal and ordinal scales of measurement, and continuous data use the interval or ratio scales of measurement. However, interval and ratio data can be either discrete or continuous.[5] For example, DMF teeth and number of sealants are discrete variables (cannot be expressed meaningfully as a fraction) and have the ratio scale of measurement (equal distance between numbers and can have no DMF teeth or sealants). However, as discussed earlier, for all practical purposes they can be identified as continuous data.

Several important points are necessary to understand that sometimes, the rules vary for how to treat the various scales of data statistically. The distinction between interval and ratio data is insignificant for our purposes. Both types of variables are handled the same way when analyzing data.[6] Interval and ratio data can be converted to nominal or ordinal data.[5] For example, subjects can be placed in nominal categories of "Controlled BP" or "Uncontrolled BP" according to their blood pressure, which is a ratio variable. Another example is to categorize subjects' gingivitis as mild, moderate, or severe (ordinal scale) according to the number of bleeding points (ratio scale). Also, when ordinal data consist of many ranks or categories, the data are customarily treated as continuous rather than discrete data.[4,5] Ordinal attitude scales (e.g., very satisfied, satisfied, neither satisfied not dissatisfied, dissatisfied, very dissatisfied) are commonly treated as interval data.[4]

DESCRIPTIVE STATISTICS

Statistics are divided into two major categories; descriptive statistics and inferential statistics. Descriptive statistics consist of the procedures that are used to summarize, organize, and describe quantitative data. Inferential statistics, on the other hand, are used to make inferences or generalizations about a population based on data taken from a sample of that population.[4] This is also called making statistical decisions. The application of descriptive statistics to a data set always precedes the use of inferential statistics. Descriptive statistics discussed here include measures of central tendency, measures of dispersion, frequency distribution tables, and graphing techniques.

Measures of Central Tendency

Statistics rarely ever speak about the average of something. Instead three distinct terms with three different meanings can be used, depending on what type of data the researcher is collecting. The mean is what is commonly meant by the average.

To arrive at it, one would add all the scores and divide by the total number. For example, the mean of the numbers 2, 3, 3, and 4 would be 3. The symbol used to denote the mean is x; the symbol M is also commonly used in journal articles.[5] The formula for the mean, Mean = $\Sigma x/n$, which can be explained as the upper case Greek letter sigma (Σ), means "the sum of." If the letter x represents a single value in the distribution, then Σx means "the sum of all the values." The letter n represents the sample size or number of observations.

The median is the point at which exactly half of the values are above and half are below. The median of the scores 2, 3, 3, 4, and 5 would be 3. If only the scores 2, 3, 3, and 4 occurred, the median would be the average of the middle two scores, which in this case would be 3. It can be used to describe ratio, interval, or ordinal data, but not nominal data.

The mode is the value that occurs the most often. The mode of the scores 2, 3, 3, and 4 would be 3. Some instances may have more than one mode, which would be referred to as bimodal, and if there would be more than two modes, it would be referred to as multimodal. In a normal distribution curve, these three values are the same. When analyzing nominal data, such as SES, the mode is the only measure of central tendency that makes sense.[6]

Measures of Dispersion

Most occurrences in this world tend to fall into a bell-shaped curve, called the normal distribution. Generally the majority of subjects will fall under the large part of the middle of the curve with a few low and high outliers. Grades are a good example of this tendency. Generally speaking if one looked at a group of people who took a class in introduction to statistics, most of them would receive a grade of C with a few getting Bs and Ds and an even fewer receiving As and Fs. When researchers want to know whether an intervention made a difference, they cannot just look at pure numbers. It isn't enough that a subject's score improved. It has to be an improvement that is "statistically significant." To report an average without a measure of dispersion can misrepresent the data. Two distributions of data can have the same central tendency and vastly different measures of dispersion.

This value is determined by looking at the range, variance, and standard deviation. The range is determined by subtracting the highest score from the lowest score. The variance is determined statistically by the square of the standard deviation. If an imaginary "score" without treatment X is 50, is a score of 40 with treatment X necessarily better? The answer depends on the standard deviation (SD). In the example, if the SD is 15, then treatment X doesn't make a statistically significant difference. If the SD is 5, however, then treatment X may suggest a significant finding. See Figure 13–1 for the steps in computing variance and standard deviation.

Figure 13–1.   Steps in Computing the Variance and Standard Deviation (SD)

1. Calculate the mean for the distribution of scores.

2. Subtract the mean from each score $(X -)$. This is called the deviation. When the mean is larger than the score, the result will be a negative value.

3. The sum of the deviations $[\Sigma(X -)]$ always equals zero. Add the deviations to check this.

4. Square each deviation $(X -)^2$.

5. Add the squared deviations to determine the sum of squares $\Sigma(X -)^2$.

6. Divide the sum of square by $N - 1$. This resulting quantity is called the variance.

7. Take the square root of the variance. This resulting quantity is the standard deviation.

The Normal Distribution

The normal distribution, or Gaussian distribution, is a population frequency distribution that yields a symmetrical, unimodal, bell-shaped curve.[4] The mean, median, and mode are of equal value. The extreme ends (called tails) of the curve do not touch the abscissa (x axis). The standard normal distribution is a theoretical normal distribution. Figure 13–2 shows the standard normal distribution.

The standard normal distribution explains why random variables tend to be normally distributed. Also, it is the foundation of the central limit theorem. Based on this statistical proposition, less sampling error will occur with a larger sample, a

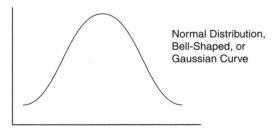

Normal Distribution, Bell-Shaped, or Gaussian Curve

Normal Distribution

Figure 13–2.   Bell Curve

sample size of 30 or more will estimate the population mean with reasonable accuracy, and we can use the normal distribution to study a wide variety of statistical problems.[4,5] Also, according to the central limit theorem, if an infinite number of randomly selected samples are drawn from a population, the means of the samples tend to be normally distributed, and the average of the sample means is very close to the actual population mean. The SD of these sample means is called the standard error of the mean. It is figured by dividing the SD by the square root of the sample size; hence, a larger sample size significantly reduces the standard error. The term error here does not signify an error made, but indicates the fact that each sample mean is likely to vary somewhat from the population mean.[4] In contrast to a normal distribution, when a distribution of scores is asymmetrical, the curve is said to be skewed (see Figure 13–3). The skew is caused by a few extreme scores in the distribution. In a positively skewed (or upper or right skewed) distribution, the infrequent or extreme scores are on the right side of the x axis, and the mean is larger (to the right) than the median. In a negatively skewed (or downward or left skewed), the infrequent or extreme scores are on the left side, and the mean is smaller (to the left) than the median. Vogt suggests a method to remember which skew is which. Remember that a skewer is pointed. When the point is on the right, it is right skewed; when the pointed end is on the left, it is left skewed. Because of the relative position of the mean and median, the skew of a curve can be determined by examining the mean and median of the distribution. Remember that the mean is highly affected by extreme scores and pulled in their direction, and the median and mode more accurately represent central tendency in a skewed distribution. This will help you determine the direction of the skew. A population variable may be skewed, for example, blood pressure among the elderly. The significance of recognizing a skewed sample distribution is that it may result from using small or homogenous samples, or failing to use random sampling or random assignment techniques.[1]

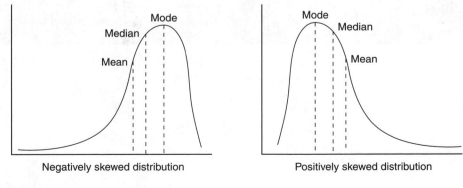

Figure 13–3.   Skewed Data

GRAPHING DATA

Data can be presented pictorially in graphs. The advantages of using graphs and tables include effective and economic communication of data, easier and quicker understanding and interpretation of data, and the ability to compare multiple distributions visually.[1]

Frequency Distribution Tables

A frequency distribution table is used to present the data in a way that shows the number of times each score occurs in the group of scores.[5] For nominal and ordinal variables, the categories are listed in a natural order, and then the frequency for each category is tabulated. Figure 13–4 illustrates a frequency distribution table for ordinal data, that is, age category of patients treated in a dental hygiene clinic.

For interval and ratio data, the values are first arranged in an array, which is an ordered display of a set of observations.[4] For these types of data, the frequency can be expressed in four ways:

1. The actual frequency or count for the category
2. The relative frequency or percent, figured by dividing the frequency by the total number in the data set
3. The cumulative frequency, which is the total up to and including that value
4. The cumulative relative frequency or cumulative percent, which is also known as the percentile rank

Figure 13–4. Number of Patients Treated in Clinic in Fall 2002 Semester by Age Category

Patient type	Frequency	%
Child	112	15
Adolescent	100	14
Adult	355	49
Geriatric	162	22
TOTAL	729	100

Frequency distribution tables can be ungrouped or grouped.[1] An ungrouped frequency distribution includes all the scores in the distribution. It is recommended for small samples with less than 30 observations. With a large data set (over 30 observations), a grouped frequency distribution can be constructed by grouping the data into class intervals. Also, if the difference between the maximum and minimum values is larger than 15, a grouped frequency distribution is recommended.[5] However, it is important to note that when the scores are widely dispersed, grouping the data can cause loss of detail in the scores reported.

To construct a grouped frequency distribution, group a set number of scores into mutually exclusive intervals called class intervals. This is also known as collapsing the data.[4] Try to choose an interval and a starting point that are divisible by 5. To determine the number of intervals, consider the total number of measurements. It is equally inappropriate to have just one or two measurements in several intervals, and to have a large number of measurements in only a few intervals. About 5–10 intervals are appropriate for most distributions.[7] Figure 13–5 illustrates an ungrouped frequency distribution for ratio data, and Figure 13–6 illustrates a grouped frequency distribution for the same data.

A frequency distribution is usually made into a graph by representing the variable on the horizontal (x) axis and the frequency on the vertical (y) axis, although the axes can be reversed. The vertical axis should have a height of one-half to three-fourths the width of the graph.[5] This will prevent expanding or collapsing

Figure 13–5.   Ungrouped Frequency Distribution for Ratio Data

X	f	X	f	X	f	X	f
100		90		80		70	
99	2	89	4	79	1	69	1
98	1	88	2	78	3	68	
97	1	87	2	77	1	67	
96		86		76	4	66	
95	1	85		75	1	65	
94	3	84	3	74	2	64	1
93	1	83	4	73		63	
92	1	82	2	72		62	
91	1	81	1	71		61	

Figure 13–6.   Grouped Frequency Distribution for the Same Data

Class interval	f	Cumulative f
99–95	5	45
90–94	6	40
85–89	8	34
80–84	12	26
75–79	10	14
70–74	2	4
65–69	1	2
60–64	1	1

of the x and y scales and minimize misrepresentation and misinterpretation of the data.[1] The construction of graphs has been facilitated by the use of computers. Some computer programs, for example, Excel, label graphs as charts. Some of the most commonly used graphs are described here, namely, the bar graph, the histogram, and the polygon.

A bar graph is used to present categorical data.[4] A space separates the bars to emphasize the discrete nature of the data. The height of each bar corresponds to the frequency of the value it represents. Figure 13–7 is an example of a bar graph. Two or more distributions can be compared by using a cluster bar graph. Figure 13–8 is an example of this type of graph.

A histogram is similar to a bar graph, but the bars appear side by side, that is, touching. A histogram is appropriate for interval or ratio variables, and sometimes for ordinal variables that are treated as continuous data.[5] Both ungrouped and grouped frequencies can be represented in a histogram. Computer programs are handy to experiment with the number and height of bars, and the width of the intervals, so that you can meet the goal of constructing a graph with a smooth appearance that accurately represents the data. See Figure 13–9.

A polygon, also known as a frequency polygon, is a line graph drawn by connecting the midpoints of the bars of a histogram, then extending the line at both ends to imaginary midpoints at the right and left of the histogram. This extension of the line assures that the total areas of both graphs are equivalent.[5] Just like histograms, polygons can be used to represent ungrouped or grouped frequency distributions, and can present frequency, percent, cumulative frequency, or

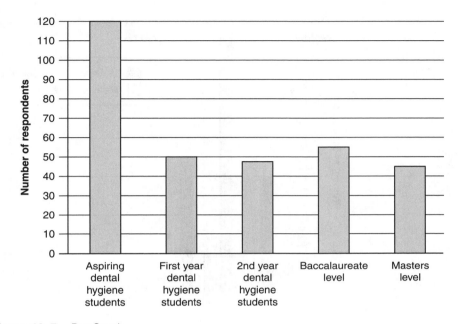

Figure 13–7. Bar Graph

Source: Koot, A. C. Values of dental hygienists in three occupational settings. Thesis, Old Dominion University, Norfolk, VA, 1978.

cumulative percent. Polygons are especially useful to compare two or more distributions visually by superimposing them in one graph, as in Figure 13–10.

Tables and graphs facilitate our understanding and interpretation of the data. They help us quickly spot the shape of the distribution, where the data cluster, and how the data scatter around the clustering points, outliers, and gaps in the data.[5] Data presented in tables and graphs should be understandable even without the written discussion of the data. Figure 13–11 presents characteristics of effective tables and graphs and appropriate ways to achieve them.[1,4,5]

CORRELATION

Correlational techniques are used to study relationships among variables. The term **correlation** is used in everyday language to mean relationship. In statistics, correlation refers to a relationship or association between variables that can be measured mathematically. The null hypothesis in a correlation analysis is one of no association between the variables.

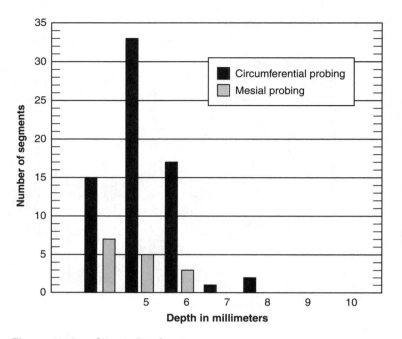

Figure 13–8. Cluster Bar Graph

The most common statistic to measure correlation is the correlation coefficient, signified by *r*, which is expressed as a number between −1 and +1. The value of *r* communicates both the direction and strength of the relationship. The sign (+ or −) determines the direction of the relationship, negative or positive. In a positive relationship, both variables vary in the same direction. In other words, as one increases in value, the other also increases in value. In the same way, as one decreases in value, the second also decreases in value. An example is the relationship between periodontal disease and heart disease. Heart disease and periodontal disease increase and decrease together in the population. When there is a negative relationship, the variables vary in opposite directions, so as one variable increases in

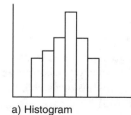

a) Histogram

Figure 13–9. Histogram

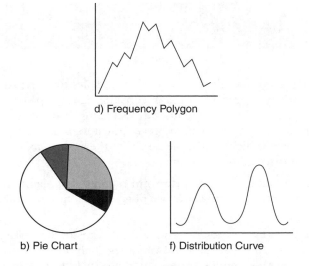

d) Frequency Polygon

b) Pie Chart

f) Distribution Curve

Figure 13–10.   Polygon and Other Graphing Techniques

value, the other decreases. This is also described as an inverse relationship. For example, as the consumption of fluoridated water increases, the caries rate decreases.

The value of *r* indicates the strength of the relationship. As the value moves closer to +1 or −1, it indicates a stronger relationship; as it moves closer to 0, it indicates a weaker relationship. This means that a value of +.90 is just as strong as a value of −.90. A value of +1 or −1 indicates a perfect relationship, and a value of 0 indicates no relationship.[1] The following provides a general interpretation of *r*: 0.00–0.25 (little if any correlation), 0.26–0.49 (low), 0.50–0.69 (moderate), 0.79–0.89 (high), and 0.90–1.00 (very high).[5]

Several correlation techniques are available. The selection is based on the number of variables to be correlated, the nature of the variable (discrete or continuous), the scale of measurement, and the linearity of the relationship between the variables.[8]

Correlation does not *necessarily* equal causality, otherwise known as a cause-and-effect relationship. This means that a strong or significant correlation between two variables does not mean that one necessarily caused the other. For example, caries and fluorosis are highly correlated, but fluorosis is not the cause of caries and caries does not cause fluorosis. The causal factor for both fluorosis and low caries rates is fluoride. It is also a mistake to think that two correlated variables cannot be causally related or that correlation provides no evidence whatsoever for cause.[4] Remember that the first evidence of a cause-and-effect relationship between caries and fluoride was correlation. Additional research demonstrated that there was indeed causation. Also, correlation provides much of the evidence in oral epidemiology.[9] When a correlation coefficient shows that two variables are related, further experimental research is necessary to provide unequivocal evidence of causality.[1]

Figure 13–11. Characteristics of Effective Tables and Graphs and Ways to Achieve Them

1. *Accuracy.* Enter data carefully. Follow basic principles for construction of tables and graphs. Select the type of table or graph considering the type of data being presented. Construct graphs that will not be misleading or open to misinterpretation. Begin the vertical axis at zero, with a break drawn in, if necessary because the frequency of scores is high. Make the height of the vertical axis one-half to three-fourths of the horizontal width of the graph.

2. *Simplicity.* Present data in a straightforward manner. Highlight only the major points of information. Minimize the use of grid lines, tics, unusual fonts, and showy patterns.

3. *Clarity.* Make them easy to understand and self-explanatory. Use brief but clear titles and headings. Label all axes and variables, including type of frequency (count, percent, cumulative). Carefully choose intervals. Include information on when and where data were collected, if appropriate, and the size of the groups. Communicate exclusions of observations from the data set, including the reasons and criteria for their exclusion. Include the basis for measurement of rates. Use textbooks on statistics and graphing, scientific writing style manuals, and samples of tables and graphs in journal articles to guide your construction.

4. *Appearance.* Pay attention to the construction so that the final result is neat and appealing.

5. *Well-designed structure.* Emphasize the important points visually. Use dark bars and light grid lines, and horizontal lettering when possible.

Pearson Product Moment Correlation Coefficient

The most common correlation coefficient is the Pearson Product Moment Correlation Coefficient. Pearson r is used when both variables are continuous, are at least interval scaled, and have a linear relationship. The linearity of the relationship is determined by plotting the scores on a scattergram. In Figure 13–12, A and B, C and D demonstrate linear relationships, E demonstrates no correlation, and F demonstrates a curvilinear relationship.

Spearman Rank-Order Correlation Coefficient

The Spearman Rank-Order Correlation Coefficient (also called Spearman rho) is a variation of r used to correlate two ordinal variables. Other correlation techniques are available for data that are nominal scaled, for data with curvilinear

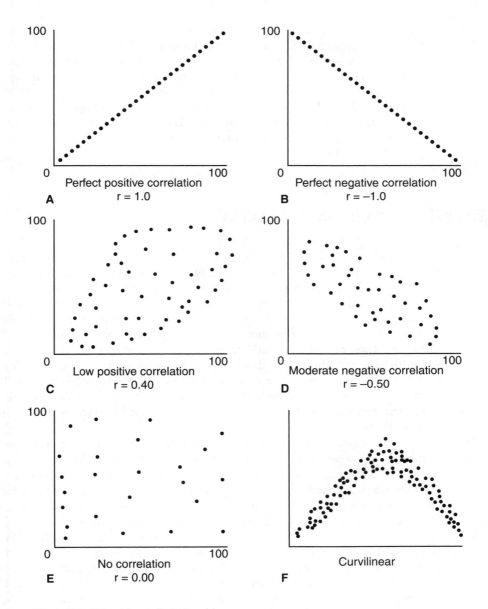

Figure 13–12.   Linear Relationships

relationships, to relate more than two variables, and for other purposes.[5] Correlation techniques can also be used to determine reliability of data collection instruments, intrarater reliability, and interrater reliability.[1] Statistical significance of correlation can also be determined. Regression analysis is the expansion of correlation to predict the score of one variable (dependent variable) based on the score of another (independent variable). Multiple regression analysis takes correlation a step further to provide a mathematical model that gives the strength of the ability of two or more variables (independent variables) to predict another variable (dependent variable).

STATISTICAL DECISION MAKING

The null hypothesis is an initial statement of belief about the value of a population parameter, for example, the means of two groups, do not differ. Basically a null hypothesis is "innocent (true) until proven guilty (false)." The alternative hypothesis (often also called the research or positive hypothesis) is the logical opposite of the null hypothesis, and can indicate a direction of difference. For example, the null hypothesis is that the retention rate of one brand of sealants does not differ from the retention rate of a second brand. The accompanying alternative hypothesis can be that the retention rates differ (no direction of difference specified) or that the first brand has a higher retention rate than the second (directional hypothesis). The object of hypothesis testing is to decide whether it is reasonable to continue believing that the null hypothesis is true, or to reject that belief in favor of the alternative hypothesis.

A statistical decision is made about the null hypothesis based on the results of inferential statistics. Remember that inferential statistics (more later) is the category of statistics used to make inferences or generalizations about a population based on data taken from the sample. These statistics are used to test a hypothesis or estimate a population parameter based on the sample data, for example, to estimate the mean of the population based on the mean of the sample.

The statistical decision to reject or accept the null hypothesis is based on probability at a set significance level, also known as the alpha α level, and expressed as a probability value or **p value**. The p value commonly accepted as statistically significant in oral health research is equal to or smaller than 0.05 ($p \leq .05$). We see p values in journal articles of $p = .05$, $p = .01$, and $p = .001$. A lower p value signifies greater statistical significance of the result. When the p value is larger than .05, the results are said to be not statistically significant, or NS. A result of hypothesis testing reported as $p < .05$ means that the probability of this result occurring by chance alone is less than (<) 5 percent. The p value is the final arithmetic solution obtained by using the calculated test statistic, the sampling distribution of the test statistic, and the size of the sample. Regardless of the inferential statistic used, the statistical decision is made this same way, using the p value to determine statistical significance.

Because the statistical decision is based on probability, there is a possibility of error. A Type I error (also called alpha α error) occurs when the null hypothesis is rejected, and it is true. The probability of a Type I error is the same as the alpha α level. For example, in the previous example of testing the retention rates of two sealants, a Type I error would be to decide incorrectly that one sealant had a better retention rate than the other. Setting an alpha level at .05 denotes a willingness to take a 5 percent chance of making an alpha error. A large sample size can lead to a Type I error.[4] A randomly selected representative sample and a good study design help to avoid making a Type I error.[7]

A Type II error (also called beta β error) occurs when the null hypothesis is accepted, and it is false (Figure 13–13). The exact probability of computing a Type II error is generally unknown; however, it is possible to design a decision rule so that the risk of making a Type I error is as small as the researcher wants. Furthermore, if the sample size is large enough, the researcher has the ability to make the risk of making a Type II error small at the same time the risk of a Type I error is small.[4] Using the same example of testing the retention rates of two sealants, a Type II error would be to decide incorrectly that the two sealants had equivalent retention rates. Using too small a sample, unreliable measuring devices, or imprecise research methods will increase the probability of making a Type II error.[6] The power of a test is its ability to reject a false null hypothesis, or detect relationships among variables. It is defined as $1 - \beta$. By increasing power, we decrease the Type II error rate. A power of .80 is considered reasonable.[4] Power can be improved by increasing the sample size, improving the measuring device, increasing the α level, or choosing a different study design.[6] Power is critically important in clinical trials using a positive control, because the differences in the groups are likely to be slight.[9] For example, if a test fluoride dentifrice is compared with a positive control of a standard fluoride dentifrice, differences in caries rates will likely be small. In this case, group sizes have to be extremely large. A power analysis is a technique used to determine the appropriate sample size considering the statistic being used, the α level, and characteristics of the data.[5]

The probability of Type I and Type II errors is inversely related; that is, the smaller the risk of one, the greater the risk of the other. Committing a Type I error can be more costly than a Type II error. Type I errors lead to unwarranted change while Type II errors maintain status quo. One example of the significance of Type I and Type II errors is if a patient could receive incorrect treatment or not receive treatment that could have been helpful, even life saving. The degree of risk relates directly to the level of significance. When planning a research project, the Type I and Type II error rates should be considered in light of the particular research problem and which type error is more serious for the situation.[1] Because it is not possible to know if a Type I or Type II error has occurred, it is important to conduct replication studies to increase the confidence that results are true.[1] Guidelines for the conduct of oral research should be followed to avoid both Type I and Type II errors.[10,11]

DENTAL HYGIENIST'S SPOTLIGHT
Ms. Lisa M. Esparza, RDH, BS

I am a graduate of the University of New Mexico Division of Dental Hygiene class of 1989. As a dental hygienist, I have worked 11 years in private practice, 1 year as Public School Based Programs Coordinator and the last 3 1/2 years as Director of ACC Consultants Inc., which specializes in portable/mobile public health dentistry throughout New Mexico. Over the years, I have also been a clinical instructor at the University of New Mexico and currently teach a geriatric rotation to the senior class every spring. I am an active member of the American Dental Hygienists' Association (ADHA), New Mexico Dental Hygienists' Association, and the American Association of Public Health Dentistry. I have held various offices in my component, at the state and national level, and enjoy being a mentor every year for our dental hygiene students. As an advocate of oral health care and community involvement, I have served as chair of the New Mexico Spe-

cial Olympics Special Smiles Program, and the chair and cofounder of the New Mexico Dental Hygienists' Association Healthy Smiles Program. The Healthy Smiles Program won the ADHA/Colgate Community Outreach Award in 1999. In 1998, I was awarded the University of New Mexico Division of Dental Hygiene's Outstanding Contributions Award, and I received the 1997–98 Special Recognition Award from the New Mexico Dental Hygienists' Association and the 2000 New Mexico Special Olympics Volunteer of the Year award. Currently, I am the director of operations for a mobile dental company, ACC Consultants Inc., which was started by a dental hygienist Ginny Berger, RDH, whose mission is to provide access to oral health care to populations that are not treated in the private sector. We are a for-profit company that is mainly a Medicaid provider, and we offer comprehensive oral health care to long-term care facilities (over 76 facili-

(continued)

Dental Hygienist's Spotlight *(continued)*

ties) and 8 school districts throughout New Mexico. We have over 5,000 patients and employ over 60 oral health care and administrative professionals. I firmly believe "you reap, what you sow," and I have been blessed to be so fortunate to receive so much fulfillment and honor from my profession as a dental hygienist.

Degrees of freedom (*df*) refers to the number of values or observations that are free to vary when computing a statistic, that is, the number of measurements taken, minus one for each population parameter estimated.[1] The number is necessary to interpret inferential statistical tests. Statistics textbooks contain clear rules to calculate and use *df* to interpret a statistic. Degrees of freedom is based on the sample size so the larger the *df*, the easier it is to obtain a statistically significant result.

Another way to infer the true value of an unknown population parameter, for example, the mean from the sample statistic, is by using confidence intervals. Typically 95 percent and 99 percent confidence intervals are used, and the standard error of the mean is used to calculate the intervals. For example, if the 95 percent confidence interval for the mean Plaque Index of 1.16 in a sample of school children is 1.08 to 1.24, then we can be 95 percent sure that the mean Plaque Index of the population is between 1.08 and 1.24.

INFERENTIAL STATISTICS

The purpose of inferential statistics is to generalize between the sample being studied and the population that it represents. Computing inferential statistics and analyzing the results require a more sophisticated understanding of statistics. Some of

Figure 13–13. Type I and Type II Errors Made When Rejecting and Accepting the Null Hypothesis

	Decision About the Null Hypothesis	
	Accepted	**Not Accepted**
True	No error made	Type I error (α)
Not true	Type II error (β)	No error made

these are fairly easy to compute using a computer program. Others are more complex. Use of computers and consultation with a statistician is advised.

Parametric Inferential Statistics

Parametric statistics are used when the data are continuous. This would include ratio and interval data, as well as ordinal data that approximate the continuous nature. Recall our discussion about continuous and discrete data. Discrete variables that have a large number of possible scores can be treated as continuous data, for example, DMF, Plaque Index, Gingival Index, most other dental indices, and many rating scales.

Student *t*-test

The *t*-test is used to compare two mean scores to determine if there is a statistically significant difference. It is formally known as the Student *t*-test, named after its inventor who published under the pseudonym Student. It is used to test a null hypothesis of differences, for example, "the mean sealant retention rates for the two groups do not differ." There are two versions of the *t*-test. First, consider the *t*-test for independent samples, also called the non-paired *t*-test. It is selected when the mean scores are from two groups drawn independently from a population, that is, two different groups of subjects. For example, if a hygienist wanted to test the effectiveness of a new model electric toothbrush compared with the existing older model of the same toothbrush, he or she would have one group of patients use the new model brush and have the second group use the older model brush. At the end of the study, the mean improvement of the two groups using the *t*-test for independent samples would be compared. The computational result of the *t*-test, called the *t* statistic, would be compared with critical values of *t* on the *t* distribution, for the predetermined *p* value and degrees of freedom for the study. The statistical decision to reject or accept the null hypothesis is based on the test *t* statistic relative to the critical values of *t*. Today, the task is made easier by the use of computers for the statistical computation and comparison to the *t* distribution.

In this same study of a new electric toothbrush model, assume the hygienist wanted to compare the pretest and posttest plaque scores for just the group that used the new model brush. In this case, the groups of data (pretest and posttest) are not mutually exclusive or independent, thereby violating one of the assumptions described earlier. To accommodate, he or she would use the *t*-test for correlated samples, also known as the *t*-test for paired samples. This *t*-test is used when the two mean scores are derived from the same group of subjects or when the experimental and control groups are matched on the basis of a variable known to be correlated with the independent variable. The results of this test would be interpreted the same way as the *t*-test for independent samples.

Analysis of Variance (ANOVA)

In the example of the study testing the new model electric toothbrush, a third of a group of patients is using a manual toothbrush. In this case there would be three mean improvement scores to compare. Analysis of variance (ANOVA) is the parametric statistic used to determine if statistically significant differences occur when comparing more than two mean scores. In journal articles sometimes similar studies are seen in which the data are analyzed using the t-test to perform multiple comparisons with different combinations of mean scores, two at a time. This is an incorrect application of the t-test as the Type I error rate will increase exponentially by the number of combinations of the t-test conducted.[2,5] When more than two mean scores are being analyzed, the ANOVA should be used.

Various forms of the ANOVA statistic are used according to the number of independent variables: one-way ANOVA for one independent variable and two-way ANOVA for two independent variables.[5] ANOVA can also be used as Multivariate analysis of variance (MANOVA) to analyze the effects of the independent variable(s) on two or more dependent variables within the same test to increase power, limit Type I errors, and control for a relationship among the dependent variables. Analysis of covariance (ANCOVA) is another variation, and it controls for the effect of an extraneous variable that equally affects all groups, called a covariate.

ANOVA is used to analyze the differences within each group, the differences between or among groups, and the interactions. The data are presented in a complex table that describes these various comparisons. The result of the ANOVA test is an F ratio, which tells us if there is a difference among the groups. However, it does not tell us which group mean significantly differs from the others. To determine which is significantly different, a posthoc analysis is done with one of a variety of available tests, including Tukey, Scheffe, Duncan, and Newman-Keuls.[4] Using the previous example of the study testing the effectiveness of a new model electric toothbrush, the use of the ANOVA allows comparison of the mean improvement of plaque scores from the three groups, new model electric brush, older model electric brush, and manual brush. The F and corresponding p value suggest that the improvement of one group is statistically different from the others, and the posthoc analysis tells us that it is the new model group. Now, assume that some of the patients are regular flossers and others are not, and we want to make sure that this extraneous variable does not affect our results. In this case, ANCOVA would be used. Finally, to measure the effect of the different brushes on plaque and gingivitis (two dependent variables that are correlated), the MANOVA would be the test of choice.

Nonparametric Inferential Statistics

Nonparametric statistics should be used when variables are discrete, sample size is small, population distributions are not normal, or group variances are not equal. There are a variety of nonparametric statistics to test a range of null hypotheses, from a question about relationships among variables to a question about group differences in outcome measures. Several nonparametric statistics are discussed.

Chi Square Test

The Chi square test (χ^2) is the most commonly used nonparametric statistic.[5] It is used to determine if a significant difference exists between frequency counts of nominal (categorical or dichotomous) data by comparing the observed frequencies to expected frequencies. It can be used to compare two groups of data (χ^2 test of the independence of categorical variables) or to compare the observed frequencies in one group to the expected frequencies (goodness of fit). McNemar's test for the significance of changes is an adaptation of chi-square used to compare dichotomous data from related or matched samples or from pretest and posttest measures on a single group.[7]

Here is an example that illustrates these two uses of χ^2. Using the same study of the new model electric toothbrush, the researcher crossed over the groups so that by the end of the study all patients have used each of toothbrushes. Then each subject was asked which brush he or she preferred using. According to probability theory, the normal (or expected) frequencies would be equal for each group. If there are 90 subjects, 30 would be expected to prefer the new model electric, 30 to prefer the old model electric, and 30 to prefer the manual brush. The observed frequencies, the patients' reported preference, are 40 for the new model electric, 30 for the old model electric, and 20 for the manual. The goodness of fit χ^2 test would reveal if the observed preference for the new model electric brush is statistically significant compared with the expected frequencies. Another example is theorizing that a dental hygienist works in two offices: one a family practice and the other a periodontal practice. This study was conducted in both offices. The expected frequencies remain the same. The observed frequencies for the family practice are 40, 30, and 20 as presented above. The observed frequencies for the periodontal practice are 47 for the new model electric, 38 for the old model electric, and 5 for the manual brush. The χ^2 test of independence will reveal if the different preferences of the two groups are statistically significant.

Other Nonparametric Tests

Various other tests provide nonparametric equivalents to parametric statistics. The Sign test for paired comparisons is used to compare ordinal or higher data from two paired samples.[7] The Wilcoxon matched pairs signed-rank test also is used to compare ordinal or higher data from two paired samples, and is considered to be the nonparametric equivalent of the paired t-test.[7] It is more powerful than the sign test because it considers the magnitude of the differences between observations, as well as the direction of the difference. The Wilcoxon rank-sum test is used to test whether two independent groups have been drawn from the same population and is an alternative to the t-test for independent samples.[7] The Mann-Whitney U test is exactly equivalent to the Wilcoxon rank-sum test.[1] It is the most powerful of the nonparametric tests because it uses most of the detail of the data. The Kruskal-Walis and the Friedman matched-pairs tests are nonparametric equivalents of two forms of ANOVA.[5]

INTERPRETATION OF DATA

Once the data have been analyzed, it requires interpretation, which involves critically thinking and rethinking about the meaning of the results in an unbiased manner. Interpretation should answer the questions presented in Figure 13–14.[1]

Results of a study can have statistical significance and not have **clinical** or practical **significance**.[2] In other words, there can be practical implications of research that may or may not be inherent in the results.[1] When study groups are large, even trivial differences in disease increments can be statistically significant.[9] This can be misleading if there is no clinical importance. One example is a study to compare the time that it takes two tooth-bleaching products to whiten teeth. The statistical decision may reveal that one product whitens teeth in less time than the

---

Figure 13–14. Questions That Should Be Answered by Interpretation of Data (DB)

1. What could these results mean?
2. What factors might be contributing to these results?
3. Were these results expected based on the theoretical framework of the study and what is known in the field?
4. Do these results agree or disagree with the findings of other researchers on the same subject area?
5. Are there any known limitations or threats to internal and external validity that could have contributed to the results?
6. What conclusions do these results lead to?
7. How do the findings relate to, contribute to, advance, or have implications for the current knowledge or practice in the field?
8. In what populations, conditions, or settings would these same results hold true?
9. What additional research questions were identified by these research results?
10. What additional research is needed to further answer this research question?

other product. However, the actual difference in time could be clinically meaningless or negligible. In this case, although the statistical significance is real, it is not useful in clinical application. Another example is the evaluation of an oral hygiene regime with a group of residents in a state mental health residential facility. Their baseline plaque score was 90 percent, and it was reduced throughout the program by one-fourth. This would mean that at the end of the program, the residents still have 67.5 percent plaque. Although these results may be statistically significant, the remaining plaque status still reflects compromised oral hygiene which will likely lead to continuing oral disease. While it may be worthwhile to continue the oral hygiene regime tested, it would be wise to also seek other measures to further reduce their plaque status. As professionals, it is important to critically interpret research results before applying them to dental hygiene practice.

RESEARCH RESULTS

Once the research project has been concluded, the subjects have been dismissed, and the data analyzed by a statistician, the investigator must turn attention to interpreting the statistics, discussing the results of the study, drawing conclusions (if any can be drawn), and disseminating the results.

Discussing the results of the study includes the narration of the course and events of the research project, including subjects who dropped out and other unforeseen occurrences such as subject death, noncompliance, or contaminated samples. The statistical analysis is also presented. Generally, raw data gathered on all the participants are not listed, but rather results are listed as a group. In addition to the actual statistical numbers, pictorial representation of those values is extremely helpful and highly recommended. The form of the picture may depend on the data or the image the researcher is trying to convey.

Once the results of the research are presented and interpreted, the investigator may then draw conclusions. The types of validity and reliability for research protocols are basically the same as for dental indexes. Validity defined means that the results of the study can be inferred to the general population. On the other hand, reliability means that the study was conducted in a controlled manner and if repeated would lend the same results; thus, the study is reproducible.

The researcher should avoid the temptation to make speculative deductions and conclude more than the numerical data indicate. Most often research projects reflect the need for continued research and give rise to new questions. A single research project rarely ever answers a question definitely. It takes many types of studies with different sample populations over time to do so. The medical literature is full of examples: one study relates caffeine intake to breast cancer risk and another finds no such relationship. Each carefully planned and executed research study is valuable, for each provides needed scientific data. Much like a jigsaw puzzle, each bit of research provides a little clue to solving a big picture.

Properly designed and executed research can be submitted for publication to a "refereed" scientific journal, that is, one with a panel of experts who review the research prior to its acceptance for publication. These reviewers should have no idea who wrote the article during their review process. Such journals are referred to as peer-reviewed publications. Dental hygienists have various such publications to share valuable information from valid and reliable studies.

SUMMARY

Volumes have been written on research, biostatistics, and even various types of statistics and specific statistical tests. The information presented serves as a guide for research conduction, assessing community projects, and understanding the oral health literature. However, participation in complex research projects may require further information or consultation with a statistician.

Once research has been completed, research needs to be disseminated to the professionals and the appropriate public if it is to be of any benefit. Without the distribution of the results to the target populations, the dental hygienist in private practice will not be able to incorporate new knowledge and techniques into daily practice that will benefit both clinician and patient. Oral health and hygienists' occupational health can and do suffer as a result. Quality research is published in peer-reviewed publications. Through this mechanism, the science of the laboratories becomes the art of patient care.

REFERENCES

[1]Darby, M. L., and D. M. Bowen. *Research Methods for Oral Health Professionals: An Introduction.* St. Louis, MO: C. V. Mosby, 1980. Reprinted by J. T. K. McCann Co., Pocatello, ID, 1993.

[2]Rose, L. Overview of biostatistics. In Gluck, G. M., and W. M. Morganstein, *Jong's Community Dental Health.* St. Louis, MO: Mosby, 2003.

[3]Darby, M. L., and M. M. Walsh. *Dental Hygiene Theory and Practice,* 2d edition. Philadelphia: W. B. Saunders, 2003.

[4]Vogt, W. P *Dictionary of Statistics & Methodology: A Nontechnical Guide for the Social Sciences.* Thousand Oaks, CA: Sage Publications, 1999.

[5]Munro, B. H. *Statistical Methods for Health Care Research.* Philadelphia: Lippincott, 1997.

[6]Wright, D. B. *Understanding Statistics: An Introduction for the Social Sciences.* London: Sage Publications, 1997.

[7]Weintraub, J. A., C. W. Douglass, and D. B. Gillings. *Biostats: Data Analysis for Dental Health Care Professionals.* Chapel Hill, NC: CAVCO Publications, 1985

[8]Darby, M. L. Community oral health planning and practice. In Darby, M. L., *Mosby's Comprehensive Review of Dental Hygiene.* St. Louis, MO: Mosby, 2002.

[9]Burt, B. A., and S. A. Eklund. *Dentistry, Dental Practice, and the Community,* 5th ed. Philadelphia: W. B. Saunders, 1999.

[10]Federation Dentaire Internationale, Commission on Classification and Statistics for Oral Conditions. Principal requirements for controlled clinical trials in periodontal diseases. *International Dental Journal* 27 (1977): 62–76.

[11]Federation Dentaire Internationale, Commission on Oral health, Research and Epidemiology. Principal requirements for controlled clinical trials of caries preventive agents and procedures. *International Dental Journal* 32 (1982): 292–310.

Get Connected

Multimedia Extension Activities

 www.prenhall.com/nathe

Use the above address to access the free, interactive companion web site created specifically to accompany this textbook. Here you will find an array of self study material to help you gain a richer understanding of the concepts presented in this chapter.

Chapter 14

EVALUATION OF SCIENTIFIC LITERATURE AND DENTAL PRODUCTS

OBJECTIVES

After studying this chapter, the student will be able to:

- describe the evolution of dental care product production.
- defend the dental hygienist's value in advocating the use of effective dental care products and treatment modalities.
- educate the public in dental care product evaluation.
- effectively critique dental research reported in dental publications.

COMPETENCIES

After studying the chapter and participating in accompanying course activities, the dental hygiene student should be competent in the following:

- recognize and use written and electronic sources of information.
- evaluate the credibility and potential hazards of dental products and techniques.
- evaluate published clinical and basic science research and integrate this information to improve the oral health of the patient.
- accept responsibility for solving problems and making decisions based on accepted scientific principles.
- promote the values of the profession to the public and other organizations outside of the dental hygiene profession.

KEY WORDS

American Dental Association Seal
   of Acceptance
Double-blind study
Food and Drug Administration

Placebo
Sample size
Washout

INTRODUCTION

Dental hygienists are recognized as consumer advocates in health care today because of the valuable information they provide to patients concerning dental hygiene treatment philosophies, oral health behavioral education, and dental care products.[1] The explosion of the dental care product aisle in supermarkets underscores the need for professionals who are able to provide consumers with valuable information about these products (Figure 14–1). Dental hygienists working in any aspect of health care are required to understand and effectively critique published research reports. For these reasons, it is necessary that the dental hygienist have a background in research as it concerns the recognition of effective and ineffective dental care products and treatment modalities.

REGULATION OF DENTAL CARE PRODUCTS

Currently dental products are under the regulation of the **Food and Drug Administration** (FDA), which is housed within the Department of Health and Human Services.[2] Figure 14–2 illustrates the regulation of dental care products.

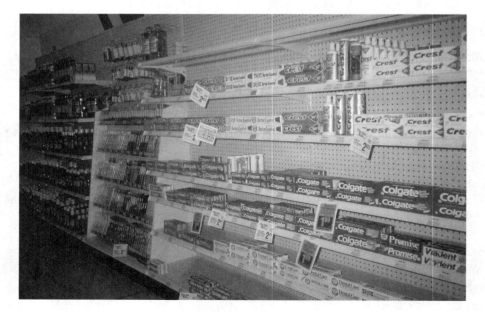

Figure 14–1. Dental Aisle of a Supermarket

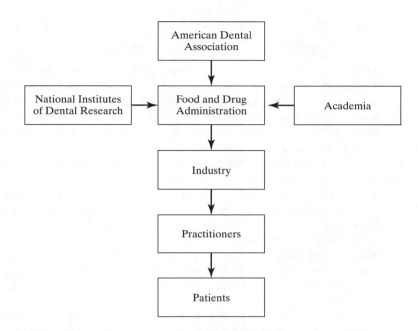

Figure 14–2. Regulation of Dental Care Products

The FDA ensures that food, cosmetics, and radiation-emitting products are safe, and that medicines and medical devices are safe and effective. If a company is found violating any of the laws that FDA enforces, the FDA can encourage the firm to voluntarily correct the problem or to recall a faulty product from the market. When a company cannot or will not correct a public health problem, the FDA has legal sanctions it can bring to bear. When warranted, criminal penalties, including imprisonment, are brought against manufacturers and distributors. The FDA periodically provides dental professionals with information concerning various products through the *FDA Medical Bulletin.* In addition, the FDA provides monographs concerning therapeutic products. FDA approval of drug products is mandated by law, and without FDA approval, a manufacturer may not legally market a product.[3]

Additionally, the American Dental Association has offered an **ADA Seal of Acceptance** Program with guidelines for testing and advertising products.[4] Although it is strictly voluntary and is not regulated by the government, about 350 companies participate in the programs. A manufacturer that applies for the seal must meet specific guidelines. Generally, the ADA seal is awarded for a three-year period. Manufacturers must reapply to continue using the ADA seal. ADA's Council on Scientific Affairs and staff scientists review and declare oral care products safe, effective, and worthy of the ADA seal. In some instances, ADA may conduct or request additional product testing.[5]

All advertising claims for any product that bears the seal are reviewed by ADA. Many times a product that has the ADA Seal will promote the dentistry profession without mention of dental hygienists in the advertisement. This omission may be due to the ADA recommendations for the advertisement. ADA has reported that it loses money on the program costs.[6] However, it is important to remember that the ADA seal is probably the most effective public relations campaign for a professional association ever initiated.

Interestingly, the American Medical Association (AMA) recently backed out of a deal with Sunbeam to endorse their product. The AMA cited credibility concerns. In fact, the American Heart Association (AHA) has received much criticism for their endorsements of products that may be low in fat but are in fact high in sugar, and therefore not recommended for a heart-healthy diet. The ADA recently was named in a lawsuit filed against toothbrush manufacturers for failing to adequately warn people about the possible dangers of brushing. Specifically, the lawsuit seeks damages on behalf of anyone who suffers from toothbrush abrasion.[7] The ADA has dodged criticism for their promotional advertising in the past, but that is changing.

As a health care professional, a hygienist should recommend a product or treatment modality based upon documented evidence, rather than a product seal. Because the ADA is not a government entity and represents the interests of the dental profession, it is important for the dental professional to base recommendations on FDA approval, scientific literature, and reported product findings. Particularly, dental hygienists must be able to understand advertisement mechanisms and effectively critique published research, so that the public receives accurate information.

WHERE TO RESEARCH DENTAL CARE PRODUCTS

Sales representatives are definitely knowledgeable about the products they carry and frequently about competitors' products as well. This contact can be especially helpful in gathering clinical reports and published peer-reviewed articles for your perusal. Companies generally have articles pertinent to their products easily accessible.

Dental hygiene and dental schools may be a great source of information. The faculty may be researching certain products or techniques and may have additional scientific information not available to clinical providers. Many faculty members have contacts around the world and can be a great resource.

In addition, attending continuing education, which is required in most states, may be a way to get information. Although some courses may not provide the information, collegial contacts and distributed resources may prove helpful.

The Internet is obviously full of information regarding dental health care. Most Internet sites are not peer reviewed and information gleaned from the Internet should be used with caution. Because it is difficult to visit the library as much as is needed in this technology-driven time period, the Internet may offer easily accessible information and guides to order periodicals.

Patients often keep the dental hygienist apprised of the products and therapies available. This information may have been obtained at the local supermarket or through a magazine advertisement, so it is helpful for the dental hygienist to constantly keep up-to-date on advertisers' claims in magazines and the supermarket aisles. Table 14–1 contains a listing of possible sources for further information concerning dental care products.

EVALUATION OF ADVERTISEMENTS

It is valuable for the dental hygienist to be able to effectively critique not just published studies, but also lay magazine advertisements and infomercials. This skill is necessary for the dental hygienist because of the ever-increasing role as a consumer advocate. The dental hygienist needs to be aware of what advertisements may be saying to patients.

One example of an influential advertisement is a mouthwash that claims to be the number one choice of hospitals. What does that claim mean to dental hygienists? Dental hygienists generally recommend a product that meets the needs of individual patients or groups. In addition, are hospitals considered experts in mouthwash choices? Certainly not. In fact, a patient who has questions about mouthwash selection is not likely to contact a local hospital. Most likely, the

Table 14–1.   Where to Locate Information on Dental Care Products

- Colleagues
- Continuing education courses/Professional meetings
- Dental hygiene and dental schools
- Lay magazines
- Library
- Internet
- Patients
- Professional magazines, journals, and newsletters
- Sales representatives
- Television

Table 14–2.   Criteria for Judging a Research Report

When was the work published?

Where was it published?

Are the qualifications of the authors appropriate?

Is the purpose clearly stated?

Is the experimental design clearly described?

Have the possible influences on the findings been identified and controls instituted?

Has the sample been appropriately selected?

Has the reliability of the scoring been assessed?

Is the experimental therapy compared appropriately to the control therapy?

Is the investigation of sufficient duration?

Is the statistical analysis appropriate to answer the research questions or hypotheses?

Have the research questions or hypotheses been answered?

Do the interpretations and conclusion logically follow the experimental findings?

Source: McCann, A. and E. Schneiderman. Interpreting and evaluating a research report. *Dent Hyg News* 5: 1997; 5–10.

patient would ask the dental hygienist and/or dentist during a dental visit. This advertisement has been notably effective, yet it says nothing about the product's effectiveness or method of efficacy.

In addition, it is important to realize what influence advertisements have on patients. Many patients now think it is necessary to purchase toothpastes that have a bubbling action. Does an advertised bubbling action prevent dental caries or remove plaque more effectively? Certainly not, but many patients are tricked into believing this myth and others. The need for hygienists to be savvy, consumer-oriented professionals has never been greater and underscores the need to be able to critically review the scientific literature. (See Table 14–2.)

HOW TO EVALUATE SCIENTIFIC LITERATURE

Within the past decade, many periodicals have been initiated that include literature reviews. Literature reviews should contain the pertinent studies conducted on a particular topics and provide the dental hygienist with the current theories and paradigms for dental hygiene practice. The literature review should contain an introduction with significance of the topic, a main body with advantages and disadvantages described, and a summary. These reviews can be valuable in helping the dental hygienists stay current with ever-changing technological advances. However, because these are merely reviews of the current literature available on a particular topic, they are not to be reviewed as actual research on that topic.

When evaluating scientific literature for product and treatment modality knowledge, it is important to recognize how to effectively critique the article. Equally as important is the ability to understand the inherent quality in a well-written study. When "abstracting" the key concepts from published studies, it is necessary to describe the purpose of the study, the problem investigated, the methodology, materials and equipment used, the results obtained, and the conclusions drawn. Please see Figure 14–3 for the current *Journal of Dental Hygiene* guidelines for the preparation of original research reports.

Purpose

It is important to first define a clear, concise purpose statement when reading a research study. This statement cannot be underscored enough, when presenting this next scenario. Suppose a plaque-removing, brushing prerinse product is touting the fact that the product removes excess plaque when compared with brushing without rinsing. The study may have clearly delineated that rinsing and brushing together does in fact remove more plaque than just brushing without rinsing. Common sense would lead us to believe this phenomenon. If the purpose were clearly stated as the investigators were trying to prove that rinsing and brushing are better than rinsing alone, this study would have met its goal. To dental hygienists, it becomes evident that this study was designed in order to help the advertising and promotion of the product.

Research Design

Design selection must be reviewed. A **double-blind study** means that neither the participant nor the researcher knows who is using which product. This format, of course, eliminates potential bias of the study results from both the investigator and the participants in terms of expectation of how a product should work.

Not all studies can be double blind because it may be necessary for the investigator to know which products or methods are being evaluated. One example would be when different types of fluoride applications are being compared such as fluoride varnish as compared to fluoride gel.

For a clinical study evaluating chemotherapeutics, a randomized clinical trial is merited.[8] This experiment is designed to test the hypothesis that a particular agent or procedure favorably alters the natural progression of a disease. The parallel group trial and the crossover trial are commonly used in clinical trials (Figures 14–4 and 14–5). The parallel (sometimes referred to as longitudinal) study

Figure 14–3.   Journal of Dental Hygiene Guidelines for Original Research Reports

Reports of basic, clinical, and applied studies that provide new information, applications, or theoretical developments. Typically include an abstract, introduction, review of the literature, methods and materials, results, discussion, and summary or conclusion.

Abstract: Approximately 250 words. Use the headings "Purpose" (purpose), "Methods" (design, subjects, procedures, measurements), "Results" (summary of findings), and "Conclusion."

Introduction: Briefly orient the reader to the given subject with an overview of the research problem studied, providing enough detail to ensure clarity.

Review of the Literature: Cite a variety of relevant, current studies. Compare findings, clearly indicating all sources of concepts and data. When a source is quoted, use quotation marks. Note the current status of the topic, and if further study is needed, provide a sound case for it. Define the variables, the hypotheses or research objectives, and how this study relates to previous research.

Methods and Materials: Describe the research instruments, equipment, procedures, and method of data analysis. Specify the measurements and statistical tests used as well as their significance. Furthermore, assure an adherence to all pertinent federal and state regulations concerning the protection of the rights and welfare of all human and animal subjects.

Results: Summarize all relevant data, including statistics and data characteristics.

Discussion: Evaluate and interpret the findings. Compare them with those of other related studies. Discuss study limitations; its implications to dental hygiene practice, education, and research; and recommendations/plans for further study.

Conclusion: State the conclusions, theories, or implications that may be drawn from the study. Discuss how they relate to dental hygiene practice, profession, education, and research. Include overall health promotion and disease prevention, clinical and primary care for individuals and groups, and basic and applied science.

Source: Reprinted with permission from the American Dental Hygienists' Association 2003.

includes participants randomly assigned to one of the study products; the participant continues to use that product for the duration of the investigation.

In this type of study, a comparison is made of different subjects using different products. On the other hand, during participation in a crossover design study all subjects use all products being evaluated. The subjects are assigned to one of the products for a given time period. Many times in this design a **washout** period is

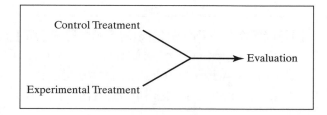

Figure 14–4.   Parallel Group Design

Source: McCann, A., and E. Schneiderman. Interpreting and evaluating a research report. *Dent Hyg News* 5 (1997): 5–10.

included, which would mean the subjects should not use any products for a given time period to "washout" any lingering effects from the product.

Sample Selection

Random selection is critical in research studies. Randomization ensures that subjects in the study are selected at chance. The assumption made is that although extraneous variables are present, the random selection of subjects and then their random assignment to the groups will tend to equalize the extraneous variables.

Sample size within the study needs to be large enough to be representative of the population. Generally, in clinical trials at least thirty subjects should be included. The subjects' gender and age should represent the population of which results are inferred.

Product Usage

Uses of the product need to be defined, including patient education protocols and the number and specific times the product was used. The study should be at least six months in duration. The longer the study period, the more valid the results. Control usage should be defined. **Placebos** may be used to substitute for the

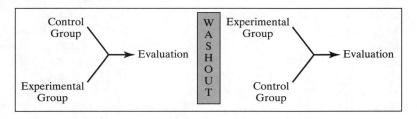

Figure 14–5.   Crossover Design

Source: McCann, A., and E. Schneiderman. Interpreting and evaluating a research report. *Dent Hyg News* 5 (1997): 5–10.

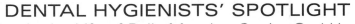

DENTAL HYGIENISTS' SPOTLIGHT

A Day in the Life of Polly Munday, Senior Oral Health Promotion Adviser, Community Dental Services, King's College Hospital NHS Trust, London, England

I work full time for the Community Dental Service in an area of South East London. We cover three London boroughs, and I manage a team of one full-time and five part-time oral health promoters in the generic team, and four Sure Start Oral Health promoters. Sure Start is similar to the American Homestart programmes. Each year we target five schools in each borough which have the highest levels of dental disease taken from school screening. We also work in preschool settings, postnatal groups, refugee groups, and so on. We work with health visitors, speech therapists, school nurses, other education and social care professionals, as well as community dental staff. The CDS treats vulnerable people in the community like children and adults with physical and learning disabilities, those with mental health problems and special needs, dental phobics, and HIV+ patients.

This is one of the schools with high levels of dental decay. It is in a socially deprived area, and many of the children are from one-parent families. I felt it was important to meet the parent/caregiver of the children, as well as the children themselves. Here, you see myself and members of the oral health promotion team talking to the children and mothers about soft, carbonated drinks in particular. This is a big problem, with children and young adults drinking fizzy drinks to excess. This causes tooth erosion as well as decay, and we try to show them, in a fun way, how to reduce consumption and substitute alternative "safer for teeth" drinks. Many of the mothers receiving social benefits (cash to support their children) find that giving cheap cans of pop to their kids keeps them quiet and fills them up so that they don't feel hungry, resulting in poor nutrition. Not surprisingly, the mothers were unaware of the danger these drinks hold

(continued)

Dental Hygienist's Spotlight   *(continued)*

for general as well as dental health. We made display boards with simple messages and encouraged mothers and children to ask questions. In our "Tooth Booth," mothers were encouraged to find out where they can get dental care for their children. Learning about teeth in this way poses no threat to the children. It was disheartening to discover the amount of caries present, and we advised mothers to make an appointment with their local dentist so that their children could get the dental care they need. All activities are evaluated to guide further planning of OHP programmes.

It is challenging working with such diverse ethnic groups and socially deprived families. Although dental treatment is free for all children and pregnant and nursing mothers, relatively few take up the offer of biannual checkups. Often mothers do not go to the dentist themselves and will only take children when they are in pain. This behavior is a poor introduction to dental care and often instills a sense of fear in their children. Dental hygienists can help make a positive change in this population by working within communities as well as in dental practice.

products, but they should have no negative or positive effect on the subject. Placebos should be identical in color, taste, packaging, and texture to the test product except for the active agent.

Examiners

The examiners should be calibrated, and the same examiners should be used throughout the study. The number of examiners should be fairly small so as to assure the calibration. The most effective way to calibrate examiners is to provide education on how to perform the given index and to use a test subject who is not even involved in the study. Also, have both examiners provide the preferred dental index and score the subjects. If the examiners are not close, more information needs to be provided to the examiners.

Statistical Significance

Statistical significance is a measure of the confidence in test results. In the scientific community, a $p \leq 0.05$ is considered the cutoff point for statistical significance, meaning that an obtained result could happen by chance only five times or less in 100. Many times manufactures might state that a product is clinically superior or clinically improves disease. These terms do not indicate statistical significance.

Results

Results may be published in peer-reviewed (sometimes referred to as nonrefereed) publications. In order to be published, several other researchers review the publication and agree with its content. Table 14–3 lists the peer-reviewed publications germane to the dental hygiene science. These reviewers should have no idea who conducted the study, thus peer review is sometimes referred to as blind review. Occasionally studies will be published in nonpeer-reviewed publications that contain valid research results.

Table 14–3. Peer-Reviewed Dental Hygiene Periodicals
Journal of Dental Hygiene
International Journal of Dental Hygiene
Contemporary Oral Hygiene
Journal of Practical Hygiene
Dimensions in Dental Hygiene
Dental Health
Probe
Compendium of Continuing Education in Dental Hygiene
Dental Hygienist News

SUMMARY

Dental hygienists should be able to clearly understand published research reports and educate consumers regarding dental care products. For practicing professionals, it is important to always be a consumer advocate and stay current with contemporary products and modalities.

REFERENCES

[1] *Six Roles of the Dental Hygienist.* Chicago: American Dental Hygienists' Association, 1993.

[2] www.hhs.gov.

[3] www.fda.gov.

[4] Rippere, J. FDA regulation of OTC oral health care drug products. *Journal of Public Health Dentistry* 52 (1992): 329–32.

[5] Whall, C. The how and why of the ADA's evaluation program for dental therapeutic products. *Journal of Public Health Dentistry* 52 (1992): 338–42.

[6] www.ama-assn.org.

[7] Toothbrush abrasion spurs suit. *Albuquerque Journal,* 1998.

[8] McCann, A., and E. Schneiderman. Interpreting and evaluating a research report. *Dental Hygiene News* 5 (1997): 5–10.

Get Connected

Multimedia Extension Activities

www.prenhall.com/nathe

Use the above address to access the free, interactive companion web site created specifically to accompany this textbook. Here you will find an array of self study material to help you gain a richer understanding of the concepts presented in this chapter.

Unit IV

PRACTICAL STRATEGIES
FOR DENTAL PUBLIC HEALTH

The dental hygiene profession is responsible for expanding the opportunities available to the public to receive quality dental hygiene care. This final unit describes the current careers available in dental public health. Moreover, this unit actually explains how a practitioner can work in a governmental position. This unit also covers how a dental hygienist can effectively create a dental hygiene position in an organizational setting or possibly a private dental hygiene practice. This entrepreneurial endeavor will undoubtedly increase the underserved populations' access to dental hygiene care.

The final chapter serves as a review of dental public health principles germane to dental hygiene. Moreover, an overview of the topics and sample test items on National Dental Hygiene Examination Boards are covered.

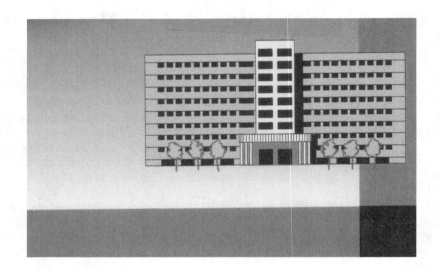

Chapter 15

CAREERS IN DENTAL PUBLIC HEALTH

OBJECTIVES

After studying this chapter, the dental hygiene student will be able to:

- define dental public health careers.
- describe various governmental opportunities.
- define dental hygiene positions in these areas.

COMPETENCIES

After studying this chapter and participating in accompanying course activities, the dental hygiene student should be competent in the following:

- provide dental hygiene services in a variety of settings, including offices, hospitals, clinics, extended care facilities, community programs, and schools.

KEY WORDS

COSTEP program
Independent contractor
National Health Service Corps

U.S. Civil Service
U.S. Public Health Service

INTRODUCTION

Dental hygienists are eligible to practice in dental public health with an entry-level associate's degree or certificate, bachelor's, master's, or doctorate degree. A plethora of positions actually exist in dental public health, including clinical dental hygiene to administrative posts in governmental agencies. A dental hygienist may contract with the U.S. Navy to work in a clinical setting in a military dental clinic providing clinical and educational services to military personnel. A dental hygienist may work as a civil servant employee or with the National Institutes of Dental and Craniofacial Research as a lead researcher in a study on the relationship of periodontal diseases to systemic conditions/diseases. A dental hygienist may hold an administrative title with the Centers for Disease Control and Prevention overseeing the agencies agenda on water fluoridation. These are just a handful of opportunities for the dental hygienist.

Dental public health governmental positions include working with the **U.S. Public Health Service**, the **U.S. Civil Service**, and contracting with a governmental agency or private placement agency. Dental hygienists may serve an entrepreneurial role, initiating dental hygiene services for the underserved, or work in positions that exist in private agencies that work directly in public health which are discussed in chapter 16.

U.S. PUBLIC HEALTH SERVICE CAREER

The mission of the Public Health Service (PHS)[1] Commissioned Corps is to provide highly trained and mobile health professionals who carry out programs to promote the health of the nation, understand and prevent disease and injury, assure safe and effective drugs and medical devices, deliver health services to federal beneficiaries, and furnish health expertise in time of war or other national or international emergencies. See Table 15–1 for the goals of the PHS. As one of the seven Uniformed Services of the United States, the PHS Commissioned Corps is a specialized career system designed to attract, develop, and retain health professionals who may be assigned to federal, state, or local agencies or international organizations to accomplish its mission.

The PHS Commissioned Corps is led by the surgeon general and consists of approximately 6,000 officers. See Figure 15–1 for a PHS Officer in uniform. Dental hygienists serve in the Health Services category of officers. The Health Services Officers (HSO) category represents approximately 10 percent of all PHS commissioned officers. The majority of HSOs are assigned to the agencies listed in Table 15–2.

In order to be eligible for a commissioned officer position with the U.S. Public Health Service, a dental hygienist must:

Table 15–1. PHS Goals

To accomplish this mission, the agencies/programs are designed to:

- Help provide health care and related services to medically underserved populations: to Americans, American Indians and Alaska Natives, and to other population groups with special needs

- Prevent and control disease, identify health hazards in the environment and help correct them, and promote healthy lifestyles for the nation's citizens

- Improve the Nation's mental health

- Ensure that drugs and medical devices are safe and effective, food is safe and wholesome, cosmetics are harmless, and that electronic products do not expose users to dangerous amounts of radiation

- Conduct and support biomedical, behavioral, and health services research and communicate research results to health professionals and the public and

- Work with other nations and international agencies on global health problems and their solutions

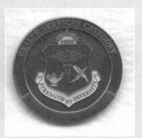

U.S. Public Health Service Health Services Category Coin

- Be a U.S. citizen
- Be under 44 years of age (age may be offset by prior active-duty Uniformed Service time and/or civil service experience in a PHS agency at a PHS site at a level commensurate with the duties of a commissioned officer)
- Have served less than 8 years of active duty if you are/were a member of another Uniformed Service
- Meet medical requirements
- Pass an initial suitability test

In addition, you must have earned a qualifying bachelor's degree from a program which, at the time the degree was conferred, was accredited by the acceptable accrediting body for your discipline. A current, unrestricted, and valid license in any of the fifty states, Washington, DC, the Commonwealth of Puerto Rico, the U.S. Virgin Islands, or Guam may be required. Compensation varies, depending on factors such as grade/rank, years of training and experience (T&E) in your profession, base pay entry data, specialty pay, geographic location of your duty station, and dependency status. The minimum starting pay grade/rank for health services

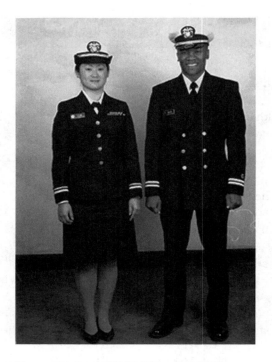

Figure 15–1. USPHS Officers in Uniform

Table 15–2. Agencies
Indian Health Service
Bureau of Prisons
Centers for Disease Control and Prevention
Food and Drug Administration
Health Resources and Services Administration
National Institutes of Health

officers in the PHS Commissioned Corps is O-2 (LTJG). T&E credit is determined by undergraduate education, graduate training, and experience considered to be professionally qualifying for appointment to the particular category. It is earned for time spent after receipt of the qualifying degree in degree-related activities. This could be

- Employment (paid or volunteer)
- Research
- Further training in your field (clinical practice, etc.)
- Teaching at the college or university level
- Allied and relevant graduate studies and/or research

U.S. CIVIL SERVICE

Dental hygienists providing clinical care can work as civil servants in a federal prison, Veteran's Affairs (VA) hospital, and military bases.[2-4] A dental hygienist must apply to a specific vacancy announcement, which may be used to fill a single vacancy or multiple vacancies over a period of time. Since vacancies can change every two weeks or so, it is suggested to visit the Web site frequently. From the list of vacancies, check on an individual dental hygiene position. The vacancy announcement provides information on specific duties, qualification requirements, ranking factors, and application forms and procedures. Complete copies of the vacancy announcement can be printed from the USAJOBS Web site. Required application materials and instructions regarding where the application must be submitted vary from announcement to announcement. For jobs that are filled through automated procedures, you must submit a resume and other specialized forms. Dental hygiene positions require copies of transcripts, licenses, or certifications.

The application submitted will be reviewed to determine whether education and/or experience requirements have been met for the position of interest, as stated in the vacancy announcement. If it meets with the basic qualification requirements, the application package will be evaluated to determine the best-qualified candidates based on job-related criteria. Evaluation procedures vary and will be specified in each announcement. In all cases, the evaluation is based on the application material you originally submitted.

The names and applications of the highest-ranking candidates are referred to the supervisor or selecting official. Selection procedures are subject to Federal Civil Service laws, which ensure that all applicants receive fair and equal treatment in the hiring process.

Almost all Civil Service positions in the U.S. Department of State require at least a secret security clearance. The clearance process considers such factors as registration for the Selective Service, failure to repay a U.S. government-guaranteed student loan, past problems with credit or bankruptcy, failure to meet tax obligations, unsatisfactory employment records, violations of the law and drug or alcohol abuse, or less-than-honorable discharge from the armed forces. Investigations, which usually take two to four months, include current and previous neighbors, supervisors, and coworkers. Depending on the nature of the job, you may begin work on a provisional basis, pending completion of the clearance process.

Working for the U.S. Department of State can be quite beneficial to you and your immediate family. Generally, you will be eligible for typical federal benefits such as federal employees' health insurance, life insurance, a retirement plan, and long-term disability insurance.

NATIONAL HEALTH SERVICE CORPS

The **National Health Service Corps** (NHSC)[3] is committed to improving the health of the nation's underserved by uniting communities in need with caring health professionals and supporting communities' efforts to build better systems of care (see Table 15–3). The NHSC provides comprehensive team-based health care that bridges geographic, financial, cultural, and language barriers. Because the NHSC is part of the "access agency"—the Health Resources and Services Administration (HRSA)—it works closely with other HRSA bureaus and programs to recruit primary care clinicians for communities in need.

Dental hygienists may work as clinicians with the NHSC, and those with qualifying educational loans may be eligible to compete for repayment of those

Table 15–3. NHSC Strategies for Meeting the Mission

- Forming partnerships with communities, states, educational institutions, and professional organizations
- Recruiting caring, culturally competent clinicians for communities in need
- Providing opportunities and professional experiences to students through Scholarship and Loan Repayment Programs and the SEARCH (Student/Resident Experiences and Rotations in Community Health) program
- Establishing systems of care that remain long after an NHSC clinician departs
- Shaping the way clinicians practice by building a community of dedicated health professionals who continue to work with the underserved even after their NHSC commitment has been fulfilled

loans if they choose to serve in a community of greatest need. In addition to loan repayment, these clinicians receive a competitive salary, some tax relief benefits, and a chance to have a significant impact on a community. The NHSC also works closely with state programs for underserved areas.

VA HOSPITAL DENTAL HYGIENE CAREERS

The Department of Veteran's Affairs[4] was created to treat the ongoing disabilities of veterans incurred during military service. Comprehensive care is delivered primarily through 172 medical centers and fifty-five outpatient clinics located nationwide, which offer a full range of primary, acute, chronic, and inpatient and outpatient health care services.

The VA Dental Services, an integral part of this health care system, are located in each medical center and in most of the major outpatient clinics. The VA employs approximately 775 full-time and 135 part-time dentists, 167 dental hygienists, and 1,600 dental assistants and other support personnel. A dental hygienist is employed as a civil service employee in the VA Dental Service Clinics.

MILITARY BASE DENTAL HYGIENE CAREERS

Dental hygienists can practice in any military branch dental clinic[5] as a civil service employee, independent contractor, professional dental management company employee, or as active duty military personnel. Each of these opportunities varies at different bases. In this setting, the dental hygienist usually works with a variety of dentists and specialists and frequently works with other health care providers.

FEDERAL PRISON DENTAL HYGIENE CAREERS

It is the mission of the Federal Bureau of Prisons[6] to protect society by confining offenders in the controlled environments of prisons and community-based facilities that are safe, humane, cost-efficient, and appropriately secure, and that provide work and other self-improvement opportunities to assist offenders in becoming law-abiding citizens. The Health Programs Section coordinates the Bureau of Prisons' medical, dental, and mental health services to federal inmates. Dental hygienists provide routine and advanced prophylactic and therapeutic dental care to the inmate population. They are also responsible for planning and directing the preventive dental health program. Qualifying applicants must be currently licensed to practice as dental hygienists in a state or territory of the United States or the District of Columbia. Applicants must also possess specialized experience performing oral prophylactic care and in providing oral health education services to patients. They must also possess experience performing advanced oral prophylactic, therapeutic, and preventive procedures in cases of periodontal diseases or inflammation or on patients with other medical or dental problems, placing temporary fillings, and finishing amalgam restorations. Dental hygienists can be hired as a civil service employee, independent contractor, U.S. Public Health Officer, or as an employee of a professional dental management firm.

INDEPENDENT CONTRACTOR

Independent contractors are dental hygienists who are in business for themselves. Independent contractors earn their livelihoods from their own independent businesses instead of depending on an employer to earn a living. Independent contractors are sometimes called consultants, freelancers, self-employed and even entrepreneurs and business owners. Dental hygienists may provide clinical services, consultative services and educational services. Independent contracting dental hygienists usually are paid more than regular employees, but do not get paid any benefits.

There is no single, clear-cut test for classifying workers as employees or independent contractors. Different legal tests for determining worker status are used by various government agencies, including:

- Internal Revenue Service
- State unemployment compensation insurance agencies
- State workers' compensation insurance agencies
- State tax departments
- U.S. Labor Department
- National Labor Relations Board

Each of these agencies is concerned with worker classification for different reasons, and each has different biases and practices. Each agency normally makes classification decisions on its own and does not have to consider what other agencies have done, which means that one agency might decide that you are an independent contractor whereas another classifies you as an employee. If opportunities exist, dental hygienists can work as an independent contractor for the Bureau of Prisons, the military, and various community dental clinics.

EMPLOYEE OF DENTAL STAFFING AGENCY

There are professional management firms[7] that provide health care personnel to federal dental and medical facilities throughout the United States. These companies will hire a dental hygienist as an employee and then place the dental hygienists in a government dental clinic. Although the dental hygienist will work in a government dental clinic, the dental hygienist will be an employee of this company. The government agency will pay the company a set fee for their dental hygiene employee, and the dental hygienist will then be paid by the company. These professional firms usually provide a variety of benefits for their dental hygiene employees.

One of these companies is the DPS, Inc. This company has administered more than ninety-four health care service contracts with the Air Force, Army, Coast Guard, Navy, and Federal Prison System. Their recruitment targets highly competent, qualified individuals who will be assets to the professional health care team. Commitment and capability make DPS one of the best firms providing government contract health care services. DPS, Inc. provides employment for dentists, dental hygienists, dental assistants, and dental lab technicians to work at federal facilities. The minimum requirements include

- Hold an unrestricted license to practice in any one of the fifty states, the District of Columbia, the Commonwealth of Puerto Rico, Guam or the Virgin Islands
- Have experience in their field in a clinical setting for at least 12 months within the preceding 24 months or be a recent graduate of an accredited program within the past 12 months
- Have a current CPR certification

STUDENT DENTAL PUBLIC HEALTH OPPORTUNITIES

In 1948 the U.S. Public Health Service (USPHS) established a summer employment program for medical students and then in 1955 other health disciplines were added to the program for participation.[1] Finally, in 1956 "COSTEP" was formally established. The **COSTEP program** introduces health disciplines for potential PHS careers and provides hands-on knowledge of PHS and its activities. If assigned to the Bureau of Prisons, the student will receive hands-on training in correctional medicine, policies, and procedures. COSTEP enables student to enhance educational background.

The Junior COSTEP provides students with an opportunity to become acquainted with the organization and mission of the U.S. Public Health Service (PHS) and with health-related career opportunities in various participating agencies.

Junior COSTEP participants are commissioned as ensigns (pay grade 0–1) in the Commissioned Corps of the U.S. Public Health Service. Assignments may

DENTAL HYGIENIST SPOTLIGHT
Carolyn Johnson, RDH, BS

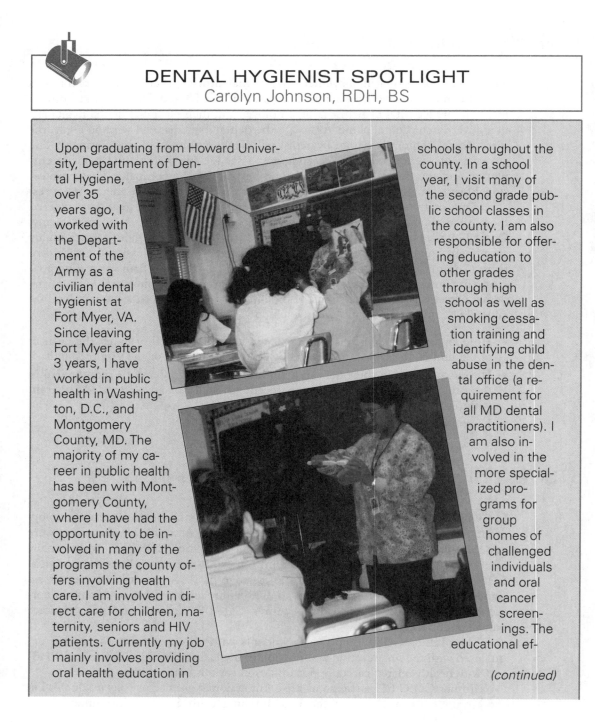

Upon graduating from Howard University, Department of Dental Hygiene, over 35 years ago, I worked with the Department of the Army as a civilian dental hygienist at Fort Myer, VA. Since leaving Fort Myer after 3 years, I have worked in public health in Washington, D.C., and Montgomery County, MD. The majority of my career in public health has been with Montgomery County, where I have had the opportunity to be involved in many of the programs the county offers involving health care. I am involved in direct care for children, maternity, seniors and HIV patients. Currently my job mainly involves providing oral health education in schools throughout the county. In a school year, I visit many of the second grade public school classes in the county. I am also responsible for offering education to other grades through high school as well as smoking cessation training and identifying child abuse in the dental office (a requirement for all MD dental practitioners). I am also involved in the more specialized programs for group homes of challenged individuals and oral cancer screenings. The educational ef-

(continued)

Dental Hygienist's Spotlight   *(continued)*

forts I have been involved in during the last three decades have been varied and exciting. I have seen the impact that education can have in improving the public's health. I have particularly enjoyed working with children, where the impact is often life-long. It is personally gratifying to know that I have made a positive difference in someone's future health.

range for thirty-one to 120 days throughout the year and are scheduled to be convenient with college enrollment. To be eligible for appointment to the Junior COSTEP program, an interested student must

- Have completed at least one year of study in medical, dental, or veterinary school; or have completed at least two years of study in a professionally accredited baccalaureate program in dietetics, engineering, medical record administration, physician assistant training, nursing, pharmacy, sanitary science, computer science, occupational therapy, or physical therapy or be enrolled in a master's or doctoral program in a health-related field.
- Expect to return to college or to a postgraduate training program in a commissionable profession immediately following participation in COSTEP.
- Be in a program of study accredited by an appropriate accrediting body.
- Be free of any obligation or responsibility that would conflict with extended active duty as a commissioned officer in the PHS (e.g., not be a member of a reserve or active duty component of any other uniformed service).
- Qualify for appointment in the PHS. This includes being a U.S. citizen, under forty-four years of age, and able to meet the physical standards of the Corps.

Participants in the Junior COSTEP program incur no obligation for future service in the U.S. Public Health Service or the selecting agency. The Senior COSTEP program was established to attract qualified students in accredited health care programs into the Commissioned Corps and service in the PHS. Effective the first day of formal studies for the last academic year, the selected student will be called to "active duty for training." The student will be paid the salary of an ensign (0–1) for that year.

To be eligible for appointment to the Senior COSTEP program, an interested student must

- Be a citizen of the United States under age forty-four
- Meet the medical fitness standards prescribed for appointment and active duty as a career officer

- Be enrolled in good standing in an accredited school of medicine, osteopathy, nursing, physician assistant training, medical records administration, pharmacy, sanitary science, computer science, dietetics, occupational therapy, physical therapy, dentistry, dental hygiene, or engineering; be eligible to enroll in the senior or final year of that school; and begin formal studies required as part of the curriculum for the senior or final year on the date of entry on active duty
- Agree in writing to serve on active duty as a commissioned officer with PHS for twice the period of training sponsored by PHS as stated in Section F of the Commissioned Corps Personnel Manual
- Be free of any obligation or commitment that would conflict with extended active duty as a commissioned officer in PHS (e.g., not be a member of a reserve or active duty component of any other uniformed service)
- Agree to waive any entitlement they may have to financial assistance (stipend or scholarship) in their final year of study other than assistance from the Senior COSTEP

The Senior COSTEP participant incurs a two-for-one commitment. For every month that the selecting agency funds the student during the final year of study, a two-month obligation for service in that agency is incurred.

STATE OPPORTUNITIES

Many state health departments employ dental hygienists to work as clinicians, educators, administrators, or researchers. Additionally, some states contract with private companies and/or independent dental hygiene contractors to provide clinical care and consulting. In many states, a dental hygienist with additional education and experience can be employed as the state dental director.

INTERNATIONAL OPPORTUNITIES

Dental hygienists have the opportunity to work in many different countries. In fact, only 23 countries educate dental hygienists, so there are ample opportunities for dental hygienists to initiate dental public health programs and dental hygiene educational programs in most of the world. Appendix G lists many opportunities for the dental hygienist overseas, including opportunities with the U.S. Peace Corps.

SUMMARY

Dental hygienists have various opportunities to work in government positions in the United States. There are also a variety of employment situations available in these positions, including U.S. Public Health Service Commissioned Officer, civil servant, independent contractor, and an employee of a professional dental management firm Additionally, opportunities for student employment exists with the U.S. Public Health Service for dental hygienists. For further information on these areas, please see Appendix C.

REFERENCES

[1] www.usphs.gov
[2] www.state.gov
[3] http://nhsc.bhpr.hrsa.gov
[4] www.va.gov
[5] www.defenselink.gov
[6] www.bop.gov
[7] www.dpsjobs.com

Note: Much of the information on the federal government was taken directly from the referenced web sites. Please see these web sites for more detailed information.

Get Connected

Multimedia Extension Activities

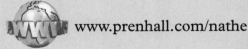 www.prenhall.com/nathe

Use the above address to access the free, interactive companion web site created specifically to accompany this textbook. Here you will find an array of self study material to help you gain a richer understanding of the concepts presented in this chapter.

Chapter 16

STRATEGIES FOR CREATING
DENTAL HYGIENE POSITIONS
IN DENTAL PUBLIC HEALTH SETTINGS

OBJECTIVES

After studying this chapter, the dental hygiene student will be able to:

- list the populations most in need of dental hygiene care.
- describe the paradigm for creating a dental hygiene position.
- develop protocol for a newly developed dental hygiene position.

COMPETENCIES

After studying the chapter and participating in accompaning course activities, the dental hygiene student will be competent in the following:

- promote the values of good oral and general health and wellness to the public and organizations within and outside the professions.
- identify services that promote oral health can prevent oral disease and related conditions.
- be able to influence consumer groups, businesses, and government agencies to support health care issues.
- assess, plan, implement, and evaluate community-based oral health programs.
- use screening, referral, and education to bring consumers into the health care delivery system.
- provide dental hygiene services in a variety of settings, including offices, hospitals, clinics, extended care facilities, community programs, and schools.
- evaluate reimbursement mechanisms and their impact on the patient's access to oral health care.

KEY WORDS

Blueprint
Contract
Legislative initiatives
Marketing

Practice management
Proposal
Public relations

www.prenhall.com/nathe

INTRODUCTION

Although dental hygiene initially began as a profession focused on public health initiatives, the professional has been positioned in the private dental office. In this setting, dental hygienists frequently have little control over the delivery of dental hygiene care. Because society is demanding a more appropriate delivery system for dental hygiene services, times are changing.[1]

It is readily apparent that not all in society are able to visit a dentist's office for a variety of reasons such as a disability, chronic illness, lack of funds, or rural location. Table 16-1 lists populations frequently in need of dental hygiene services. For them, access to dental hygiene services has been virtually unattainable. This unfortunate situation is all the more significant when it is likely that those who have the least access to dental hygiene services are the ones who would benefit most from the care that emphasizes prevention.[2]

Significant interest is being shown by members of the public, government agencies, and other health care professionals, as well as the dental hygiene profession itself, in establishing dental hygiene programs in settings other than private dental offices. The provision of dental hygiene services in these settings may require the dental hygienist to establish a distinct dental hygiene business.

Although most states have a difficult time containing health care costs while delivering quality care to all members of the population, access to preventive health care should undoubtedly improve costs while increasing autonomy for the dental hygiene practitioner. Moreover, quality and accountability should be improved by care delivered by the educated dental hygiene professional. Few would argue that the practitioner specifically educated in dental hygiene sciences best provides the

Table 16-1. Populations in Need of Dental Hygiene Care
Homebound
Institutionalized
Populations with Disabilities
Rural Area Residents
Population with Dental Phobia
Populations Faced with Language or Cultural Barriers
Inmates
Patients without Financing

optimum level of dental hygiene care.[3] This chapter focuses on the strategies for implementing dental hygiene positions within the health care delivery systems.

LEGISLATIVE PERSPECTIVE

Many states do not allow the public the opportunity to subscribe to dental hygiene services in any way other than with the private dental practice. In fact, in a few states dental hygienists can work only in a private dental setting directly supervised by a dentist. **Legislative initiatives** may be necessary to increase the accessibility of dental hygienists to the entire population.

Fortunately, forty-five states allow the dental hygienist to work without a dentist present in a variety of settings. The provision of dental hygiene care in alternative settings enables the dental hygienist to interact with those population segments currently underserved.

PROPOSED PLAN FOR ACTION

In order to effectively establish a dental hygiene position, it is necessary to follow the dental public health program planning paradigm discussed in Chapter 9. It is important to identify the various aspects dental hygienists would have to consider regarding the feasibility of an alternative delivery of dental hygiene care and to establish the parameters for setting up a dental hygiene position.

Assessment

During the assessment phase, it is vital to conduct a needs assessment of the population at hand. Moreover, a needs assessment of the facility and funding should commence during this phase. Information to be obtained may include the number, ages, and medical needs of individuals within the population; specific dental needs of the population; administrative support and values toward dental hygiene care; and facility space, staff support, and reimbursement mechanisms.

It is necessary to ascertain whether dental hygienists in the specific state can be reimbursed directly by Medicaid, SCHIPS, and/or dental insurance companies. If not, how can this avenue of reimbursement be achieved: By legislation or possibly a rule change? Is the organization amiable toward hiring a dental hygienist as an employee and completing all collection services? These questions require answers during this phase.

As a dental hygienist, never underestimate the importance of understanding what organizations will value in dental hygiene services. Many individuals still do not know what a dental hygienist is and many individuals do not value preventive dental care. For these reasons, it is necessary for the dental hygienist to completely define what services will be "sold."

Dental Hygiene Diagnosis

At this stage the dental hygienist should develop a comprehensive dental hygiene diagnosis for the target population. An example looks at a dental hygiene diagnosis directed at a population employed by a major company (4,000 employees). The company survey revealed that only 25 percent of the employees were currently seeking dental treatment (dental demand), either preventive or restorative, and that more than 500 days were lost to sick days due to toothaches (dental need). In addition, the company's on-site registered nurse calculated that 25 percent of visits made to her are for dental problems (dental need). A diagnosis of the population would read that the population has tremendous dental needs (toothaches) and is not currently accessing dental care.

Planning

The planning stage includes prioritizing goals and objectives and development of strategies and involves the development of a program blueprint. Items to include would be staff support, space availability, reimbursement mechanisms, patient management systems, dental health promotional activities, and **public relations** initiatives. During this stage evaluation mechanisms should be developed. These mechanisms may include the use of dental indexes, dental records, surveys, and interviews. Meeting with administrators and/or other interested parties should be done to assist in effective and efficient planning. See Table 16–2 for a detailed business plan of action for dental hygienists starting their own business.

Implementation

This stage involves the actual operations and generally includes constant revisions. During implementation it is necessary for the dental hygienist to effectively manage the program, which entails dealing with people, both in collaboration and many times in supervisory roles. Specific management skills needed are listed in Table 16–3.

Evaluation

The evaluative stage additionally includes measurement of the intended outcomes and possibly revisions to the program. Measurement can be obtained through dental indexes, records, and surveys. Moreover, departments within the program may be quite helpful at providing information concerning unmet needs.

Furthermore, it is vital to provide documented written and oral reports to administrators. These reports emphasize the importance of the dental hygiene program, as well as maintain visibility and testify to the value of the program. Equally

Table 16-2.   ADHA's Business Plan

Business Plan	What It Really Means
Service Development	Continually refining what you're selling to meet the changing needs of your potential clients.
Marketing	Continually taking action to become more aware of your clients' needs and informing your potential clients why your service is meant for them.
Sales	Talking face-to-face with your potential clients and getting them to say, "Yes, I'll retain your services."
Operations	Doing the work of the business. This includes everything from answering the telephone, to working directly with patients.
Personnel	Managing the people who work with you.
Finance	Measuring the financial results of your business, comparing them with your desired results and using this comparison to identify critical business issues.
Management	Making sure the above six areas are working in concert to meet your goals for the business.

Source: Reprinted with permision from the American Dental Hygienists' Association. 2003.

Table 16-3.   Management Skills

- Establish short- and long-term goals
- Participate in strategic planning
- Formulate policies and procedures
- Coordinate personnel, material, and financial resources
- Motivate and evaluate workers
- Solve problems and make decisions
- Resolve conflicts
- Effect change

Source: Darby, M., and M. Walsh. *Dental Hygiene Theory and Practice.* Philadelphia: W. B. Saunders, 1995.

DENTAL HYGIENIST'S SPOTLIGHT
Sandy Roe, RDH, MS, Public Relations Director, Participa!, Inc. Dental Services

After twenty years practicing clinical dental hygiene, never in my wildest dreams would I have thought I would be helping pioneer efforts to provide dental care to underserved children in a school-based program throughout rural New Mexico.

In 1983, at the age of twenty, I received my Associate of Arts Degree in Dental Hygiene from Johnson County Community College in Overland Park, Kansas. I worked five years in private practice in rural Kansas for my childhood dentist before moving to Albuquerque, New Mexico. In New Mexico, I continued working in private practice for several local dentists in the Albuquerque area. In 1997, after many years of dental hygiene practice, I found the courage to return to school and finish my bachelor degree in the Dental Hygiene Bachelor Degree Completion Program at the University of New Mexico. Upon completion of my bachelor degree, I continued my studies at the University of Missouri-Kansas City School of Dentistry, Kansas City, Missouri, and received my master of science degree in dental hygiene education in May 2000. I feel this accomplishment was the best career decision I could have ever made.

I began working with Participa!, Inc. Dental Services as the administrative director in May 2001. Participa!, Inc. Dental Services is a nonprofit community service organization in New Mexico whose mission is to provide dental services to the underserved children of the state via a portable school-based program. We are trying to address the problem of the tremendous lack of access to care for the children of this state. Participa is a Medicaid provider only, and our intention is to provide dental services for children who are Medicaid eligible *and* who do not have a family dentist or access to dental care.

Our school-based dental services program works directly with school personnel to help provide parents with information and children with dental health education. School administrators, school nurses, and program directors collaborate with us to provide dental services while the child is in school. For Medicaid eligible children who return a completed consent form, we provide comprehensive dental exams, diagnostic x-rays, dental cleanings, topical fluoride treatments, dental sealants, and selective restorative care as appropriate in a school setting.

If the Medicaid eligible child notes on a consent form that they have a family dentist, but the parent still requests services from Participa!, Inc. Dental Services, we will provide a visual screening exam at no charge. Any dental sealants recommended by our dentists will be

(continued)

Dental Hygienist's Spotlight *(continued)*

placed, and the sealant fee will be billed to Medicaid. By doing this, the child can continue seeing their regular dentist, and we can place the necessary sealants to prevent decay. For uninsured children who return a completed consent form, we will also provide a visual screening exam at no cost to the parents, school, and/or Medicaid. If needed, parents will receive a referral note to a dentist that offers reduced prices for dental services.

Each child will receive a completed treatment form of what services Participa!, Inc. Dental Services has provided to be taken home by the child and given to the parents. Furthermore, if the child needs follow-up care (i.e., restorations), we send home our referral for follow-up care form.

We utilize a centralized billing and management infrastructure that allows us to ensure consistency in operations and quick analysis of results. Our field operations are decentralized in order for our employees to serve their communities and surrounding areas. Our dental personnel are responsible for contacting school personnel, scheduling work assignments, providing services, and reporting results.

Our ultimate goal is to find each child a dental home while increasing dental awareness and education to school age children in rural and underserved areas of the New Mexico. We have developed partnerships with eighteen rural Medicaid providers throughout the state who will provide follow-up restorative care for our children and their families. Furthermore, we currently employ six dentists on a regular basis who perform exams and restorative care and supervise the work of our teams that provide the preventive services. These teams consist of a minimum of one registered dental hygienist and one dental assistant. For larger school populations, two prevention teams are assigned. The number of service personnel employed for any given work assignment varies with the numbers of children to be served and the number of services to be provided. Teams expand to greater numbers and different types of personnel as required. In addition to our dentists, we employ nine dental hygienists, ten dental assistants, and three administrative staff members.

In this past school year, our Medicaid business grossed over a million dollars. Participa!, Inc. Dental Services's teams provided 5,435 comprehensive dental exams, 2,970 diagnostic x-rays, 4,049 dental cleanings, and 3,933 fluoride treatments throughout the state. We have placed 17,110 sealants on permanent teeth and provided 739 fillings. We have extracted many abscessed deciduous teeth and removed several supernumerary anterior teeth. Children who were diagnosed with extensive dental disease were referred to local Medicaid providers we have partnered with.

My current job requirements as the public relations director of Participa!

(continued)

Dental Hygienist's Spotlight   *(continued)*

Inc. Dental Services is to develop policies, growth, and global decision making; ensure that Participa! complies with the Dental Practice Act and Medicaid requirements, along with ensuring compliance with federal and state laws such as Occupational Safety and Health Administration (OSHA); and Health Insurance Portability and Accountability (HIPPA) requirements. I also promote Participa! and Participa!'s mission to state legislators. I work with legislators to develop policies and funding that will promote our mission. This year, I lobbied the forty-sixth New Mexico State Legislature with Senate Bill 408, sponsored by Senator Mary Kay Pappen of Dona Ana County. This bill would allow a $100,000 appropriation from the general fund to provide dental screening examinations and dental sealants for uninsured children in rural school districts of New Mexico.

I am the contact person for new schools and new growth of our program. I provide presentations about our organization to many different groups, including school boards, dental hygiene educators and students, and Head Start programs along with health committees and alliances. I meet with community stakeholders and fraternal organizations throughout the state in order to encourage local financial support of our program. I participate and serve in various committees that promote children's dental health, and I am also the cochair of the New Mexico Oral Health Council. Daily, I interface with vendors, school personnel, and customers to promote Participa! and resolve issues that may arise.

Also, part of my job description includes actively recruiting dentists, dental hygienists, and dental assistants. I work with our payroll company developing and maintaining our employee manual, determining appropriate employee benefits, distributing literature to our regional directors regarding benefits and worker's compensation, and advise regional directors on reporting work-related injuries. Finally, I ensure that personnel records are up to date with such items as CPR, OSHA requirements, and updated liability insurance to secure proper licensure of each employee.

Variety is the spice of life! Every day offers me new challenges, and I find satisfaction in helping access care for low-income children, speaking with school nurses, or educating parents about their child's dental needs. In addition, as another different touch to my career, I also continue teaching as a part-time assistant professor at the University of New Mexico. Furthermore, I am certified to administer local anesthesia in Kansas and New Mexico, and I am one of twenty-one dental hygienists in New Mexico to receive my certification for Collaborative Practice of Dental Hygiene.

necessary is the constant communication and reporting to patients and fellow health care providers. By providing ongoing communication, needed revisions can be made, thus encouraging ongoing evaluation.

PRACTICE MANAGEMENT ISSUES

Practice management issues should be defined during the planning stages and further refined during the implementation and evaluation stages. These issues may include patient tracking, appointment scheduling, practice promotion, and collection of fees. Written patient records are extremely important in dental hygiene treatment. Information within these records should include patient contact information such as address, phone numbers, and pertinent information; health history; dental hygiene assessments, diagnoses, planning, implementation, and evaluative documentation; and financial records. Maintaining accurate records enhances the operation and serves as a comprehensive record of each patient.

Effective appointment scheduling will improve practice operations by decreasing patients' wasted time and increasing productivity. Appointment scheduling may become more complicated in health care settings, when patients have commitments for health care treatment many times during the day. Therefore, it may be beneficial to integrate appointment scheduling procedures within the institution.

Practice promotion occurs when the practice is effectively marketing its service. **Marketing** is an organized approach to selecting and servicing markets and a research approach to inform the public of a service as distinct from an impromptu approach to selling a service. The purpose of marketing a dental hygiene practice is to select and service patients. The four Ps of marketing include product/service, price, plan for distribution, and promotion. See Table 16–4 for more information on marketing strategies for a dental hygiene practice.[4]

PROPOSAL DEVELOPMENT AND PRESENTATION

Figure 16–1 presents an example of a **proposal** for a dental hygiene position within a nursing facility. The proposal should always include an introduction and the purpose of the dental hygiene program as well as the significance of such a position. The significance section should be the place where the importance of the dental hygiene position is discussed. This section is meant to motivate the administrators and persuade them to open a dental hygiene position. After reading this section, they should wonder why they have not been offering this program before and feel it is a positive step for the organization.

The **blueprint** of the program, possibly described in a diagram, should be defined with a detailed budget and financing section included. The reader should

Table 16–4.   The Four Ps of Marketing Adapted to a Dental Hygiene Practice

Product/Service

- Quality dental hygiene services
- Decrease in plaque, acute pain, and dental diseases
- Increase in value of dental health
- Positive feedback from patients and institution

Price

- Assist in reimbursement mechanisms
- Competitive with local private dental practices
- Policies and procedures describing all types of reimbursement mechanisms

Distribution Plan

- Practice location and hours
- Appointment scheduling
- Labor force
- Flexible conditions within an institution

Promotion

- Quality image of program
- Creative and legal advertising techniques
- Publicity
- Dental health education and promotion strategies

Source: Kotler, P. *Marketing for Nonprofit Organizations.* Upper Saddle River, NJ: Prentice Hall, 1982.

Figure 16–1.   Example Proposal to Fones Nursing Facility for the Establishment of a Dental Hygiene Program

Introduction

This proposal addresses the recognition of oral health care needs of elderly people, the institution of a preventive dental program, and the addition of a contract dental hygienist. Dental hygienists have the scientific background and clinical skills to initiate dental programs in long-term care facilities; therefore, it is the intention of this proposal to clarify the procedures necessary to establish a dental hygiene position.

Significance

Certain physiological changes occur in the oral cavities of the elderly, including loss of teeth, recession of gums, and teeth becoming brittle and more prone to chipping and cracking. Due to the loss of muscle-tone about the face and mouth, other

(continued)

Figure 16–1. *(continued)*

conditions occur such as cheilosis (cracking in the corners of the mouth), flacid tongue, and epulis fissuratum (growths due to ill-fitting dentures). As a result of aging or due to certain medication, xerostomia, or drying of the oral tissues, also occurs causing discomfort, difficulty in speaking, loss of taste sensations, high incidence of gum-line cavities, and discomfort in denture wearers, to mention only a few problems.

In addition, dentures may cause serious conditions if they do not fit properly and can be a factor in oral cancer, which comes from the continual irritation of the soft tissue. The importance of examining the soft tissues of the face, neck, lips, as well as all the structures inside the mouth cannot be stressed enough. The incidence of oral cancer among elderly people is alarming. Early detection and prompt treatment make a significant difference in the prognosis of this dreaded disease.

Dental Hygiene Program

As a member of the health team, and in collaboration with the dentist, the dental hygienist performs necessary procedures for total patient care. These services include counseling and instruction to patients, regularly scheduled in-service programs for the nursing staff, and preventive clinical services such as intra- and extra-oral examinations, scaling (teeth cleaning), nonsurgical periodontal therapy, radiographs, fluoride treatments to desensitize exposed roots, denture care, denture labeling, and referral either to the patients' private dentist or to the facility's dental consultant. Moreover, the dental hygienist formulates a recall system by which annual and admission exams will be performed to meet federal and state health requirements.

A dental hygienist registered in the State of New Mexico may be licensed to work in collaboration with a dentist. Therefore, a dental hygienist employed in a nursing home is ethically and legally permissible in New Mexico. Many dental hygienists are employed in nursing homes in different states. A contract dental hygienists may be reimbursed through Medicaid or charge fees directly to the patient for services provided, eliminating cost to the nursing home.

Conclusion

The quality of care that is provided to the residents of an institution is a priority to both administration and staff. However, dental care often is not a priority and sometimes neglected. The dental hygienist contracted to work would improve and expand the quality of care, which would be beneficial to the staff, administration, and most importantly, the residents of a nursing facility. This contract position, which provides necessary preventive dental care, can become an integral part of existing interdisciplinary comprehensive services.

be able to read a paragraph or two and understand the basic premise of the program. The conclusion should summarize the important points and sell the reader on the organizational need for this type of program.

Specific strategies should be employed to effectively present the proposal. Generally, the dental hygienists will be given ten to fifteen minutes for this presentation. Utilization of the proposal handout and slides or transparencies can greatly enhance the position attractiveness. As dental hygienists continually sell the service, it is necessary to be prepared, organized, and make use of effective and appropriate media. See Chapter 7 for more tips on effective presentation strategies.

DENTAL HYGIENE CONSULTATION AND POLICIES

Figure 16–2 depicts a sample agreement between a dental hygienist and nursing facility. This example will be helpful in the development of an employment **contract** for a dental hygienist working as an employee of an agency. Figure 16–3 is a sample

---

Figure 16–2.   Employment Agreement—Dental Hygienist

This agreement entered into on this _____ day of _____, _____, between _____, registered under the dental laws of this state, hereinafter referred to as the Registered Dental Hygienist, (RDH), and the Fones Long-Term Care Facility, hereinafter referred to as Facility.

Whereas Facility desires to employ the services of RDH and whereas RDH is desirous of offering certain services, it is therefore mutually agreed that Facility does employ and RDH agrees to offer services on the following mutual terms and conditions:

A. Facility assumes the professional responsibility and administrative responsibility for services rendered.

B. RDH will perform services within the realm of the dental hygiene profession for Facility.

C. Insurance (individual terms to be determined).

D. As compensation, therefore, Facility agrees to pay RDH a salary of _____.

E. Irene Newman, RDH, is the licensed dental hygienist for Fones Long-Term Care Facility.

F. The RDH in conjunction and cooperation with the dental consultant is responsible for:

(continued)

Figure 16–2.   *(continued)*

1. Formulating, establishing, and continually making revisions in the policies for dental services in her role as a member of the Dental Advisory Board.
2. Coordinating and implementing in-service programs designed for the staff, which will include daily oral hygiene care for the residents, nutritional requirements related to dental health, and identifying pathology relevant to the geriatric patient.
3. Recording and/or updating the dental history, maintaining one copy in the dental facility and placing one copy in the resident's medical file.
4. Evaluating the residents' oral health status by completing intra- and extra-oral examinations.
5. Providing the administration with written quarterly reports and recommendations and plans for the implementation of those recommendations.
6. Assisting the nursing staff in carrying out the dental consultants' and RDH's recommendations.
7. Retaining on a continuing basis proper membership credentials in the American Dental Hygienists' Association and other affiliated associations. She is required to maintain the highest level of affiliation for the profession, including periodic participation in special workshops and continuing education, particularly those related to the dental care of the geriatric patient.

G. Nursing personnel are responsible for notifying dentist/dental hygienist of any resident with a dental problem. A request for their services is left in Nursing Office.

H. In cooperation with the Facility, the RDH, when necessary, will arrange for residents to be brought to the dental facility.

Source: Modified from Employment Agreement, Suzann C. Chenery, RDH, BS, Ashlar of Newtown, CT, 1990.

Figure 16–3.   Policy for Dental Hygiene Services

Fones Long-Term Care Facility has arrangements to assist residents to obtain emergency and routine dental care.

The dental hygienist will hold office hours on a designated day each week or more often if necessary.

Services provided by the dental hygienist are:

A.   Obtaining medical clearance from resident's physician prior to treatment.

(continued)

Figure 16–3.   *(continued)*

B.   In emergencies and/or to relieve pain:

In the absence of the dental consultant, the RDH examines the resident clinically and/or radiographically and refers the resident for immediate treatment to private dentist, dental consultant, or physician.

C.   Perform periodic oral cancer screenings on all residents.

D.   Compile dental indexes for all residents and submit results to the administration in report form with the quarterly report.

E.   Document all examinations and treatment rendered.

F.   Maintain communications between the nursing staff (especially the nurse's assistants), the dental consultant, and herself.

G.   Initiate and reevaluate the dental recall system.

H.   The RDH will render appropriate preventive clinical services, i.e.:

1. obtain medical clearance and review medical history.

2. record dental history.

3. perform intra- and extra-oral exam.

4. design a treatment plan.

5. take radiographs if necessary.

6. perform oral prophylaxis: removal of calculus (tartar), dental plaque and stains from natural teeth and/or artificial teeth by scaling and polishing.

Source: Modified from Dental Hygiene Services, Suzann C. Chenery, RDH, BS, Ashlar of Newtown, CT, 1990.

policy for dental hygiene services. It can serve as an example for the dental hygienist in developing specific institutional policy. Figure 16–4 defines an advisory role for a dental hygienist to an institution. Finally, a beneficial addition to the dental hygiene program is the use of dental hygiene students, which can bring motivation and a learning initiative to the program. Figure 16–5 depicts a sample affiliation agreement.

SUMMARY

When deciding whether to start a dental hygiene practice in a public health setting, do not give consideration only to the clinical skills that dental hygienists' possess; also remember that as a dental hygienist, one also possesses communication skills,

---

Figure 16–4. Dental Advisory Role to Fones Long-Term Care Facility

A. The RDH serves on the facility's Dental Advisory Board in addition to the Facility's Administrator, Dentist or Dental Consultant, Patient Care Coordinator, and one faculty member of UNM Division of Dental Hygiene.

B. The RDH serves as an in-house dental advisor to the staff and is responsible for guidance and instruction in the care of residents' individual oral health.

Source: Modified from Dental Advisory Role, Suzann C. Chenery, RDH, BS, Ashlar of Newtown, CT, 1990.

---

motivation skills, knowledge of health and wellness, assessment and treatment planning skills, and an interdisciplinary team approach to the provision of care. These skills are adaptable to working with the public in a wide variety of settings.

Author's Note

For dental hygienists interested in creating their own position, the ADHA document entitled *Marketing Dental Hygiene Services in Alternative Practice settings: Starting and Growing Your Own Dental Hygiene Business* can be downloaded at http://www.adha.org.

Figure 16–5. Coordination of Affiliation with University of New Mexico (UNM) Division of Dental Hygiene

A. The RDH in cooperation with the supervising faculty of UNM Division of Dental Hygiene plans and implements a minimum of two annual visitations of the dental hygiene students, which include
   1. orientation.
   2. tour of facility.
   3. individualized screening and counseling sessions.
   4. submitting problem-oriented data on each resident screened to the RDH.
   5. In-service programs to the nursing staff.

Source: Modified from Affiliation Agreement, Suzann C. Chenery, RDH, BS, Ashlar of Newtown, CT, 1990.

REFERENCES

[1]Nathe, C. *Dental Hygiene: A Career for the Future Manual.* Albuquerque: University of New Mexico, 1999.

[2]*A Resource Guide for Dental Hygienists in Non-traditional Settings.* Ontario Dental Hygienists' Association, 1998.

[3]Nathe, C. Dental hygienists: A needed reality (editorial). *Contact International* 12 (1998): 3.

[4]Kotler, P. *Marketing for Nonprofit Organizations.* Upper Saddle River, NJ: Prentice Hall, 1982.

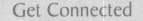

Get Connected

Multimedia Extension Activities

 www.prenhall.com/nathe

Use the above address to access the free, interactive companion web site created specifically to accompany this textbook. Here you will find an array of self study material to help you gain a richer understanding of the concepts presented in this chapter.

Chapter 17

DENTAL PUBLIC HEALTH REVIEW

with contributions from Meg Zayan, RDH, MPH

OBJECTIVES

After studying the chapter, the dental hygiene student will be able to:

- describe the National Board Dental Hygiene Examination dental public health format.
- list topics that may appear on this examination.
- list strategies to aid in studying for the dental public health section of boards.
- review sample test items.

COMPETENCIES

After studying the chapter and participating in accompanying course activities, the dental hygiene student should be competent in the following:

- provide health education and preventive counseling.
- promote the values of good oral and general health and wellness to the public and organizations within and outside the professions.
- identify services that promote oral health can prevent oral disease and related conditions.
- be able to influence consumer groups, businesses, and government agencies to support health care issues.
- assess, plan, implement, and evaluate community-based oral health programs.
- use screening, referral, and education to bring consumers into the health care delivery system.
- provide dental hygiene services in a variety of settings, including offices, hospitals, clinics, extended care facilities, community programs, and schools.
- evaluate reimbursement mechanisms and their impact on the patient's access to oral health care.
- recognize and use written and electronic sources of information.
- evaluate the credibility and potential hazards of dental products and techniques.
- evaluate published clinical and basic science research and integrate this information to improve the oral health of the patient.

- recognize the responsibility and demonstrate the ability to communicate professional knowledge verbally and in writing.
- accept responsibility for solving problems and making decisions based on accepted scientific principles.
- expand and contribute to the knowledge base of dental hygiene.

KEY WORDS

Joint Commission on National Dental
  Examinations
Licensure Requirements
  Clinical examination requirement
  Educational requirement

Jurisprudence requirements
Written examination requirement
National Board Dental Hygiene
  Examination
Testlet

INTRODUCTION

Specific dental hygiene **licensure requirements** vary among states, but all states have four types of requirements: (1) an **educational requirement**, (2) a **written examination requirement**, (3) **jurisprudence requirements**, and (4) a **clinical examination requirement**. The **National Board Dental Hygiene Examination** is intended to fulfill or partially fulfill the written examination requirements, but acceptance of a National Board score is completely at the discretion of the states. Alabama is the only state that does not require a dental hygiene candidate to pass the National Board Dental Hygiene Examination.

This chapter focuses on reviewing the community health/research principles section of the National Dental Hygiene Board Examination given by the American Dental Association's **Joint Commission on National Dental Examinations**.[1] The commission includes representatives of dental and dental hygiene schools, dental and dental hygiene practice, state dental examining boards, and the public. The purpose of the exam is to assist state boards in determining qualification of the dental hygienist who seeks licensure to practice dental hygiene.

For more information on the national examination for dental hygienists, please contact the American Dental Association at (312) 440-2678 or www.ada .org. Students can use this chapter in an effective manner after the class has been completed and during the crucial period of studying for boards.

STUDY GUIDE

The exam is comprehensive and consists of approximately 350 multiple-choice test items. The format of the exam is separated into two components. The discipline-based component includes 200 items addressing scientific basis for dental hygiene practice (anatomic sciences, physiology, biochemistry, nutrition, microbiology, immunology, pathology, and pharmacology); provision of clinical dental hygiene clinical services (patient assessments, radiology, dental hygiene care, periodontology, dental biomaterials); and community health/research principles (dental public health science). The second component includes 150 case-based items that refer to patient cases. Table 17–1 displays the breakdown of items in the community dental health/research principles category for the exam. This section of the exam is written using a **testlet** format. Each testlet introduces an issue pertinent to dental public health. The testlets are written in paragraph form followed by a series of multiple choice questions. The target populations often mentioned in these testlets may include but are not limited to the following clients: Head Start, preschool/ elementary/middle/high school, substance abuse, geriatric (nursing homes, senior day cares, senior centers), physically challenged, mentally challenged, pregnant teens, veterans, immigrants, ethnic groups, sport teams, care givers, forensic, and special needs.

As in all areas of dental hygiene, the most important factor in taking the exam is being prepared. The best methods for preparation may include the suggestions provided in Table 17–2.

Key concepts are generally covered by the community dental activities section on the exam. These concepts are provided in the following section in outlined format.

Promoting Health and Preventing Disease Within Groups
Including media and communication resources

- The overall goal of dental public health programs is to reduce oral disease.
- The major aspect of dental public health programs is promotion and prevention. This is done through activities to enhance positive behavior, education, and clinical services.
- Dental health education is defined as the teaching of oral health behaviors whereas dental health promotion is defined as informing and motivating individuals to adopt healthy behaviors.

Table 17–1.   Breakdown of Examination Specifics

Community Health Research Principles (20)

A. Promoting Health and Preventing Disease Within Groups (including media and communication resources) (4)

B. Participating in Community Programs (8)

   1. Assessing populations and defining objectives (3)

   2. Designing, implementing, and evaluating programs (5)

C. Analyzing Scientific Information, Understanding Statistical Concepts, and Applying Research Results (8)

Table 17–2. Preparation Suggestions
Be prepared! It will undoubtedly increase confidence!
Organize notes from dental hygiene school and prerequisite classes.
Outline notes in a manner that works well for you.
When perusing old notes, look up information in textbooks that is still unclear.
Review key concepts from professors.
Review old boards.
Study with groups and by yourself.

- In areas where dental public health programs are indicated, the demand for dental care is low and the need is high. It is the intent of public health programs to achieve a higher demand for dental care and to decrease the need.
- Dental public health dental hygienists should concentrate on teaching those individuals who work closely with the target population, including teachers, caregivers, nurse's aides, and so on.
- State dental health departments' primary purpose is to serve as a consultant for public and private and in state dental issues.
- When teaching a population to adopt positive dental health behaviors, it is necessary to change the values they may hold toward oral health.
- Behavior change will not commence until value adoption is complete; providing dental health education to a population does not assure behavior change.
- When distributing educational materials, be careful to critique them beforehand to make sure they are not blatantly promoting a dental care product, and, most important, that they have factual information that is not misleading.
- Water fluoridation has proven cost effective, although opponents claim that fluoridation itself violates their human rights.
- Advocates of water fluoridation may find it beneficial to develop long-term strategies for adoption.

Participating in Community Programs
   Assessing populations and defining objectives
   Designing, implementing, and evaluating programs
- Planning consists of determining consumer needs, which can be diagnosed by a dental professional, as compared with consumer demands, which can be defined as the frequency of dental visits or attempted dental visits.

- Program planning involves the dental hygiene process of care, including assessment, dental hygiene diagnosis, planning, implementation, and evaluation. Many public health paradigms place the diagnosis stage within the planning stage.
- Prioritizing is a necessary component during the dental hygiene diagnosis and planning stages of program development.
- When planning a program it is necessary to develop measurable objectives so that the program can be effectively evaluated.
- In order to increase participation in a program, it is beneficial to have personal contact with your target population.
- Dental hygienists should include the target population or its representatives when planning the dental public health program.
- When working with programs targeted at minority groups, it is helpful to have minority leaders supporting your program.
- When initiating a dental public health program, it is necessary to first contact the head administrator for approval and support.
- When planning a dental sealant program, the children involved should be in the second and sixth grade to ensure fully erupted molars for placement of the sealants.
- If a program involves parents, it is necessary to have parental support. Always have support from the target group.

Analyzing Scientific Information, Understanding Statistical Concepts, and Applying Research Results

- Prevalence is the expression of the number of existing cases of a specific disease or condition in a population at a specific point in time.
- Incidence is the expression of the new number of cases of a disease or condition in a population at a specific point in time.
- Mortality is the ratio of the number of deaths from a specific disease to the total number of cases of that disease.
- Morbidity is the ratio of sick to well persons in a population.
- Reliability is the consistency or degree to which an instrument will produce the same results within the same population every time the characteristic is measured.
- Validity is the degree to which an instrument measures the variable that it is designed to measure.
- A pilot study is a trial run of a research study so those variables can be best controlled during the long-term study.
- Dependent variable is the measure expected to change as a result of the manipulation of the independent variable.
- Independent variable is the manipulated measure controlled by the investigator.
- Measures of central tendency, including mean, median, and mode, measure what is typical in the sample group.

DENTAL HYGIENIST'S SPOTLIGHT
Susan Sanzi-Schaedel, RDH, MPH

I have always loved the science of dental hygiene. However even as a student I knew that I was not meant to provide dental hygiene services in a traditional private office setting. I knew that I could never provide services to all the people needing care if I was working with only one person at a time. Many years later, I still cannot provide services to all who are in need, but the profession of dental public health has given me the tools to be able to look at the community as my patient, assess what the needs are, and to be able to target services and strategies where they can be most effective.

My career as a dental hygienist started in 1969 in a large metropolitan children's hospital, where I had the opportunity to work with a variety of children, and families. Working with both healthy and developmentally disabled children was a real opportunity to expand my skills while supporting families.

From the children's hospital, I moved to a community health center (CHC). I was a clinician as well as an oral health educator in the local schools. I also had the opportunity to mentor dental hygiene students who were at the CHC for rotation. It was at the community health center that I learned about the richness brought to the work environment and life in general, by being in a culturally and ethnically diverse community. It was an experience that drove my desire to work in public health.

A community dentistry department in a dental school was my next stop. I taught a prevention course for dental assistants, supervised dental hygiene rotations, and set up a program for preventive services and referral in a local elementary school. The department developed a master's of science degree program in dental public health for which I became an advisor to one of the students. It was then that I knew that having experience in public

(continued)

Dental Hygienist's Spotlight *(continued)*

health was only part of the picture. I also needed the theory for what I was trying to teach. This was the time I realized I needed to return to graduate school myself.

In 1975, I found myself back in graduate school studying dental public health/health education and health behavior. I knew I was finally in the "right" place for me. My desire to work with people and communities with limited resources was being given structure and a theoretical framework. It gave me the tools to implement and evaluate successful approaches to prevention, education and health promotion, and treatment services. Graduate school also introduced me to many of the experts in the area of dental public health. These introductions have proven useful over and over again.

Following receipt of a master's in public health, I took a job with a large county health department. Twenty-five years later, I still find excitement and space for creativity in that position. I have worked to ensure our activities fall under the core functions of public health, that is, assessment, policy development, and assurance. Our programs are implemented based on community needs, so assisting in the planning and implementation and communicating the results of oral health needs assessment is a critical role. I have worked on many coalitions, advocacy groups, and interdepartmental groups whose focus was policy development or modification. The focus of my efforts has been developing, budgeting, implementing, and eval-

uating community-based strategies for the prevention of tooth decay. No two days are the same, and my days may encompass a variety of activities and functions. I supervise a staff of eleven who provide a school-based fluoride program, dental sealant program, and an oral wellness program in the classroom. We partner with local Early Head Starts and have a large component within the dental clinics in the health department. We also provide an early childhood cavity prevention program for pregnant women, parents, and infants. Using a local dental van in partnership with the school nurses, urgency care is provided for uninsured children in one school district in the County. Again, I have the opportunity to mentor dental hygiene and nursing students and work with a broad spectrum of volunteers and agencies in the community. It is a dynamic job where change is the status quo.

Throughout my career, I have found great growth through the sharing and networking that occurs when you participate and become involved in professional organizations. I have pushed myself and stretched myself to be president of the state dental hygiene association and participate on the Council on Public Health for ADHA. I have chaired a committee for the local dental association, and I have taken leadership positions in both local and national public health organizations. Each of the positions has added to my skills as a public health dental hygienist.

Thirty-four years and it is still exciting and fulfilling!

- Measures of dispersion, including range, variance, and standard deviation, are used to describe the variability of score in a distribution. If a relation has a normal distribution, it is depicted as a normal bell curve. If a relationship has a few extreme scores, it will be skewed.
- Correlation is the determination of the strength of the linear relationship between two variables. The closer the number is to one the stronger the relationship.
- Research studies utilize different approaches to sampling the population.

In addition to these concepts, please see the student web site for more study suggestions.

SAMPLE QUESTIONS

This section provides the reader with sample questions that may be asked on the national examination. It is intended to familiarize the student with necessary information about the items that may appear on the exam.

TESTLET I (questions 1–6)

A team of dental hygienists was approached by the board of education to establish a dental health education curriculum for the students enrolled in the public school system. The board was concerned that the only dental health education students received was during Children's Dental Health month. The teachers were interested in discussing dental health education in the student's health class. The school system consists of 6,000 students, grades K–12. Health care facilities are available at each school, including a nurse, who was available twice a week.

1. What is the first step in developing a pilot dental health education program?
    a. contacting the State Department of Education
    b. identifying the students who will participate in the pilot study
    c. meeting with the parents to identify the student's oral hygiene habits
    d. develop a data collection instrument
    e. obtain informed consent from the parents

2. Possible negative reactions and conflict could be avoided by obtaining which of the following:
    a. permission from the board of dentistry
    b. permission from the State Department of Education

    c. support of the school nurse and teachers

    d. permission from the local dental hygiene association

    e. permission from the governor

3. To determine the oral hygiene knowledge of the target population the dental hygienists should

    a. perform DMFS on all students

    b. conduct a caries-activity test

    c. perform clinical examinations and radiographs

    d. conduct a discussion group with all teachers

    e. conduct a dental questionnaire for all students

4. The BEST way to evaluate the effectiveness of oral hygiene home care instruction is by

    a. interviewing the students regarding oral hygiene habits

    b. utilizing an oral hygiene index

    c. conducting a DMFT survey

    d. conducting a questionnaire

5. The BEST way to determine the target population's actual dental needs for treatment is for the dental hygienist to

    a. send a survey out to the parents

    b. perform an oral cancer exam and radiographs

    c. conduct a dental questionnaire

    d. conduct a discussion group with teachers and parents

    e. perform a DMFT

6. After the program is developed, the MOST effective role for the community dental hygienists would be as a (an)

    a. major provider for classroom instruction

    b. consultant for the parents

    c. chairside instructor

    d. evaluator of the success of the program

    e. clinical hygienist

TESTLET 2 (questions 7–13)

Several community dental hygienists are involved in conducting a 5-year study on the use of sealants in conjunction with fluoride. The study involves all the public schools in Tooth County, and the grades consist of students K–12. At the begin-

Answers: 3. (e) 4. (b) 5. (e) 6. (d)

ning of the study, none of the public schools had fluoridated water, and fewer than 20 percent of the children attending these public schools had sealants. The total number of students in the county is 5,000. To decrease the number of subjects involved in the study a random sample was taken from the 5,000 students; however, students who did not have their first molars could not participate. The sample size then consisted of 2,000 students K–12.

The sample was then further divided into two groups: Group 1 received sealants at the start of the study and professional fluoride treatments every 6 months for 5 years. Group 2 only received fluoride treatments every 6 months for 5 years.

In addition the dental caries and plaque accumulation indexes were performed on both groups.

A mean plaque index score of 2.6 (based on a 3.0 scale) was recorded for both Group 1 and Group 2 and at the end of the 5 years the plaque index for Group 1 was 2.0 and the plaque index for Group 2 was 2.3. There was high interrater reliability between the dental hygienists.

7. What type of research study did the dental hygienists conduct?
   a. historical
   b. experimental
   c. cross-sectional
   d. descriptive

8. The mean plaque index score for both groups at the beginning of the study revealed the students having
   a. no plaque
   b. slight plaque
   c. moderate plaque
   d. severe plaque
   e. cannot be determined

9. A random sample suggested that the
   a. subjects were total volunteers
   b. every nth name on a list was selected
   c. every student had equal chance to be included in the study
   d. a person in Group 1 will not be a member of Group 2

10. The BEST way to gather information about the students' knowledge of dental health care is by
   a. interviewing the students and parents regarding oral hygiene habits
   b. utilizing a plaque and calculus index

    c. conducting a DMFT survey

    d. conducting a questionnaire

11. What is the MOST cost-effective way to add fluoride to these public schools?

    a. fluoride tablets; .25 mg sodium fluoride

    b. fluoride tablets; .5 mg sodium fluoride

    c. fluoride rinse; .5 mg sodium fluoride

    d. fluoridated water; 2.0 ppm

12. When evaluating the study, what dental index would help compare the effectiveness of sealants and fluoride versus fluoride alone?

    a. DMFT

    b. deft

    c. gingival index

    d. demineralization index

13. When the researcher claims a high interrater reliability between the dental hygienists, it means

    a. results were acceptable and can be generalized back to the population the sample came from

    b. two or more observers measured the students in the same way

    c. the index measured what it intended to measure

    d. results were similar each time the same dental hygienist observed the students

TESTLET 3 (questions 14–17)

A group of dental hygienists are devoting one day a week to the elementary schools in their community. A grant was given by the state for the public health department to purchase a van with portable dental equipment and supplies. The dental hygienists will conduct in-service workshops for the parents and teachers. The students will receive information on the importance of oral hygiene care and the development of dental diseases. The hygienists also have designed a dental clinic, which will allow the dental hygienists to conduct oral exams, place sealants, and administer fluoride.

14. The scenario BEST describes which type of community-based program being conducted in the elementary schools by the dental hygienists?

    a. fluoride

    b. preventive

    c. therapeutic

    d. sealants

    e. education

Answers: 11. (c) 12. (a) 13. (b) 14. (b)

15. The dental hygienists are going to discuss the importance of good oral hygiene habits and the prevention of dental disease. Which of the following is the BEST technique(s) for teaching this material?
   a. lecture and question-answer session
   b. distribution of brochures and class activities
   c. lecture only
   d. lecture with slides and posters
   e. lecture with slides, posters, and class activities

16. Select the BEST and SIMPLEST combination method of dental indexes to determine the dental needs and formation of debris on the teeth.
   a. DMFT and GI
   b. DMFT and CPITN
   c. DMFT and OHI-S
   d. DMFT and DI-S

17. The FIRST step the dental hygienists need to complete before starting clinical procedures such as exams and sealant placement is
   a. identifying dental insurance reimbursement
   b. determining the students' daily schedule
   c. identifying the students that do not need dental treatment
   d. gathering informed consent from the parents

TESTLET 4 (questions 18–31)

A high school class of 12 physically challenged students, 14 to 19 years of age; show a need for improved oral hygiene. The district dental hygienist has been asked by the high school nurse to assess their needs and to work with the nurse to implement a dental public health program to this class. The dental hygienist plans to set up a portable dental unit to orally screen the students and to implement an evaluative tool to understand the dental health knowledge of the group. In addition, she plans to provide oral hygiene instruction each month during the remaining of the school year, and the nurse will follow up with the instructions each Tuesday. The Patient Hygiene Performance (PHP) scores during the initial assessment of the class were 2.5, 2.75, 1.5, 3.0, 2.5, 2.0, 2.5, 2.75, 2.5, 2.5, 2.0, and 3.0. The mean OHI-S score of the 12 individuals was 4.8.

18. A complete dental assessment of the class should include all of the following EXCEPT one. Which one is the EXCEPTION?
   a. plaque and gingival scores
   b. dental hygiene treatment needs

   c. individual dexterity skills
   d. familial income and education level
   e. level of physical disabilities

19. Based on the severity of the physical disabilities, the dental hygienist may need to make accommodations for all of the following EXCEPT one. Which one is the EXCEPTION?
   a. oral hygiene instruction
   b. transportation to area dentists if needed
   c. utilization of the portable dental chair
   d. selection of dental indices

20. Which of the following students is most likely to require a two-man transfer technique from wheelchair to portable dental chair?
   a. mild multiple sclerosis
   b. cerebral palsy
   c. spinal cord injury at C-6
   d. myasthenia gravis

21. Which of the following represents the mean PHP score?
   a. 2.45
   b. 2.0
   c. 2.75
   d. 2.25
   e. 2.95

22. Which of the following PHP scores represents the mode?
   a. 1.5
   b. 2.0
   c. 2.5
   d. 2.75
   f. 3.0

23. When performing a correlation test between the debris and calculus scores of this class, the correlation coefficient was +.94 The relationship between gingival disease and plaque accumulation according to this test is statistically
   a. strong
   b. moderate
   c. weak
   d. no correlation

24. The results of a dental health knowledge exercise showed scores ranging from 68 percent to 82 percent. Ranking the class from the highest dental health knowledge score to the lowest dental health knowledge score is an example of what type of measurement?
    a. ordinal
    b. nominal
    c. interval
    d. ratio

25. The program plan should be based primarily on which of the following?
    a. recommendations of the students
    b. amount of funding available
    c. assessment of the student needs
    d. guideline of the public health department

26. The best approach to improving the dental health status of these students is to:
    a. reinforce brushing techniques already practiced by the group
    b. educate the students parents on reinforcement of oral hygiene habits at home
    c. introduce flossing through demonstrations in each student's mouth
    d. initiate a plaque control education program starting with disclosing and basic brushing

27. What is the best rationale for the school nurse to follow up with oral hygiene instruction each Tuesday instead of Monday or Friday?
    a. school attendance is higher on Tuesday than Monday or Friday
    b. the school nurse most likely works on Tuesday and not Monday or Friday
    c. studies have shown that physically challenged persons have greater dexterity on Tuesdays than any other day of the week

28. During oral hygiene instruction, which of the following activities is most likely to lead to learning retention?
    a. listening to the dental hygienist discuss the importance of toothbrushing
    b. viewing a videotape on oral hygiene instruction and dental disease
    c. reading a pamphlet about the prevention of oral disease and flossing
    d. participating in individual instruction using various toothbrush techniques

29. Efforts to encourage daily brushing at home by providing samples of toothbrushes with various adaptations is an example of:
    a. health prevention
    b. disease prevention
    c. health promotion

Answers: 24. (a) 25. (c) 26. (d) 27. (a) 28. (a) 29. (c)

30. After working on oral hygiene instruction for three months, the dental hygienist decides to perform a second PHP index to determine the effectiveness of instruction. The mean now becomes 1.5 with a standard deviation of .5. Which of the following interpretations can be made?
    a. the highest score is 2.0
    b. the most common score is 1.5
    c. most of the scores are between 1.0 and 2.0

31. The evaluation of this dental health program should be concerned primarily with the
    a. effectiveness of the program in reducing dental disease problems
    b. number of students who seek dental treatment
    c. teamwork established between the dental hygienist and the school nurse
    d. ability of each student to use a power operated toothbrush

TESTLET 5 (questions 32–41)

Three state public health dental hygienists are identifying oral health needs of persons residing in state subsidized drug and alcohol rehabilitation centers. One study performed was comparing oral lesions present in those persons who smoke cigarettes to those who do not smoke cigarettes. This study was performed in all of the three state rehabilitation centers and patient selection was done in alphabetical order by choosing every third individual when going down the patient list. The two dental hygienists who worked jointly for one day at each of the three sites performed calibration of the index.

32. This research is an example of what type of epidemiological study?
    a. cross sectional
    b. prospective cohort
    c. case control
    d. retrospective cohort

33. Which of the following is characteristic of the type of sampling used in these data?
    a. stratified
    b. simple random
    c. convenience
    d. systematic

34. The research hypothesis the dental hygienists established is, "there is no significant correlation between cigarette smoking and oral lesions." This is an example of what type of hypothesis?
    a. positive
    b. correlational
    c. null

35. When the dental hygienists select the most effective index to measure oral lesions which of the following is necessary criteria?
    a. predictability of outcome
    b. ease in calibration
    c. flexibility in measurement

36. In order to assure high interrater reliability, the dental hygienists must do which of the following?
    a. select only one of the hygienists to do the dental index calibrations
    b. thoroughly review the index criteria with each other so that the subjects are evaluated the same way.
    c. guarantee that the factor measured is the factor intended to be measured.
    d. determine that the results of the sample can be generalized to the population from which the subjects were drawn.

37. Which of the following tests can best measure the strength of the relationship between cigarette smoking and oral lesions?
    a. chi-square
    b. correlation
    c. students t-test
    d. probability test

38. Which of the following symbols of a test of significance would most likely indicate to the reader that the researcher's results were due most likely to their independent variable rather than chance occurrences?
    a. $p < 2.0$
    b. $p > .1$
    c. $p > .05$
    d. $p < .001$

39. If part of the program implementation includes smoking cessation, which sequence of the adoption process must an individual undergo to successfully move from smoking to smoking cessation?
    a. awareness, interest, appraisal, and trial
    b. awareness, interest, trial, and appraisal

    c. interest, awareness, appraisal, and trial
    d. interest, awareness, trial, and appraisal

40. To generate participation in this group, the dental hygienists most likely used which of the following communication strategies?
    a. pamphlet distribution
    b. radio and television announcements
    c. face-to-face exchanges
    d. church bulletin insertions
    e. mass mailings

41. Which of the following allows for the study to be regarded as having external validity?
    a. amount of variable control the researchers maintained over the study
    b. generalization of the results are applicable to other settings
    c. the change in the dependent variable is due to the independent variable
    d. full participation of the subjects when calibrating results

TESTLET 6 (questions 42–51)

A dental clinic has been built to meet the dental needs of a community. Assessment data are as follows: The community has a population of 12,142 people with 2 percent mobility. The SES of the community is considered to be low to low middle class (median income of $14,800). Drinking water is fluoride deficient, and most homes have well water. There are five practicing dentists, resulting in a dentist to patient ratio of 1:2,428. Dental survey data indicate that 65 percent of the population brush daily, 10 percent floss on a regular basis, and 80 percent of emergency dental cases are due to toothaches. Medicaid funds are limited, and few people are eligible or applying for public assistance. Within the one school district, there are two elementary schools, one middle school, and one high school. It was determined that health education; including dental health, is limited both in content and effectiveness. In the middle and high school, vending machines contain cariogenic foods, and protective mouth appliances often are not worn in contact sports.

42. To further ascertain the dental needs of the community, it is recommended that which of the following be utilized?
    a. pre-indice scores for dental caries, plaque, and periodontal conditions
    b. a survey regarding dental knowledge, values, and attitudes of the community
    c. the amount of demand for dental care by the community
    d. financial resources in planning treatment within the dental clinic
    e. access to care in regard to clinic hours, transportation, and payment plans

43. Taking into consideration the assessment of the community, which of the following actions will be most effective in reducing dental disease?
   a. implementing fluoridation of the community water supply
   b. initiating a plaque control program in the schools
   c. removing cariogenic food from the schools' vending machines
   d. requiring the use of athletic mouth protectors during all sports

44. The overall goal of this community dental clinic is to
   a. reduce the amount of dental disease
   b. increase the number of people seeking dental treatment
   c. increase the amount of practicing dentists
   d. provide more affordable dental care
   e. implement a dental health education program in the schools

45. When a questionnaire was sent to help assess oral hygiene practices of the respondents, all of the following EXCEPT one maximized the response rate. Which one is this EXCEPTION?
   a. limiting the length of the questionnaire
   b. indicating that responses are confidential
   c. including a cover letter with a deadline date
   d. increasing the time in which to respond

46. The recently built community dental clinic should have all of the following characteristics except one. Which one is this exception?
   a. payment options available to patients
   b. easy access to dental care
   c. more than one dentist employed
   d. located in an area with a high dentist to population ratio

47. The statistics regarding brushing, flossing, and emergency dental care visits, implies
   a. the need for dental care is lower than the demand for dental care
   b. the need for dental care is higher than the demand for dental care
   c. the need and the demand for dental care are equal

48. Efforts to exclude highly sugared snacks from school vending machines is an example of which of the following?
   a. health prevention
   b. disease progression
   c. health promotion
   d. health services

49. Medicaid is part of the Social Security Act. It is designed to provide funds to meet the health care needs of the indigent and medically indigent persons.
    a. the first statement is true and the second statement is false
    b. the first statement is false and the second statement is true
    c. both statements are true
    d. both statements are false

50. A deft index was performed on children in all four of the elementary schools. All of the following are true regarding the deft index EXCEPT one. Which one is this EXCEPTION?
    a. indicated for children with primary dentition
    b. measures observable caries experience
    c. the "e" indicates extracted teeth or a need for extracted teeth
    d. a tooth meeting criteria for "d" and "f" is recorded as "d"

51. In this nonfluoridated community, which preventive dental health program would have the maximum cost benefit for the control of caries in elementary schoolchildren?
    a. dental health education program
    b. fluoride mouth rinse program
    c. restorative care program
    d. parent-teacher education program
    e. pit and fissure sealant program

TESTLET 7 (questions 52–60)

A dental hygienist was asked to plan an in-service to a group of nursing assistants in a 200-bed nursing home. The dental hygienist first surveyed the nursing assistants concerning their understanding of dental health concepts using a written questionnaire. Following compilation and evaluation of the answers, the dental hygienist planned the in-service. The planning process included writing goals and objectives to be met during the in-service.

52. These activities parallel which of the following private practice activities?
    a. history taking and diagnosis
    b. diagnosis and treatment planning
    c. history taking, diagnosis, and treatment planning
    d. history taking, diagnosis, and treatment
    e. history taking, treatment planning, implementation, and evaluation

Answers: 49. (c) 50. (c) 51. (b) 52. (c)

53. Before initiating this dental in-service training program, it is recommended that the dental hygienist confer with whom?
    a. nursing home residents
    b. family members of the residents
    c. nursing home administrator and consulting dentist
    d. local dental hygienist association board members

54. As in the cognitive learning model, the intended outcome for this in-service is:
    a. knowledge
    b. behavioral change
    c. attitude

55. The most effective way to provide oral hygiene instruction in a nursing home is to
    a. distribute oral hygiene pamphlets to all residents and staff
    b. educate the nurses and other caregivers about proper oral hygiene care
    c. teach the nursing home residents the importance of brushing and flossing
    d. discuss with the administrators the necessity of educating the staff in oral care

56. In writing a behavioral objective, it is important to include the verb that depicts what the learner is expected to do. Which of the following is the best learner performance term?
    a. to believe
    b. to know
    c. to demonstrate
    d. to understand
    e. to feel

57. The more specific the objectives, the more effective the intent will be communicated to the nursing assistants. In-service evaluation is more effective without objectives.
    a. the first statement is true and the second statement is false
    b. the first statement is false and the second statement is true
    c. both statements are true
    d. both statements are false

58. Which of the following best describes an in-service designed for these nursing assistants?
    a. orally reviewing the results of the dental health survey and answering questions
    b. providing a slide presentation on geriatric oral health and demonstrating proper oral hygiene techniques on themselves

c. showing toothbrush adaptations indicative to nursing home residents and having each nursing assistant practice making sample adaptations

d. discussing proper communication techniques to improve oral hygiene self-care of the residents

59. To reinforce the skills necessary for toothbrushing the nursing home residents teeth, it is important to have the nursing assistants do which of the following?

a. describe the technique

b. read about the technique

c. watch the dental hygienist brush

d. use a disclosing agent for evaluation

e. practice toothbrushing on themselves

60. Prior to the in-service, the dental hygienist visited with some nursing home residents. When communicating with them, she was conscious to do all of the following EXCEPT one. Which one is this EXCEPTION?

a. speak loudly and into their ears

b. directly face the resident when speaking

c. use gestures and visual aids when indicated

d. repeat and write oral instructions

TESTLET 8 (questions 61–70)

A high incidence of dental caries has been detected in a group of Head Start children. A team of public health dental hygienists has been asked to design a dental health education program to reduce the incidence of dental caries among this population. The team has decided to conduct an in-service to the teachers, implement classroom activities, perform indices, implement a fluoride tablet program, and refer children for dental treatment when indicated.

61. What is the primary focus of this public health program?

a. assessment and evaluation

b. service and educational

c. therapeutic and promotional

d. referral and treatment

62. During the in-service, which of the following would be most helpful for the teachers in conveying dental health knowledge?

a. reviewing lesson plans

b. discussing appropriate media

c. explaining indice results

d. role-playing the fluoride tablet regimen

63. When the team explains the goal of the program to parents and staff, which of the following is most appropriate?
    a. services will be available for dental emergencies
    b. dental health education will be provided monthly
    c. the incidence of dental decay will be reduced
    d. fluoride tablets will reduce dental caries

64. The dental index most appropriate to use for this population is the:
    a. deft
    b. CPITN
    c. OHI-S
    d. DMFT
    e. PI

65. To assure interrater reliability of examiners when performing indices on the children, it is necessary that:
    a. a double-blind scoring mechanism be utilized
    b. each examiner be responsible for one age group
    c. procedures of calibrating scores are discussed among examiners
    d. different indices be used for pre and post scores

66. When providing classroom activities to the children, which of the following will be most effective?
    a. reading a story about dental cavities to the children
    b. showing a video on the importance of brushing teeth
    c. having the children participate in brushing a large mouth model
    d. giving the children a sticker each time they brush their teeth after lunch

67. The primary purpose of referring indicated children to a dentist for treatment is to:
    a. provide a follow up activity to the program
    b. assure that parents are aware of their child's dental needs
    c. increase the probability that dental disease will be reduced
    d. create an environment where dentists are treating more patients

68. All these financial assistance programs would be resources for payment in treating the children's teeth at local dental offices except one. Which one is the EXCEPTION?
    a. Medicare
    b. Medicaid
    c. Head Start
    d. private insurance

Answers: 63. (c) 64. (a) 65. (c) 66. (d) 67. (c) 68. (a)

69. The goal of this dental health education program is to
   a. define the dental needs of this population
   b. provide factual information to all participants
   c. motivate individuals to take positive action to reduce dental disease
   d. emphasize the importance of dental health as a daily routine

70. If funding is a problem, what strategy is the most effective in obtaining needed financial support?
   a. partnering with other community agencies to develop a collaborative request to local foundations
   b. approaching local business and industries requesting program funds
   c. engaging community churches to conduct fund-raising efforts
   d. sending high school students door-to-door in the affluent parts of the community to solicit funds

REFERENCE

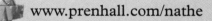

[1]*National Board Dental Hygiene Examination Guidelines.* Chicago: American Dental Association, 2004.

Get Connected

Multimedia Extension Activities

www.prenhall.com/nathe

Use the above address to access the free, interactive companion web site created specifically to accompany this textbook. Here you will find an array of self study material to help you gain a richer understanding of the concepts presented in this chapter.

Answers: 69. (c) 70. (a)

Appendix A

∙∙

ORGANIZATIONS INVOLVED WITH DENTAL PUBLIC HEALTH

The following is a list of commonly used private and public organizations for dental public health issues:

American Association for Dental Research (AADR)
1619 Duke Street
Alexandria, VA 22314
Telephone: (703)548-0068
http://www.iadr.com/

American Association of Public Health Dentistry (AAPHD)
National Office
1224 Centre West, Suite 400B
Springfield, IL 62704
Telephone: (217) 391-0218
http://www.aaphd.org

American Dental Association (ADA)
211 East Chicago Avenue
Chicago, IL 60611
Telephone: (312) 440-2500 or (800) 621-8099
Fax: (312) 440-2707
http://www.ada.org

American Dental Hygienists' Association (ADHA)
444 North Michigan Avenue
Chicago, IL 60611
Telephone: (800) 243-2342
http://www.adha.org

American Public Health Association
800 I. Street, NW
Washington, DC 20001
Telephone: (202) 777-2742
E-mail: comments@apha.org
http://www.apha.org

Association of State and Territorial Dental Directors
322 Cannondale Road
Jefferson City, MO 65109
Telephone: (573) 636-0453
http://www.astdd.org

Dental Hygiene Research Center
Old Dominion University
School of Dental Hygiene
Norfolk, VA 53259
(757) 683-5150
http://www.odu.edu/webroot/orgs/HS/dental.nsf/pages/research

The Hesperian Foundation
1919 Addison Street, Suite 304
Berkeley, CA 94704
Telephone: (888) 729-1796
http://www.hesperian.org/

Hispanic Dental Association
188 W. Randolph Street, Suite 1811
Chicago, IL 60601-3001
Telephone: (800) 852-7921
Fax: (312) 577-0052
http://www.hdassoc.org

HIV/AIDS Treatment Information Service
Telephone: (800) HIV-0440
http://www.aidsinfo.nih.gov

Institute of Medicine
500 Fifth Street NW
Washington, DC 20001
Telephone (202) 334-2352
http://www.iom.edu

National Center for Dental Hygiene Research
USC School of Dentistry
925 West 34th Street, Room 4330
Los Angeles, CA 90089
Telephone: (213) 740-8669
http://www.usc.edu/hsc/dental/dhnet
Project HOPE

Appendix B

∷∷∷∷∷∷∷∷∷∷∷∷∷∷∷∷∷∷∷∷∷∷∷∷∷∷∷∷∷∷∷∷∷∷

RESOURCES FOR DENTAL SAMPLES AND PAMPHLETS

The following is a list of companies that may be able to deliver samples or information about their products to aid you in presentations or upcoming events.

BreathAsure, Inc.
  Web site: www.breathasure.com
  Telephone: (800) 727-3284

Cheesebrough-Ponds USA Co.
  Web site: www.mentadent.com
  Telephone: (800) Mentadent (636-8233)

Church & Dwight Co., Inc.
  www.myoralcare.com
  Telephone: (800) 524-1328

Colgate-Palmolive
  Web site: www.colgate.com
  Telephone: (800) 763-0246

Dental-Resources
  www.dental-resources.com

Dentsply
  Web site: www.dentsply.com
  Telephone: (800) 989-8826

Discus Dental
  Web site: www.discusdental.com
  Telephone: (800) 826-9711

Hu-Friedy
  Web site: www.hu-friedy.com
  Telephone: (800) HU-FRIEDY

Johnson & Johnson
   Web site: www.johnsonandjohnson.com

Laclede, Inc. Health Care Products
   Web site: www.laclede.com
   Telephone: (800) 922-5856

Oral-B Laboratories
   Web site: www.oralb.com
   and www.braun.com
   Telephone: (800) 765-2959

Palmero Health Care
   Web site: www.palmerohealth.com
   Telephone: (800) 344-6424

Procter & Gamble
   Web site: www.dentalcare.com
   Telephone: (800) 492-7378
   (800) 543-2577 (technical questions)

Phillips Sonicare
   Web site: www.sonicare.com
   (800) 676-SONIC (800-676-7664)

Snore Guard
   Fax: (209) 545-3533
   Web site: www.snoreguard.com

Teledyne Waterpik
   Web site: www.waterpik.com

Warner–Lambert Consumer Health Care/Pfizer
   Web site: www.pfizer.com
   Telephone: (800) 223-0182

W.L. Gore & Associates, Inc.
   Web site: www.gore.com/glidefloss
   Telephone: (800) 645-4337

Appendix C

∴∴

GOVERNMENT DEPARTMENTS SERVING DENTAL NEEDS

U.S. Department of Agriculture
Office of Inspector General
P.O. Box 23399
Washington, DC 20026-3399
Telephone: (800) 424-9121
Web site: http://www.usda.gov

U.S. Department of Health and Human Services
200 Independence Avenue SW
Washington, DC 20201
Telephone: (202) 619-0257 or (877) 696-6775
Web site: http://www.hhs.gov/

Centers for Disease Control (CDC)
U.S. Public Health Service
1600 Clifton Road
Atlanta, GA 30333
Telephone: (404) 639-3311
Web site: http://www.cdc.gov/

Centers for Medicare and Medicaid Services
7500 Security Boulevard
Baltimore, MD 21244
Web site: http://www.cms.hhs.gov/

Health Resources and Services Administration
Parklawn Building
5600 Fishers Lane
Rockville, MD 20857
Web site: http://www.hrsa.gov/

National Institute of Dental and Craniofacial Research (NIDCR)
National Institutes of Health
9000 Rockville Pike
Bethesda, MD 20892
Web site: http://www.nidr.nih.gov/

U.S. Public Health Service Corps
Telephone: (800) 279-1605
Web site: http://www.usphs.gov/

U.S. Department of Defense
Telephone: (703) 697-5737
Web site: http://www.defenselink.mil/

U.S. Department of Education
400 Maryland Avenue SW
Washington, DC 20202-0498
Telephone: (800) USA-LEARN
Web site: http://www.ed.gov/index.html

U.S. Department of the Treasury
Office of Public Correspondence
1500 Pennsylvania Avenue NW
Washington, DC 20220
Telephone: (202) 622-2000
Web site: http://www.ustreas.gov/

U.S. Department of State
Secretary of State
Washington, DC 20520
Fax: (202) 647-7120
Web site: http://www.state.gov/index.html

U.S. Department of Justice
950 Pennsylvania Avenue NW
Washington, DC 20530-0001
Web site: http://www.usdoj.gov/

U.S. Department of Veterans Affairs
Consumer Affairs Service (075B)
810 Vermont Avenue NW
Washington, DC 20420
Telephone: (202) 273-5771
Fax: (202) 273-5716
Web site: http://www.va.gov/

Peace Corps
1990 K Street NW
Washington, DC 20526
Telephone: (202) 606-3886
Web site: http://www.peacecorps.gov/

Appendix D

STATE PUBLIC HEALTH AGENCIES

Alabama

Donald E. Williamson, MD
State Health Officer
Alabama Dept. of Public Health
The RSA Tower
201 Monroe St., Suite 1552
P. O. Box 303017
Montgomery, AL 36130
Phone: (334) 206-5200
Fax: (334) 206-2008
Web site: www.adph.org
E-mail: donwilliamson@adph.state.al.us

Alaska

Douglas Bruce, MBA
Director of Public Health and
State Health Officer
Alaska Division of Public Health
350 Main St., Room 503
P. O. Box 110610
Juneau, AK 99811-0610
Phone: (907) 465-3090
Fax: (907) 586-1877
Web site: http://health.hss.state.ak.us/
E-mail: dougbruce@health.state.ak.us

Arizona

Catherine R. Eden, PhD, Director
Arizona Dept. of Health Services
1740 W. Adams St., Room 407
Phoenix, AZ 85007

www.prenhall.com/nathe

Phone: (602) 542-1025
Fax: (602) 542-1062
Web site: www.hs.state.az.us
E-mail: ceden@hs.state.az.us

Arkansas

Dr. Faye Boozman, MD, MPH, Director
Arkansas Department of Health
4815 W. Markham St.
Little Rock, AR 72205
Phone: (501) 661-2111
Fax: (501) 671-1450
Web site: www.HealthyArkansas.com
E-mail: fboozman@HealthyArkansas.com

California

Ms. Diana Bontá, RN, Dr PH, Director
California Department of Health Services
714 P St., Room 1253
Sacramento, CA 95814-6401
Phone: (916) 657-1425
Fax: (916) 657-5183
Web site: www.dhs.ca.gov
E-mail: dbonta@dhs.ca.gov

Colorado

Douglas H. Benevento, Executive Director
Colorado Department of Public Health & Environment
4300 Cherry Creek Dr. South
Denver, CO 80246-1530
Phone: (303) 692-2000
Fax: (303) 691-1979
Web site: www.cdphe.state.co.us

Connecticut

Dr. Joxel Garcia, MD, MBA
Commissioner
Connecticut Dept. of Public Health
410 Capitol Ave.,
MS#13COM P. O. Box 340308
Hartford, CT 06134
Phone: (860) 509-7101
Fax: (860) 509-7111
Web site: www.state.ct.us/dph/

Delaware
Maureen E. Dempsey, MD, Director
Delaware Department of Public Health
Jesse Cooper Bldg., Federal Street
P. O. Box 637
Dover, DE 19903
Phone: (302) 739-4700
Fax: (302) 739-6659
Web site: www.state.de.us/_dhss/dph/index.htm
E-mail: maureendempsey@state.de.us

District of Columbia
James A. Buford, Chief Health Officer
District of Columbia Dept. of Health
825 N. Capitol St., NW, Suite 4400
Washington, DC 20002
Phone: (202) 442-5999
Fax: (202) 442-4788
Web site: www.dchealth.com
E-mail: james.buford@dc.gov

Florida
John O. Agwunobi, MD, MBA, Secretary
Florida Department of Health
4052 Bald Cypress Way, Bin #A07
2585 Merchants Row Boulevard
Tallahassee, FL 32399-1701
Phone: (850) 245-4321
Fax: (850) 487-3729
Web site: www.doh.state.fl.us

Georgia
Dr. Kathleen E. Toomey, MD, MPH,
Director
Division of Public Health
Georgia Dept. of Human Resources
2 Peachtree St. NW, Rm. 7-300
Atlanta, GA 30303
Phone: (404) 657-2700
Fax: (404) 657-2715
Web site: http://health.state.ga.us/
E-mail: ket1@dhr.state.ga.us

Hawaii
Loretta Fuddy, MSW, MPH
Acting State Health Official
Hawaii Department of Health
1250 Punchbowl St.
Honolulu, HI 96813
Phone: (808) 566-4410
Fax: (808) 586-4444
Web site: www.state.hi.us/health
E-mail: lfuddy@hawaii.edu

Idaho
Mr. Karl Kurtz, Director
Idaho Dept. of Health & Welfare
450 W. State St.
P. O. Box 83720
Boise, ID 83720
Phone: (208) 334-5945
Web site: www2.state.id.us/dhw/
E-mail: kurtzk@idhw.state.id.us

Illinois
Eric E. Whitaker, MD, MPH
Director
Illinois Department of Public Health
535 W. Jefferson St.
Springfield, IL 62761
Phone: (217) 782-4977
Fax: (217) 782-3987
Web site: www.idph.state.il.us
E-mail: ewhitake@idph.state.il.us

Indiana
Dr. Gregory A. Wilson, MD
State Health Commissioner
Indiana State Department of Health
2 N. Meridian St.
Indianapolis, IN 46204
Phone: (317) 233-7400
Fax: (317) 233-7387
Web site: www.IN.gov/isdh/
E-mail: gwilson@isdh.state.in.us

Iowa

Mary A. Hansen, Director
Iowa Department of Public Health
Lucas State Office Building
321 East 12th St.
Des Moines, IA 50319
Phone: (515) 281-5605
Fax: (515) 281-4958
Web site: www.idph.state.ia.us
E-mail: mhansen@idph.state.ia.us

Kansas

Roderick L. Bremby
Secretary of Public Health
Kansas Department of Health &
Environment
Curtis State Office Building
1000 SW Jackson, Suite 300
Topeka, KS 66612
Phone: (785) 296-1500
Fax: (785) 368-6368
Web site: www.kdhe.state.ks.us

Kentucky

Rice C. Leach, MD, Commissioner
Kentucky Cabinet for
Health Services
Department for Public Health
275 East Main St.
Frankfort, KY 40621
Phone: (502) 564-3970
Fax: (502) 564-6533
Web site: http://publichealth.state.ky.us/
E-mail: rice.leach@mail.state.ky.us

Louisiana

Mr. David Hood, Secretary
Louisiana Department of Health &
Hospitals
P. O. Box 3214
Baton Rouge, LA 70821
Phone: (225) 342-8093
Fax: (225) 342-8098
Web site: www.oph.dhh.la.us/

Maine
Mr. Kevin Concannon
Commissioner
Maine Department of Human Services
157 Capital St.
Augusta, ME 04333
Phone: (207) 287-8016
Fax: (207) 287-9058
Web site: www.state.me.us/dhs/boh
E-mail: kevin.w.concannon@state.me.us

Maryland
Arlene Stephenson, Deputy Secretary
Maryland Department of Health
& Mental Hygiene
201 W. Preston St., Suite 500
Baltimore, MD 21201
Phone: (410) 767-6500
Fax: (410) 767-6489
Web site: www.dhmh.state.md.us/
E-mail: stephensona@dhmh.state.md.us

Massachusetts
Christine C. Ferguson, JD Commissioner
Massachusetts Dept. of Public Health
Executive Office of Health & Human Services
250 Washington St., 2nd Floor
Boston, MA 02108-4619
Phone: (617) 624-6000
Fax: (617) 624-5206
Web site: www.state.ma.us/dph/dphhome.htm
E-mail: christine.c.ferguson@state.ma.us

Michigan
Mr. James K. Haveman Jr., Director
Michigan Dept. of Community Health
3423 N. Martin Luther King Jr. Blvd.
P. O. Box 30195
Lansing, MI 48909
Phone: (517) 335-8024
Fax: (517) 335-9476
Web site: www.michigan.gov/mdch
E-mail: mdch.state.mi.us

Minnesota

Dianne Mandernach
Commissioner
Minnesota Department of Health
85 East 7th Place, Ste. 400
P. O. Box 64882
St. Paul, MN 55164
Phone: (651) 215-5800
Fax: (651) 215-5801
Web site: www.health.state.mn.us/
E-mail: dianne.mandernach@health.state.mn.us

Mississippi

Brian W. Amy, MD, MHA, MPH
State Health Officer
Mississippi Department of Health
2423 N. State St., Box 1700
Jackson, MS 39215
Phone: (601) 576-7634
Fax: (601) 576-7931
E-mail: barry@msdh.state.ms.us
Website: www.msdh.state.ms.us

Missouri

Richard C. Dunn, Director
Missouri Department of Health &
Senior Services
912 Wildwood Dr.
Jefferson City, MO 65102
Phone: (573) 751-6001
Fax: (573) 751-6041
Web site: www.health.state.mo.us
E-mail: dunn1@dhss.state.mo.us

Montana

Ms. Gail Gray, EdD, Director
Montana Department of Public Health & Human Services
111 Sanders St., 3rd Floor
Helena, MT 59604
Phone: (406) 444-5622
Fax: (406) 444-1970
Web site: www.dphss.state.mt.us/
E-mail: ggray@state.mt.us

Nebraska

Richard Nelson, Director
Nebraska Department of
Regulation & Licensure
P. O. Box 95007
Lincoln, NE 68509
Phone: (402) 417-8566
Fax: (402) 471-9449
Web site: www.hhs.state.NE.us

Nevada

Ms. Yvonne Sylva, State Health Administrator
Nevada State Health Division
505 E. King St., Room 201
Carson City, NV 89710
Phone: (775) 684-4200
Fax: (775) 684-4211
Web site: www.state.nv.us/health
E-mail: ysylva@nvhd.state.nv.us

New Hampshire

Kathleen A. Dunn, Director
Office of Community & Public Health
New Hampshire Department of
Health & Human Services
6 Hazen Dr.
Concord, NH 03301-6527
Phone: (603) 271-8560
Fax: (603) 271-8705
Web site: www.dhhs.state.nh.us/

New Jersey

Clifton R. Lacy, MD, FACC, FACP
Commissioner
New Jersey Department of
Health & Senior Services
P. O. Box 360, Rm. 805
Trenton, NJ 08625-0360
Phone: (609) 292-7837
Fax: (609) 292-0053
Web site: www.state.nj.us/health
E-mail: clifton.lacy@doh.state.nj.us

New Mexico

Patricia T. Montoya, RN, MPA
New Mexico Department of Health
1190 St. Francis Dr.
Santa Fe, NM 87502
Phone: (505) 827-2613
Fax: (505) 827-2530
E-mail: vickimtz@doh.state.nm.us
Web site: www.health.state.nm.us/

New York

Dr. Dennis P. Whalen,
Executive Deputy Commissioner
New York State Dept. of Health
Corning Tower Bldg., 14 Floor
Empire State Plaza
Albany, NY 12237
Phone: (518) 474-2011
Fax: (518) 474-5450
Web site: www.health.state.ny.us
E-mail: dpw03@health.state.ny.us

North Carolina

Carmen Hooker Buell, Secretary
Department of Health &
Human Services
101 Blair Dr.
Raleigh, NC 27626
Phone: (919) 733-4261
Fax: (919) 715-4645
Web site: www.state.nc.us/DHR

North Dakota

Terry L. Dwelle, State Health Officer
North Dakota Department of Health
600 E. Boulevard Avenue
Bismarck, ND 58505
Phone: (701) 328-2372
Fax: (701) 328-4727
E-mail: tdwelle@state.nd.us
Web site: www.health.state.nd.us

Ohio

J. Nick Baird, MD, Director
Ohio Department of Health
246 North High St., P. O. Box 118
Columbus, OH 43266-0118
Phone: (614) 466-2253
Fax: (614) 644-0085
Web site: www.odh.state.oh.us/
E-mail: nbaird@gw.odh.state.oh.us

Oklahoma

Leslie M. Beitsch, MDJD, Commissioner
Oklahoma Department of Health
1000 Northeast 10th
Oklahoma City, OK 73117-1299
Phone: (405) 271-5600
Fax: (405) 271-3431
Web site: www.health.state.ok.us/
E-mail: LMBeitsch@health.state.ok.us

Rhode Island

Patricia A. Nolan, MD, MPH, Director
Rhode Island Department of Health
3 Capitol Hill, Room 401
Providence, RI 02908
Phone: (401) 222-2231
Fax: (401) 222-6548
E-mail: pnolan@doh.state.ri.us
Web site: www.healthri.org

Oregon

Grant K. Higginson, MD, MPH
State Public Health, DHS Officer
Oregon Health Division
800 NE Oregon St., Ste. 930
Portland, OR 97232-2162
Phone: (503) 731-4000
Fax: (503) 731-4078
Web site: www.ohd.hr.state.or.us
E-mail: grant.k.higginson@state.or.us

Pennsylvania

Robert S. Muscalus, DO
Acting Secretary of Health
Pennsylvania Department of Health

Health & Welfare Bldg.
P. O. Box 90, Room 802
Harrisburg, PA 17108
Phone: (717) 787-6436
Fax: (717) 787-6959
Web site: www.health.state.pa.us
E-mail: rmuscalus@state.pa.us

South Carolina

C. Earle E. Hunter, Commissioner
South Carolina Department of
Health & Environmental Control
2600 Bull Street
Columbia, SC 29201
Phone: (803) 898-3300
Fax: (803) 898-3323
Web site: www.scdhec.net/
E-mail: hunterce@dhec.state.sc.us

South Dakota

Ms. Doneen B. Hollingsworth
Secretary
South Dakota Department of Health
600 E. Capitol Avenue
Pierre, SD 57501
Phone: (605) 773-3361
Fax: (605) 773-5683
E-mail: doneen.hollingsworth@ state.sd.us
Web site: www.state.sd.us/doh

Tennessee

Kenneth S. Robinson, MD, Commissioner
Tennessee Department of Health
Cordell Hull Bldg., 3rd Fl.
425 5th Ave. North
Nashville, TN 37247
Phone: (615) 741-3111
Fax: (615) 741-2491
Web site: www.tennessee.gov/health
E-mail: kenneth.s.robinson@state.tn.us

Texas

Nick Curry, MD, MPH
Executive Deputy Commissioner
Texas Department of Health
1100 W. 49th St.
Austin, TX 78756
Phone: (888) 963-7111
Fax: (512) 458-7477
E-mail: nick.curry@tdh.state.tx.us
Web site: www.tdh.state.tx.us

Utah

Mr. Rod L. Betit
Executive Director
Utah Department of Health
P. O. Box 141000
Salt Lake City, UT 84114-1000
Phone: (801) 538-6111
Fax: (801) 538-6306
Web site: health.utah.gov/

Vermont

Paul E. Jarris, MD
Commissioner
Vermont Department of Health
108 Cherry St.
P. O. Box 70
Burlington, VT 05402
Phone: (802) 863-7280
Fax: (802) 865-7754
Website: www.healthyvermonters.info/

Virginia

Robert B. Stroube, MD, MPH
Commissioner
Virginia Health Department
P. O. Box 2448
1500 E. Main St.
Richmond, VA 23218
Phone: (804) 786-3561
Fax: (804) 786-4616
E-mail: rstroube@vdh.state.va.us
Web site: www.vdh.state.va.us

Washington
    Ms. Mary C. Selecky, Secretary
    Washington State Department of Health
    1112 SE Quince Street
    Mail Stop 47890
    Olympia, WA 98504-7890
    Phone: (360) 236-4010
    Fax: (360) 586-7424
    E-mail: mary.selecky@doh.wa.gov
    Web site: www.doh.wa.gov

West Virginia
    Mr. Paul Nusbaum, Secretary
    West Virginia Bureau for Public
    Health
    350 Capitol Street
    Room 702
    Charlestown, WV 25301
    Phone: (304) 558-2971
    Fax: (304) 558-1035
    Web site: www.wvdhhr.org/bph

Wisconsin
    Kenneth Baldwin, Interim Administrator
    Wisconsin Division of Public Health
    1 West Wilson St.
    P. O. Box 2659
    Madison, WI 53701
    Phone: (608) 266-1251
    Fax: (608) 267-2832
    Web site: www.dhfs.state.wi.us
    E-mail: baldwk@dhfs.state.wi.us

Wyoming
    Deborah K. Fleming, PhD, Director
    Wyoming Department of Health
    117 Hathaway Bldg.
    Cheyenne, WY 82002
    Phone: (307) 777-7656
    Fax: (307) 777-7439
    Web site: www.wdhfs.state.wy.us
    E-mail: dflemi@state.wy.us

Source: StatePublicHealth.org May 16, 2003

Appendix E

TABLE CLINIC PRESENTATION
···

A table clinic is a presentation using both verbal communication and visual aids to inform and discuss material on a specific topic. The clinic is presented at a tabletop booth setting including a visual component and verbal communication (Figure E–1). The presentation may include slides, graphs, or pictures that are displayed on the board. The length of a typical table clinic presentation is five to seven minutes. The topic chosen may be a technique, theory, service, trend, or career opportunity in the practice of dental hygiene. Table E–1 provides tips on preparing a table clinic.

RESEARCH
· ·

Research that is learned can be shared with patients, employees, or peers. It is inevitable that as health care professionals we will be questioned about oral care products, as well as specific techniques. The information gathered during a table clinic is a perfect way to formulate recommendations about issues that may arise.

After choosing your topic, it is important to next choose a theme. Brainstorm for ideas. When researching your topic use all available resources. Your public or school library is a great place to gather information. Don't limit yourself to books—try journals, newspapers, and videotapes; contacting companies directly is a fantastic way to get information. Remember to keep a list of all your resources because you will need to provide a bibliography on your pamphlet. In addition, other professionals may inquire where you obtained your information.

VISUAL DISPLAY
· ·

Next, you will need to prepare your poster board. The visual media is aimed at informing, clarifying, and/or reviewing specific material. Begin by looking at arts and crafts stores or at stores that cater to

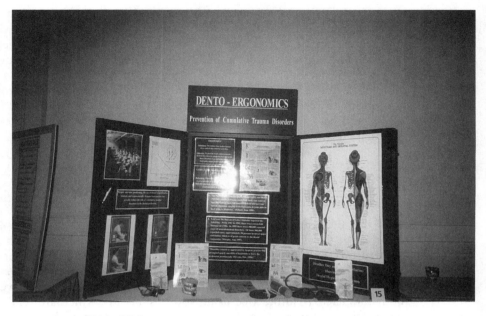

Figure E–1. Table Clinic

Table E–1. Tips on Preparing Your Table Clinic

- **Getting Started:** Choose a topic that is interesting to you.
- **Research:** Determine a theme for your presentation and work toward developing it.
- **Research:** Do thorough research of your topic and have documentation of your findings available.
- **Research:** Be prepared for questions and discussion.
- **Visual Aids:** Use visual aids effectively to reinforce what you are saying.
- **Presentation:** Limit your presentation to approximately 7 minutes.
- **Presentation:** Practice your communication skills, i.e. voice projection, body language, eye contact.
- **Presentation:** Practice your presentation in front of friends and family; ask for constructive criticism.
- **Handouts:** Prepare handouts to outline, summarize, or supplement your presentation.

teachers. Items such as foam board, stick-on lettering, artwork, and crepe or construction paper can usually be found in these types of stores. Also a visit to a copying center can be a great way to have pictures or graphs enlarged, copied, or colored. The display board can be bifold or trifold by taping or gluing two or three pieces of poster board/foam board together. In addition, if slides are planned, a slide projector can be easily fit into the display board by cutting around the slide projector and placing it within the display. The poster board should be neat, organized, and easy to read from a distance. Your board should be eye-catching and stimulate the audience's curiosity.

PRESENTATION

Now that the visual component is completed, it is time to begin the verbal section. First, if two speakers will present you need to decide how the speech is going to be divided up. Next write your part of the speech on note cards. Then just practice, practice, practice. Present your speech to friends and family members. Besides just the verbal section be sure to practice voice projection and control, eye contact, and body language. Also practice using your visual aids, which are reinforcing what is being said. It is best when the time comes to do the actual presentation that you have your speech memorized. This shouldn't be hard, and remember, between the two of you, your speech should only be five to seven minutes. In addition to preparing for your speech, also be prepared for questions and controversial feedback. The best way to promote confidence about your topic is to be well versed in your topic as well as other areas that closely relate to your topic.

HANDOUTS

In addition to the display, visual aids, and presentation, handouts should be available.[1] The information in a handout is used to outline, summarize, and/or supplement your presentation. The handout should include the table clinic's title and date of presentation, the name of the presenter(s), dental hygiene affiliation, and bibliography. The audience should be able to use your handout as a reference guide concerning your topic and, if needed, as a way to contact the presenter at a later date.

ADHA GUIDELINES

Every year, at the American Dental Hygienists' Association Annual Session, students from around the country compete in the table clinic presentations (please see Table E–2). ADHA current guidelines are available for more information at

Table E–2.   ADHA Rules and Regulations

- Handouts must be available and should include title of clinic, date, bibliography, and dental hygiene affiliation.
- Only one 3 ft. × 6 ft. table will be permitted for each table clinic.
- All clinics are conducted at individual tables; no more than two clinicians are permitted to present at one time.
- Advertising matter, commercial promotion, solicitation of sales of any type is prohibited.
- Drugs should be identified by their generic or chemical formula, rather than the commercial trade name.
- Any trade name on instruments must be covered.
- Clinicians must supply all equipment, except for the table, cloth cover, identification sign, and two chairs. Electrical outlets, AV equipment, etc., must be ordered directly from the supplier. An order form will be forwarded to each accepted table clinic presenter. The charges for this equipment are the responsibility of the clinicians.
- Clinicians are not permitted to use patients or live models for treatment or demonstration.
- Sound devices of any kind are not permitted.
- Clinicians must have completed setup of their table clinic 30 minutes prior to commencement of judging.
- Clinicians must remain at their clinics at all times, as judging times may overlap with the public viewing time.
- Charts or diagrams must be constrained to the tabletop. Easels will not be provided and no materials are allowed on the floor or in the aisles.

Source: ADHA Guidelines. Chicago: ADHA, 1997.

(800) 243-ADHA. Table E-2 shows basic guidelines developed by ADHA for table clinic presentations.[2] These guidelines change slightly every year, so it is a good idea to contact ADHA for current guidelines.

SUMMARY

By preparing a table clinic dental hygienists have the opportunity not only to expand their knowledge of a specific topic but also to inform other individuals. A table clinic is also an excellent way to meet other health care professionals and possibly new employment contacts. Many times sponsors of the table clinics present awards to the best-prepared and presented table clinic. Have fun and be creative!

REFERENCES

[1]George, P. Preparing a table clinic. *Dental Hygienist News* 8 (1994): 20–23.
[2]*ADHA Guidelines*. Chicago: ADHA, 2003.

Appendix F

POSTER SESSION PREPARATION

A poster session is a method utilized to describe a dental hygiene research study. It is a presentation of an original research study. Basically, a poster session is a method to disseminate the results of a research study, whereas a table clinic is a method to disseminate a review of the literature on a specific topic of study. Poster sessions actually incorporate visual media that reflects an area of dental hygiene research (please see Figure F–1).

Figure F–2 depicts an outline that should be used for the poster session. The research should have been conducted in this order.

As with all professional endeavors, organization is the key. Faculty members should serve as mentors during research, and it is rec-

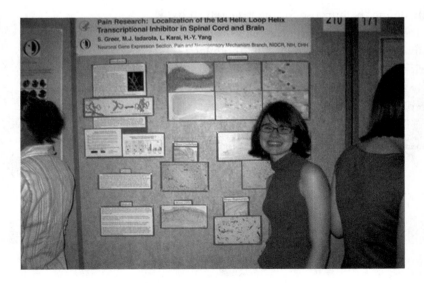

Figure F–1. NIH Poster Day

Figure F–2. Poster Session Outline Format

1. Purpose of study or hypothesis tested
2. Statement of the problem and significance of the study
3. Brief overview of methodology
4. Statistical tests employed
5. Results of the study, including statistical data analysis
6. Conclusion

ommended that all research conducted have numerous reviews before, during, and after the process to ensure success in presenting the information. The ADHA has set criteria for prepaing a poster session which are depicted in Figure F–3.

Please see www.adha.org for the rules and regulations for research poster sessions at the American Dental Hygienists' Association Annual Sessions.

Figure F–3. ADHA Poster Session Criteria

- Clearly define the purpose for the research study
- State the problem and significance of the study
- Identify and outline the research methodology
- Describe the results, including statistical data analysis
- Clearly state how the conclusions or findings are supported by the results
- Be prepared for questions and discussions

Source: Reprinted with permission from the American Dental Hygienists' Association. 2003.

Appendix G

INTERNATIONAL DENTAL CARE OPPORTUNITIES

Dental Health International
Postbus 3185
3760 DD Soest
Nederland
Postbank 4735988, Borne
+31 35 60 32 536 or

847 South Milledge Avenue
Athens, GA 30605
Telephone: (404) 546-1715
http://www.dhin.nl

Fédération Dentaire Internationale (FDI)
13 Chemin du Levant, l'Avant Centre
F-01210 Ferney-Voltaire
France
+33 450 40 50 50
www.fdiworldental.org

Christian Medical and Dental Associations
P.O. Box 7500
Bristol, TN 37621 USA
Telephone: (808) 231-2637
www.cmds.org

Health Volunteers Overseas
c/o Washington Station
P.O. Box 65157
Washington, DC 20035 USA
www.hvousa.org

www.prenhall.com/nathe

International Association for Dental Research (IADR)
1619 Duke Street, Alexandria, VA 22314-3406
Telephone: (703) 548-0066
Fax: (703) 548-1883
www.iadr.com

International Dental Health Foundation
Telephone: (800) 368-3396
http://members.aol.com/idhf

International Federation of Dental Hygienists
Ornäsgatan 4
79162 Falun
Sweden
Telephone: +46 23 778428
Fax: +46 23 778401
www.ifdh.org

Mercy Ship
P.O. Box 2020
Garden Valley, TX 75771-2020
Telephone: (903) 939-7000
www.mercyships.org

Mission Finder
P.O. Box 356
Sunol, CA 94586
Telephone: (208) 723-4657
www.missionfinder.org

Operation Smile
6435 Tidewater Dr.
Norfolk, VA 23509 USA
Telephone: (757) 321-7645
www.operationsmile.org

Peace Corps
1990 K Street NW
Washington, DC 20526
Telephone: (202) 606-3886
http://www.peacecorps.gov/

Smiles Foundation
Telephone: (423) 239-9525
www.smilesclub.org

United Nations (UN)
Publications, Room DC2-0853
New York, NY 10017
Telephone: (212) 963-8301
www.un.org

U.S. Agency for International Development (USAID)
Bureau for Europe and Near East
Office of Technical Resources
Population Health and Nutrition Area
State Department
Washington, DC 20523
www.usaid.gov

World Federation of Public Health Associations (WFPHA)
Headquarters
P.O. Box 99
1211 Geneva 20, Switzerland
World Health Organization
Avenue Appia
CH-1121 Geneva 27, Switzerland
Telephone: 791 21 11
Fax: 791 07 46
Telex: 415416OMS
Telegram: UNISANTE-GENEVA
http://www.who.int

World Health Organization Publications Center USA
49 Sheridan Avenue
Albany, NY 12210
Telephone: (518) 436-9686
World Health Organization Regional Office for the Americas
c/o Pan American Sanitary Bureau
525 Twenty-Third Street NW
Washington, DC 20037
Telephone: (202) 861-3200
Fax: (202) 223-5971
www.who.int

Appendix H

DENTAL TERMS AND PHRASES TRANSLATED TO SPANISH AND VIETNAMESE

English	Spanish	Vietnamese
dentist	dentista	Nha sĩ
tooth	diente	Răng
throat	garganta	Cuống họng
neck	cuello	Cổ
mouth	boca	Miệng
head	cabeza	Đầu
face	cara	Mặt
ear	oido	Tai
nose	nariz	Muỗi
tongue	lengua	Lưỡi
tonsils	amigdalas	Hạch
denture	dentadura	Hàm răng
toothbrush	cepillar(v), cepillo(n)	Bàn chãy đánh răng
show me	enseneme	Chỉ cho tôi
relax	relajese	Bình tỉnh, thông thả
don't move	no se muera	Đừng nhúc nhích
look straight ahead	vea derecho	Nhìn thẳng phía trước
swallow	trague	Nuốc vào
open your mouth	abra la boca	Mở miệng ra
stick out your tongue	saque la lengua	Lè lưỡi ra
close	cerra	Đóng lại
spit	escupir	Nhổ ra
abscess	abceso	Ung, nhọt
asthma	astma	Bệnh suyễn
bleeding	sangrado	Nhảy máu
cold	frio	Lạnh
diabetes	diabetes	Bệnh tiểu đường

English	Spanish	Vietnamese
edema	edema	Chứng phù thủng
fracture	fractura	Chỗ nứt, chỗ gãy
headache	cefalea	Nhức đầu
high blood pressure	presion alta	Chứng cao huyết áp
hot	caliente	Nóng
infection	infeccion	Nhiễm trùng
injured	herido	Bị thương
pregnant	embarazada	Mang thai
stitches	puntadas	Khâu, vá
swelling	inflamacion	Bị sưng
trauma	trauma	Chấn thương
wound	herida	Vết thương
mild	suave	Nhẹ, êm
moderate	moderado	Vừa phải
severe	severo	Nghiêm khắc
earache	dolor de oido	Bệnh đau tai
sore throat	dolor de garganta	Đau họng
difficulty swallowing	dificultad al tragar	Khó khăn khi nuốt
tooth ache	dolor de muela	Nhức răng
neck pain	dolor de cuello	Đau cổ
sensitive	sensible	Nhạy cảm
disease	enfermedad	Bệnh tật
medications	medicamentos	Bốc toa thuốc (dùng thuốc)
antibiotics	antibioticos	Kháng sinh
pain pills	calmantes	Thuốc đau nhức
narcotics	narcoticos	Thuốc mê
penicillin	penicilina	Thuốc trụ sinh
right	derecho (m.) derecha (f.)	Phải
left	izquierdo (m.) izquierda (f.)	Trái

GOOD DAY! HOW ARE YOU?
BUENOS DIAS! COMO ESTA?
(boo-eh-nus dee-ass) (kum-muh estah)

DOES IT HURT?
LE DUELE?
(leh doo-eh-leh)

WHEN DOES IT HURT?
CUANDO LE DUELE?
(kwan-doh leh doo-eh-leh)

ALL THE TIME?
TODO EL TIEMPO?
(toh-doh el tee-m-poh)

WHERE DOES IT HURT?
DONDE LE DUELE?
(dun-deh leh doo-eh-leh)

DOES THE COLD WATER OR AIR HURT YOU?
LE MOLESTA EL AGUA O EL AIRE FRIO?
(leh muh-les-tah el ah-goo-ah oh el i-reh free-oh)

DOES IT HURT WHEN YOU BITE?
LE DUELE CUANDO MUERDE?
(leh doo-eh-leh kwan-doh moo-erdeh)

OPEN YOUR MOUTH.
ABRA LA BOCA.
(ahbra lah bokah)

CLOSE YOUR MOUTH A LITTLE.
CIERRE LA BOCA UN POCO.
(see-ehreh lah bokah oon poh-koh)

BITE SLOWLY.
MUERDA DESPACIO.
(moo-erdah des-pah-see-oh)

BITE AGAIN.
MUERDA OTRA VEZ.
(moo-erdah oh-trah vez)

SPIT OUT PLEASE.
ESCUPA, POR FAVOR.
(ess-coo-pah por favor)

TURN YOUR HEAD TO THE RIGHT.
—TO THE LEFT.
VOLTE LA CABEZA A LA DERECHA.
—A LA IZQUIERDA.
(vol-teh lah ka-beh-zah ah lah deh-reh-chah
—ah lah eez-kee-erdah)

DO NOT EAT OR DRINK FOR 30 MINUTES.
NO COMA NI BEBA POR 30 MINUTOS.
(noh koh-mah nee beh-bah por trentah mee-nuh-tohs)

DO NOT CHEW ON THIS SIDE FOR 24 HOURS.
NO MASTIQUE EN ESTE LADO POR 24 HORAS.
(no mahs-teekeh en esteh lahdoh por ven-tee kwah-troh o-rahs)

DO NOT BRUSH TONIGHT.
NO SE CEPILLE ESTA NOCHE.
(no seh seh-peeyeh ess-tah no-cheh)

DO NOT RINSE TONIGHT.
NO SE ENJUAGE ESTA NOCHE.
(noh seh en-huah-ghe ess-tah no-cheh)

Appendix I

∙∙

STANDARDS FOR DENTAL HYGIENISTS IN DENTAL PUBLIC HEALTH EDUCATION

COMMISSION ON DENTAL ACCREDITATION, DENTAL PUBLIC HEALTH STANDARDS

Dental hygiene students attend programs that have been accredited by the Commission on Dental Accreditation, which is part of the American Dental Association. The Commission is comprised of twenty members and includes a representative from the American Dental Hygienists' Association. The Commission has been accrediting dental hygiene educational programs since 1953.

The Accreditation Standards for Dental Hygiene Education Programs includes mandatory curriculum content. Dental hygiene students must prove competency in dental public health. Specifically, dental hygiene graduates must include and advocate the evaluation of current literature to prepare the student for lifelong learning in dental hygiene practice. Faculty should integrate these principles of lifelong learning throughout the curriculum.

Moreover, content in community dental health and public health dentistry must be included in the curriculum to provide students with background in the procedures of assessing, planning, implementing, and evaluating community oral health programs. Experience in oral health education and preventive counseling for groups must be included in the curriculum. A mechanism for planning, supervising, and evaluating community field experiences must be implemented by the dental hygiene faculty.

This information can be found in the Accreditation Standards for Dental Hygiene Education Programs, Commission on Dental Accreditation. Chicago, IL: American Dental Association, 1993. Please see http://www.ada.org for these standards.

JOINT COMMISSION ON NATIONAL DENTAL EXAMINATIONS NATIONAL BOARD DENTAL HYGIENE EXAMINATION

The information that dental hygienists in all states, except Alabama, are tested on during the National Board Dental Hygiene Examination for dental public health include the following topics under the section entitled community health/research principles.

- Promoting Health and Preventing Disease within Groups (including media and communication resources)
- Participating in Community Programs
  1. Assessing populations and defining objectives
  2. Designing, implementing, and evaluating programs
- Analyzing Scientific Information, Utilizing Statistical Concepts, and Applying Research Results

Chapter 17 further discusses the National Board Dental Hygiene Examination.

Appendix J

::

GUIDE TO SCIENTIFIC WRITING

The following guidelines to writing can be used when writing scientifically based papers for table clinic presentations or poster presentations.[1]

TITLE PAGE

The title page should include the title of the manuscript in boldface; the name, credentials, and rank or title and organizational affiliation of each author; the mailing address; and telephone, e-mail, and fax number for the primary author. In addition, if the investigation has been funded by an organization, it should be noted on the bottom of the title page.

LENGTH

Manuscripts should be six to ten pages in length, excluding references, tables, figures, and photographs.

PRESENTATION

The English language should be utilized in all manuscripts. Manuscripts must include an abstract and the following:

- Original research should include an introduction, methods and materials, results, and discussion and conclusion.

- Case studies should include an introduction and case as described in the dental hygiene process of care; assessment, dental hygiene diagnosis, treatment planning, implementation, and evaluations; and summary.
- Literature reviews should include an introduction, significance, main body, and conclusions.
- Position papers should include an introduction, significance, main body, and summary.

REFERENCES

All references should be numbered in the order they are cited. The following style of citation should be used. Examples are as follows: Periodical: Nelson, MJ and Newell, KJ: A career development program from graduate dental hygienists. *J Dent Hyg* 1993;67:398–402. Textbook: Darby, ML and Walsh, MM: *Dental Hygiene Theory and Practice*. Philadelphia: W.B. Saunders Co., 1994:8–10.

TABLES, FIGURES, AND PHOTOGRAPHS

All tables, figures, and photographs should follow the manuscript and not be inserted into the manuscript. Written permission for the use of copyrighted material must be included with the manuscript and is the author's responsibility.

ACKNOWLEDGMENTS

The authors may acknowledge one to two individuals for their assistance in manuscript preparation.

AUTHORS

Primary authors of all manuscripts must be dental hygienists or dental hygiene students; secondary authors may represent any discipline.

CONTENT

Manuscripts may be original research, case studies, literature reviews, or position papers.

REFERENCE

[1]Author Guidelines. *Contact International.* 14(2000):4.

GLOSSARY

•••

A

Administrative law: The delegation of legislative power to an administrative agency.

Affective domain: The learning domain that includes feelings, attitudes, and values; it is not easily measured.

Agent factors: Biological or mechanical means for causing diseases or conditions.

American Association of Public Health Dentistry (AAPHD): The organization that represents American public health dentists, dental hygienists, and the science of dental public health.

American Association of State and Territorial Dental Directors: The organization that represents state dental departments.

American Dental Association (ADA): The organization that represents American dentists and the science of dentistry.

American Dental Hygienists' Association (ADHA): The organization that represents American dental hygienists and the science of dental hygiene.

Atraumatic Restorative Treatment (ART): A dental sealant placed on a tooth surface with demineralization that has been removed by hand. This preventive/restorative dental method is utilized when a patient will have difficulty accessing restorative dental care.

Assessment: The part of the dental hygiene process of care that carefully analyzes the program's target group and resources.

B

Barrier: Something that prevents an individual or a group from receiving dental care.

Benefits: The amount that the insurance entity will pay for covered dental services described in their policy.

C

Calibration: Ensuring consistency within and among examiner(s).

Capitation: A dental provider gets paid a specified dollar amount, for a given time period, to take care of the dental needs of a specified group of people.

Change agent: A person who lobbies to change laws, increasing access to care for the underserved populations.

Civilian Health and Medical Program of the Uniformed Services (CHAMPUS): Health care services for military personnel and dependents.

Civil service employee: An employee of the federal government. A hygienist may work as a civil servant at various government entities.

Claims processing: The entire process of entering the procedures rendered until payment is collected or denial is determined.

Clinical evaluation: Any clinical method utilized to evaluate a dental public health program or research.

Clinician: A person who provides dental hygiene clinical care to the population.

Control: A group in a study that does not receive treatment or therapy.

Cognitive domain: The learning domain that consists of intellectual skills.

Collaborative practice: The science of the prevention and treatment of oral disease through the provision of education, assessment, preventive, clinical, and other therapeutic services in a cooperative working relationship with a consulting dentist, but without general supervision as practiced in the state of New Mexico.

Commercial insurance plans: An insurance plan that operates for a profit.

Common law: A law that is created and changed only by the courts.

Community dental health: *See* dental public health.

Component organizations: The local components of the American Dental Hygienists' Association.

Congressman: *See* representative.

Constituent organizations: The state or regional components of the American Dental Hygienists' Association.

Constitutional law: Law that is created and changed by the people.

Consumer advocate: A person who provides dental health consultation to various target populations.

Continuous variable: A variable that can be expressed by a large and infinite number of measures along a continuum, can be expressed in fraction, and is considered quantitative.

Contract: The insurance contract between the insurance entity and the group.

Copayment: A portion of the costs of each service that is paid by the patient.

Correlation: The linear relationship between variables.

Cultural diversity: The integration of an individual's or population's socioethnocultural background into dental hygiene care.

Culture and cycle of poverty: Exploration of the culture of poverty and the cyclical change of poverty.

D

Data: The information that is collected by a researcher.

Deductible: The amount an individual enrolled in the insurance plan must pay toward covered services before the insurance entity begins paying.

Defluoridation: The process of removing excessive natural fluorine from water supplies.

Demand: The particular frequency or desired frequency of dental care from a population.

Dental assistant: The professional who assists the dental hygienist and/or dentist.

Dental claim: A claim for payment made by the patient for a dental procedure that was rendered.

Dental claim form: The standard form utilized to file a claim or request authorization for a procedure.

Dental hygiene: The art and science of preventive oral health.

Dental hygiene diagnosis: The formal diagnosis of a population's current dental hygiene status.

Dental hygiene process of care: The assessment, dental hygiene diagnosis, planning, implementation, and evaluation of dental hygiene care of a target population.

Dental hygiene treatment: Periodontal debridement and oral hygiene instruction.

Dental hygienist: The professional who provides clinical and educational dental hygiene services to the public.

Dental indexes: The standardized methods used to describe the status of an individual or group with respect to an oral condition.

Dental necessity: A service provided by a dental provider that has been determined as a generally acceptable dental practice for the diagnosis and treatment of an individual.

Dental public health: The oral health care and education, with an emphasis on the utilization of the dental hygiene sciences, delivered to a target population.

Dentist: The professional who provides clinical and educational dental services to the public.

Dentistry: The art and science of restorative oral health.

Dependent variable: In a clinical study, the variable that is being tested.

Descriptive statistics: Consist of the procedures that are used to summarize, organize, and describe quantitative data.

Determinants of health: The factors that interact to create specific health conditions, including physical, biological, behavioral, social, cultural, and spiritual.

Developmental disability: A disability that occurs during uterine development.

Discrete (categorical) variable: A variable that is made up of distinct and separate units or categories, also referred to as mutually exclusive, and is counted only in whole numbers.

Disease rates: The number of disease cases or deaths among a population or target group during a given time period expressed as a ratio.

E

Early and Periodic Screening, Diagnosis and Treatment (EPSDT): Persons under 21 years of age must be covered by Medicaid for medical, dental, and vision care.

Early childhood caries: Dental caries that affects children, sometimes referred to as nursing bottle decay or baby bottle decay.

Early Head Start: The federal program that promotes the economic and social well-being of pregnant women and their children up to age three.

Educator: The person who educates and promotes dental health issues to various target populations.

Endemic: A relatively low, but constant level of occurrence of a disease or health condition in a population.

Epidemic: A disease or condition occurring among many individuals in a community or region at the same time and usually spreading rapidly.

Epidemiology: *See* oral epidemiology.

Ethnocentrism: The belief that one's culture is superior.

Etiology: The theory of causation for a disease or condition.

Evaluation: The part of the dental hygiene process of care that encompasses evaluation of a dental public health program.

Exclusive Provider Arrangement (EPA): Dental care providers contracts with an employer (which eliminates the third party) and negotiates the fees for services offered to the employer's employees.

Explanation of benefits: A form sent to the patient and provider explaining the payment for procedures or denial of payment for procedures rendered.

F

Federal: National; of or pertaining to the United States of America.

Federation Dentaire Internationale (FDI): The organization that represents the international community of dentists.

Fee slip: Form utilized by the dental provider that details the services rendered.

Fluoridation: The addition of fluoride to drinking water.

Fluoride: A salt of hydrofluoric acid.

Fluoride varnish: A varnish of fluoride that is applied to teeth to prevent dental caries; particularly effective in the prevention of early childhood caries.

Fluorosis: A form of enamel hypomineralization due to excessive ingestion of fluoride during the development of the teeth.

Formative evaluation: An evaluation of the program during implementation; evaluating the process.

Frontier: A geographic area that is even more sparsely populated than a rural area.

G

Government: A method or system of controlling people.

Group: *See* target population.

H

Head Start: The federal program that promotes the economic and social well-being of families and children from three to five years of age.

Health behavior: An action that helps prevent illness and promote health.

Health education: The education of health behaviors that bring an individual to a state of health awareness.

Health promotion: The promotion of healthy ideas and concepts to motivate individuals to adopt health behaviors.

Healthy People 2010:   The report released from the federal government which states the goals and objectives necessary to improve the health and quality of life for individuals and communities.

I

Implementation: The part of the dental hygiene process of care that includes the actual operation of a program.

Incidence: The number of new cases of a disease in a population over a given period of time.

Independent contractor: A person who works for him-, or herself in a governmental or private capacity.

Independent practice: The practice of dental hygiene without the supervision of a dentist, although the dental hygienist refers all dental needs to a dentist; sometimes called unsupervised practice or collaborative practice.

Independent variable: In a clinical study, the variable that is being manipulated.

Index: *See* dental indexes.

Inferential statistics: Used to make inferences or generalizations about a population based on data taken from a sample of that population.

International Federation of Dental Hygienists (IFDH):   The organization representing the international community of dental hygienists.

Interval scale of measurement: Has equal distance between any two adjacent units of measurement, but there is no meaningful zero point.

L

Learning domain: The domains of learning, a way to differentiate the individual types of learning.

Lesson plan: A written document used in planning a presentation.

Long-term care facility: A facility that provides live-in care for patients with medical complications.

M

Managed care: Refers to the integration of health care delivery and financing.

Manager: The developer and coordinator of dental public health programs; sometimes referred to as an administrator.

Manpower: The available personnel to do a job; referred to as labor force.

Manpower shortage: Inadequate availability of personnel to perform a job.

Mean: The average of scores.

Measurement: A particular method utilized to evaluate a dental public health program based upon the program objectives.

Median: The midpoint of scores.

Medicaid (Title XIX): Money from federal, state, and local taxes pays bills for certain groups of people, including low-income, aged, blind, disabled, and member of families with dependent children.

Medicare (Title XVIII): A federal insurance program from trust fund to pay medical bills of all people over age sixty-five.

Metropolitan: A large population nucleus, consisting of a city and surrounding suburban areas.

Modality: A clinical or educational dental hygiene treatment.

Mode: The score that occurs most often.

Morbidity: The ratio of "sick" (affected) individuals to well individuals in a community.

Mortality: The ratio of the number of deaths from a given disease or health problem to the total number of cases reported.

Motivation: The will of the individual to act.

N

Need: A normative, professional judgment as to the amount and kind of health care services required to attain or maintain health.

Nonclinical evaluation: A method utilized when evaluating a dental public health program that does not measure clinical changes.

Nominal scale of measurement: Organizes data into mutually exclusive categories, but the categories have no rank order or value.

Normal bell curve: A normal distribution of the mean, median, and mode.

Nursing home: *See* long-term care facility.

O

Oral epidemiology: The study of the amount, distribution, determinant, and control of disease and health conditions among given populations.

Ordinal scale of measurement: Organizes data into mutually exclusive categories which are rank ordered based on some criterion but the difference between ranks is not necessarily equal.

P

P.A.N.D.A.: An acronym for Prevent Abuse and Neglect through Dental Awareness. An educational program aimed at helping dental providers recognize and report child abuse.

Paradigm: A model used to explain a concept or theory.

Parameter: Numerical characteristic of the population.

Planning: The part of the dental hygiene process of care that includes the development of a program.

Poster session: A method utilized to disseminate original research findings.

Practice Act: A statute that defines the practice of dental hygiene or dentistry.

Preceptorship: The on-the-job training of dental hygienists, sometimes referred to as alternative education.

Preexisting condition: The condition of the mouth that exists prior to the patient being covered by an insurance entity.

Premium: The monthly amount due to the insurance entity by the group or the individual.

Prepaid group practice: A large group of dental providers that contract to groups of patients.

Prevalence: A numerical expression of the number of all existing cases of a disease in a population measured at a given point.

Procedure number: The number given to a specific procedure as designated in the *Codes on Dental Procedures and Nomenclature* published by the ADA.

Program planning: The process of developing a dental public health program.

Promulgate: To put a law into practice as done by state dental boards.

Provider: A legally licensed dental hygienist or dentist that is operating within their scope of practice.

Psychomotor domain: The learning domain that describes actions.
Public health: *See* dental public health.
Public health officer: *See* U.S. Public Health Service Officer.
***p*-value:** The probability that the findings from study are due to chance.

Q

Qualitative evaluation: Answering the why and how of a dental public health program or research project.
Quantitative evaluation: A numerical evaluation of a dental public health program or research project.
Quasi-experimental research design: A research design that does not include a control group.

R

Range: The range is determined by subtracting the highest score from the lowest score.
Ratio scale of measurement: Contains all the characteristics of the preceding scales, but also has an absolute zero point determined by nature.
Regulation: The state dental boards' procedure which further defines the law.
Reliability: The reproducibility of a research study.
Representative: An elected member of the U.S. or individual state House of Representatives.
Researcher: A person who conducts research germane to the study of health and disease.
Research types: The way of categorizing research studies.
Risk factors: The characteristics of an individual or population that may increase the likelihood of experiencing a given health problem.
Rural: A geographic area that is sparsely populated.
Rules: The state dental boards' interpretation of a law.

S

Self-regulation: The governing of dental hygiene practice by dental hygienists.
Senator: An elected member of the U.S. or individual state senate.
Single procedure: a specific procedure designated by a specific code.
Skew: The tail of a distribution formed by a few extreme scores.
Social worker: A professional who works at helping individuals or the community enhance their capacity for social functioning.
Socioeconomic status (SES): An individual's comparative status in social and economic standing within a community.

Sound natural teeth: Teeth that are either primary or permanent that have adequate hard and soft tissue support.

Standard deviation: The measure of dispersion.

State Children Health Insurance Program (SCHIP): A federal program that was created by the federal government to cover individuals that have incomes too high to qualify for state medical assistance but cannot obtain private insurance. All states participate, but some do not cover dental.

Statute: A law, sometimes in the form of a practice act.

Statutory law: The law that is created and changed by the legislature.

Summative evaluation: An evaluation of all parts of an implemented program.

Supply: The quantity of dental care services available.

Surgeon general: The appointed administrator of the U.S. Public Health Service.

Surveillance: The methods or systems used to monitor disease and morbidity in a population periodically or on an ongoing basis.

T

Table clinic: A method utilized to disseminate past research studies and literature reviews of a specific topic.

Target population: A representation of a certain segment of the population.

Therapeutic services: The services the dental hygienist provides that benefit the patient. These may include periodontal debridement, polishing, fluoride application, local anesthesia, dental sealants, education, and behavior modification interventions.

Three-party system: The dental provider renders the service and a sponsor of the patient pays for the service; insurance company or employer pays the dental provider for the service.

Two-party system: The dental providers render the service and the patient pays the dental provider for the service.

U

UCR (Usual, customary, and reasonable fee): The fee that reflects the average dentist fee per service in the immediate local region.

Urban: A concentrated human settlement, usually consisting of at least 2,500 people.

U.S. Public Health Service Officer: A dental hygienist or dentist that is a commissioned officer of the U.S. Public Health Services.

Utilization: The number of dental care services actually consumed.

V

Validity: The degree to which the research study measured what it was supposed to measure.

Variance: The squared deviation of each score from the mean's sum.

W

Water fluoridation: *See* fluoridation.

INDEX

Page numbers followed by a *t* indicate table. Page numbers followed by *f* indicate figure.